DRUGS
HANDBOOK
2007

Glyn Volans   **Heather Wiseman**

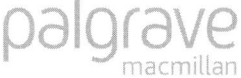

DEDICATION

To the memory of our colleague Professor Paul Turner, in recognition of his role in establishing and maintaining this book over a period of 18 years, and in appreciation of his experience and teaching that formed the basis for this work.

GLYN N. VOLANS
HEATHER M. WISEMAN

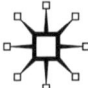
Twenty-eighth revised edition published 2007 by
PALGRAVE MACMILLAN
Houndmills, Basingstoke, Hampshire RG21 6XS and
175 Fifth Avenue, New York, N. Y. 10010
Companies and representatives throughout the world

PALGRAVE MACMILLAN is the global academic imprint of the Palgrave Macmillan division of St. Martin's Press, LLC and of Palgrave Macmillan Ltd. Macmillan® is a registered trademark in the United States, United Kingdom and other countries. Palgrave is a registered trademark in the European Union and other countries.

ISBN 0–2305–1674–2

This book is printed on paper suitable for recycling and made from fully managed and sustained forest sources.

A catalogue record for this book is available from the British Library.

10   9   8   7   6   5   4   3   2   1
16   15   14   13   12   11   10   09   08   07

Printed and bound in Great Britain by
Creative Print & Design (Wales), Ebbw Vale

CONTENTS

INTRODUCTION

We continue to respond to changes in the prescribing and use of medicines and the recent innovations in drug development.

This book has always been intended for the many health professionals other than clinicians who need information about the mechanism of action, therapeutic indications and unwanted effects of medicines. Certain groups of nurses are now authorized to prescribe and there are proposals to extend authority still further to new groups of professionals to prescribe in specific clinical areas. With such a wide range of drugs available, we believe that individuals will most appreciate this handbook as a source of information about medicines used in fields outside their areas of expertise.

Non-prescription Medicines

Originally we concentrated on medicines prescribed by doctors, but over the years we have included a growing number of non-prescription medicines to take account of their increasing significance in the consideration of effectiveness and safety. Our teaching now emphasizes the need for health professionals to be aware of the diversity of medicines available for self-treatment and keep adequate records of patients' self-medication in their medical notes.

Non-prescribed medicines include:

1. General Sales List (GSL) medicines that can be supplied by any shop such as a supermarket or garage. This category covers only a very limited range of active drugs supplied in small amounts.
2. Licensed non-prescription medicines that must be supplied or sold by a pharmacist or in a pharmacy. This list continues to grow, and following extensive monitoring of their safety and efficacy, many drugs that were previously prescription-only medicines (POM) are now available for self-medication. We fully support these developments which acknowledge the ability of many patients to treat themselves effectively and give pharmacists a greater role in advising on both effectiveness and safety.
3. Complementary medicines, many of which at present are not adequately covered by the licensing process, including:
   - herbal products
   - homeopathic preparations
   - food supplements
   - herbal and other traditional medicines, including medicines from other non-European cultures.

Innovations in Drug Development

The most striking new drugs are those that have been developed to treat specific conditions with more accurately targeted activity. We have attempted to describe complex drugs and new delivery systems briefly but clearly, providing definitions when needed.

Cost-effectiveness

New drugs are expensive, as manufacturers seek to recover the costs of developing them. In some cases the resulting products seem to have relatively small health benefits compared with existing treatments or even with no treatment. Since the funds for healthcare are limited, there are restrictions on the range of medicines which may be provided and publicly funded through NHS prescriptions. In 1985 the government issued a 'blacklist' of drugs and preparations that cannot be prescribed or dispensed under the NHS but only on private prescriptions, the patient having to pay for them in full. The *British National Formulary* distinguishes these drugs with a symbol against their names.

Decisions on prescribing are also guided by the National Institute for Clinical Excellence (NICE), which provides authoritative guidance on current 'best practice'. Guidance on the use of new and existing medicines and the appropriate treatment and care of people with specific diseases and conditions within the NHS in England and Wales can be viewed on the NICE website (www.nice.org.uk). Short summaries and information for the public are published in addition to the full assessments.

Interactions

The potential for interactions between drugs is common and is extended by use of unlicensed drugs and even some foods. In this text we can only comment on the most significant interactions. Readers who are concerned about the safety of co-prescribed drugs should consult a pharmacist or doctor.

Drugs and Medicines

A doctor usually prescribes a *drug*, but the patient receives a *medicine*. The medicine is the whole formulation in which the drug, that is, the active substance, is combined with other ingredients to form a convenient form of administration, such as a tablet, capsule, suppository, inhalation, ointment or injection. We have not included all constituents of the medicines listed in this book, but have mentioned only those substances which we believe may contribute to the therapeutic or adverse effects of the medicine involved. It must be stressed that the mention of a medicine in this book, and statements about its indications, do not imply that it is necessarily an effective treatment, or that the authors believe it to be such; in fact we believe that for large numbers of drugs there is no good evidence of their effectiveness.

Names of Drugs

Most drugs have at least three names. The first is the full chemical name, which is too long and complicated to use regularly. Drugs are usually identified by their generic or approved name. In the past, the same substance sometimes had different approved names in different countries. Recently, however, it has been recognized that there would be scientific, clinical and commercial advantages if such inconsistencies were removed, and European law now requires the use of the Recommended International Non-proprietary Names (rINN) for medicinal substances. In most cases the British Approved Name (BAN) and rINN were the same, but where the two differed, the BAN has been changed. Finally there is the brand or trade name, given by the pharmaceutical manufacturer for its own particular brand or formulation. For example, 4-amino-5-chloro-*N*-(2-diethylaminoethyl)-2-methoxybenzamide hydrochloride is the chemical name for metoclopramide hydrochloride, the approved name of the drug marketed at present by at least two drug firms under the brand names Maxolon and Primperan.

The book has two sections. The first is an alphabetical list of drugs under their approved names. The main entry for each substance is under the BAN/rINN. However, where the BAN has changed to conform to the rINN, the old name is still listed with a cross-reference to the new entry. Where a number of drugs have essentially similar effects, in order to avoid duplication and keep the handbook a manageable size, the main entry is under the name of the most typical and most frequently prescribed, with cross-references to it from the names of the similar drugs. The second section is an alphabetical list of brand names with cross-references to the appropriate approved names. Thus all cross-references refer to the list of approved names and are shown in small capitals, for example TETRACAINE.

Entries are included for some obsolete drugs that are no longer included in prescribed medication in the UK but are still of therapeutic, toxicological or pharmacological interest.

Drugs Safety Monitoring

When a new medicine comes onto the market, it will have been tested in clinical trials in order to demonstrate not only its effectiveness but also its safety. However, since these trials generally involve quite small numbers of carefully selected patients, they may not detect the full range of possible adverse reactions, particularly those that occur only rarely. In order to compensate for this lack of information, drug safety monitoring programmes have been developed throughout the world, and the information thus gathered is shared internationally through regulatory agencies and the WHO.

In this small book we can only include the most important findings from this critical surveillance but we aim to ensure that any necessary revisions are made as part of the annual update. We have indicated those medicines that are currently being intensively monitored by the UK monitoring agency, the Commission on Human Medicines (CHM), which replaced the Committee on Safety of Medicines in 2005. Intensive monitoring of all new active substances and also new combinations of active substances, new routes or systems of delivery and significant new indications for use is undertaken for at least two years until safety is well established. The CHM revises its list monthly, so our annual publication can never be completely up to date. Nevertheless we hope our readers will find this helpful. Now that not only doctors but also pharmacists and other healthcare professionals are being encouraged to report adverse reactions, and direct patient reporting is also to be tested, we hope that readers may be able to contribute to safety monitoring either directly or through others.

Drugs in Pregnancy

Several drugs are known to be hazardous to the developing foetus and for most drugs there is no definite information on their safety in pregnancy. We have avoided constant repetition of this but would stress that in pregnancy all drugs should be used with caution and only when essential.

Drug Combinations

Many of the preparations listed in this book are combinations of drugs rather than individual ones. The majority are rather crude attempts at what might be called 'blunderbuss treatment' of a variety of signs and symptoms, but some have been developed on scientific grounds to exploit the interaction of two or more drugs working together. Others, by combining drugs that are commonly used together, offer, if correctly used, a means of simplifying treatment for patients on long-term multiple drugs and thus improve compliance, for example combination drugs for hypertension. Several approved names have now been coined for such combinations. These are identified by the prefix 'co-', and usually include syllables from the approved names of the ingredient drugs. For example, co-trimoxazole is a combination of trimethoprim and sulphamethoxazole.

Other Reference Sources

This book has not been written for the general public. Its primary purpose is to provide information for groups within the health professions. It assumes a basic knowledge and understanding of human biology and disease. For readers who wish to refer to books with more complete and detailed information we would recommend:

1. For information on drugs

Brunton, L., Lazo, J. and Parker, K. *Goodman & Gilman's The Pharmacological Basis of Therapeutics*. 11th edition, 2005. McGraw-Hill, New York.
Humphries, J. L. and Green, J. (eds) *Nurse Prescribing*. 2nd edition, 2002. Palgrave Macmillan, Basingstoke.
Bennett, P. N. and Brown M. J. *Clinical Pharmacology*. 9th edition, 2003. Churchill Livingstone, London.
Reid, J. L., Rubin, P. C. and Walters, M. *Lecture Notes: Clinical Pharmacology and Therapeutics*. 7th edition, 2006. Blackwell Science, Oxford.
Ritter, J. M., Lewis, L. D. and Mant, T. G. K. *A Textbook of Clinical Pharmacology*. 4th edition, 2000. Hodder & Stoughton, London.
Sweetman, S. C. (ed.) *Martindale. The Complete Drug Reference*. 35th edition, 2006. Pharmaceutical Press, London.
Trounce, J., Greenstein, B. and Gould D. *Trounce's Clinical Pharmacology for Nurses*. 17th edition, 2004. Churchill Livingstone, London.

2. For information on diseases and their management

Kumar, P. J. and Clark, M. L. (eds) *Clinical Medicine*. 6th edition, 2005. Saunders, Philadelphia.
Warrell D. A., Cox T. M., Firth, J. D. and Benz, E. J. (eds) *Concise Oxford Textbook of Medicine*. 4th edition, 2005. Oxford Unversity Press, Oxford.

3. For information on treatment of poisoning

Bates, N., Edwards, J. N., Roper, J. and Volans, G. N. (eds) *Paediatric Toxicology*. 1997. Macmillan – now Palgrave Macmillan, Basingstoke.
Dart, R. C. (ed.) *Ellenhorn's Medical Toxicology*. 3rd edition, 2004. Lippincott, Williams & Wilkins, Philadelphia.
Jones, A. L. and Dargan, P. I. *Churchill's Pocket Book of Toxicology*. 2001. Churchill Livingstone, London.

GLYN N. VOLANS
HEATHER M. WISEMAN

ABBREVIATIONS

The following abbreviations have been used throughout the book:

(b)   indicates a borderline substance, that is, a substance which may only be prescribed as a drug under certain conditions.

(c)   indicates a drug whose prescription is controlled under the Misuse of Drugs Act.

(d)   discontinued by the manufacturers during the year prior to publication. As supplies will still be available from pharmacies until stocks run out, these products have not yet been deleted from our lists.

(m)   indicates a drug that is misused or abused, although prescription is not controlled by the Misuse of Drugs Act.

(r)   indicates intensive monitoring by the Commission on Human Medicines (CHM) that may be limited to a specific brand or preparation, or extend to all available forms of the drug.

CNS   central nervous system.

rINN   Recommended International Non-proprietary Name.

DEFINITIONS OF DRUG GROUP NAMES AND MEDICAL TERMS

abortifacient. Used to produce abortion.

adjuvant. Something added to a drug which aids or modifies the main ingredient.

adrenergic. Has similar actions to ADRENALINE.

adrenoceptor. Receptor for ADRENALINE, NORADRENALINE, which mediates sympathetic activity in the body.

adsorbent. Material which binds drugs and other chemicals and prevents or reduces their absorption.

agonist. Has an observable effect within the body, resulting from a direct action upon a specific receptor.

alpha-adrenoceptor. Subgroup of adrenoceptors that mediates some of the effects of sympathetic stimulation including vasoconstriction, increase in blood pressure and mydriasis.

amino acids. Simple molecules from which peptides, polypeptides and proteins are formed.

aminoglycoside. Drug with a chemical structure related to STREPTOMYCIN.

anabolic. Stimulates cell metabolism causing increased tissue growth.

analgesic. Relieves pain.

angiotensins (I and II). Angiotensin I is an inactive peptide molecule that is produced in the kidneys and converted by an enzyme, angiotensin-converting enzyme (ACE), to form angiotensin II, a potent vasoconstrictor which plays a role in controlling blood pressure. In patients with hypertension, control of blood pressure may be improved by drugs that inhibit the ACE enzyme (ACE inhibitors) or by blocking the action of angiotensin II at its receptor sites in the blood vessel walls (angiotensin receptor antagonists).

anorectic. Appetite suppressant used in obesity.

antacid. Neutralizes acid produced by the stomach.

antagonist. Opposes the action or blocks the effect of another drug.

antiandrogen. Acts to block the effects of the male sex hormones (androgens).

antiarrhythmic. Suppresses arrhythmias.

anticholinergic. Blocks the action of ACETYLCHOLINE or cholinergic (acetylcholine-like) drugs.

anticholinesterase. Blocks the action of cholinesterase – a naturally occurring enzyme which breaks down ACETYLCHOLINE bringing its action to an end. The effect of the anticholinesterase is therefore to prolong and intensify the action of acetylcholine.

anticholinesterase inhibitors. Centrally acting drugs which reduce breakdown of brain acetylcholine by cholinesterase. Used to increase central acetylcholine levels (and thus cognitive function) in mild to moderate Alzheimer's dementia. Includes DONEPEZIL, GALANTAMINE, RIVASTIGMINE.

anticoagulant. Prevents blood from clotting.

anticonvulsant. Stops or prevents epileptic seizures.

anticytokine. A drug which blocks the action of the pro-inflammatory cytokine, tumor necrosis factor alpha (TNF-α), which has been shown to play a major role in inducing severe inflammatory disease in rheumatoid arthritis.

antidysrhythmic. *See* antiarrhythmic.

antiemetic. Prevents nausea and vomiting.

antihistamine. Blocks the action of histamine, a chemical released from body cells in response to exposure to allergic substances, e.g. plant pollens. Used both topically and systemically to treat allergic reactions including seasonal allergic rhinitis (hay fever), allergic skin rashes, drug allergies and allergic emergencies. Also used to treat and prevent nausea and vomiting caused by motion sickness or adverse drug reactions. Many antihistamines, e.g. PROMETHAZINE, have sedative effects which may be helpful in some therapeutic uses but are undesirable when the patient needs to be alert, e.g. to drive a car or operate machinery. In these circumstances a nonsedating antihistamine, e.g. ACRIVASTINE, should be used.

antihypertensive. Lowers blood pressure.

antipruritic. Relieves pruritus.

antipsychotics. (also known as tranquillisers or major tranquillisers). A group of drugs used in short-term management to quieten disturbed patients, whatever the underlying psychopathology, and in longer term treatment to relieve and prevent the psychotic symptoms of schizophrenia, such as delusions, hallucinations and thought disorders. Thought to act by blocking dopamine receptors in the brain and, by the same mechanism, may also cause abnormal parkinsonion-like movements. Their effects on cholinergic, adrenergic, histaminergic and serotinergic receptors give a wide range of possible uses (e.g. as anti-emetics) and adverse effects (e.g. postural hypotension and epilepsy). The original antipsychotics included, amongst others, phenothiazines e.g. CHLORPROMAZINE and butyrophenones, e.g. HALOPERIDOL. Although effective at controlling psychotic symptoms, they cause many troublesome adverse affects, notably movement disorders. More recently, the atypical antipsychotics have been developed, e.g. CLOZAPINE and OLANZEPINE, which have been shown to have a much lower incidence of movement disorders and other adverse effects.

antipyretic. Lowers body temperature in febrile conditions.

antiserotonin. Blocks the action of serotonin.

antispasmodic. Relieves spasm of muscles, for example, in the gastro-intestinal tract (gastro-intestinal colic).

antitussive. Suppresses cough.

anxiolytic. Reduces anxiety.

arrhythmia. Disorder of rhythm, generally of the heart.

arthralgia. Pain in the joints.

asthenia. General feeling of physical weakness.

astringent. Precipitates protein to form a protective layer over damaged skin or mucous membranes.

bactericidal. Kills bacteria.

bacteriostatic. Inhibits growth of bacteria but does not kill them.

benzodiazepines. A group of chemically related hypnotics, sedatives, anxiolytics and anticonvulsants including DIAZEPAM.

beta-adrenoceptor. Subgroup of adrenoceptors that mediates some of the effects of sympathetic stimulation including increase in heart rate and force, and bronchodilation.

beta-lactam. An antibiotic with a chemical structure which includes a beta-lactam ring. Cephalosporins, PENICILLINS, and CEFOXITIN are betalactam antibiotics.

beta-lactamase. Enzyme produced by some bacteria, capable of breaking down the beta-lactam ring of the betalactam antibiotics. Leads to bacterial resistance to the antibiotic. Some betalactam antibiotics are beta-lactamase resistant, e.g. CLOXACILLIN.

biguanides. A group of drugs which reduce blood glucose levels by reducing the release of glucose stored in the liver and by increasing the use of glucose by body tissues. METFORMIN is the only biguanide in current use as an oral antidiabetic, particularly in overweight patients, and in combination with other drugs.

bioavailability. Extent to which and rate at which the active substance in a drug is taken up by the body in a form that is physiologically active.

biphosphonates. A group of drugs which act on bone cells to reduce the rate of cell turnover. Used to treat and prevent disease where there is thinning of the bones with consequent risk of deformities and fractures. May also be used to reduce high blood calcium levels.

bradycardia. Slow heart rate.

bronchodilator. Increases the diameter of the airways in the respiratory system and thus reduces the physical resistance to breathing.

buffer. Solution that opposes changes in acidity or alkalinity.

cardioselective. Acts on the heart without the other effects usually found in drugs of a particular group, for example beta-adrenoceptor blocking drugs. In practice, the cardioselectivity is usually relative and the other effects can be traced, although in a less pronounced form.

carminative. Facilitates the eructation of gas from the stomach.

cathartic. Relieves constipation.

cephalosporins. A group of broad-spectrum antibiotics used for the treatment of a wide range of infections including septicaemia, pneumonia, meningitis and urinary tract infections. Their chemical structures are similar to PENICILLINS but they are relatively resistant to penicillinase. Hypersensitivity is the most common adverse reaction and about 10 per cent of patients who are sensitive to PENICILLINS are also sensitive to cephalosporins.

chelating agents. Bind heavy metals to increase their excretion.

chemotherapy. Treatment using drugs rather than other measures such as surgery, radiation or vaccines.

cholinergic. Has actions similar to ACETYLCHOLINE.

corticosteroids. Hormones (natural or synthetic) with actions on metabolism and against tissue inflammation. The natural hormones are produced by the adrenal gland.

COX-2 inhibitors (Cycloxygenase-2 selective inhibitors). A group of non-steroidal anti-inflammatory drugs (NSAIDs) which were developed because their gastro-intestinal tolerability was improved by comparison with non-selective (COX-inhibitor) NSAIDs such as DICLOFENAC and IBUPROFEN. In long-term use they have been found to be associated with increased problems from cardiac, renal and hepatic disease. ROFECOXIB has been withdrawn because of an adverse risk-benefit ratio and the others have had their indications more tightly defined while safety surveillance continues.

cutaneous. Relating to the skin.

cycloplegic. Paralyses muscle of the eye controlling accommodation. Leads to blurred vision.

cytokines. Small protein molecules secreted by cells involved in inflammatory responses and regulation of the immune system, usually by a local effect on itself or adjacent cells. The group includes INTERFERONS, and interleukins such as ALDESLEUKIN.

cytotoxic. Has toxic effects upon living cells which reduce growth or cause destruction of the cells.

decongestant. Reduces congestion (i.e. swelling) of the nasal mucosa.

delirium. A state of impaired consciousness and mental confusion.

demulcent. Supposed to coat and smooth mucous membranes of the gastro-intestinal tract (e.g. milk, raw egg white).

dermatitis. General term to describe inflammation of the skin, which may be due to many causes.

diuretic. Increases urine output.

DMARDs. Disease-modifying anti-rheumatoid drugs. Drugs which, when used to treat rheumatoid arthritis, have effects on the immune response and may suppress the inflammatory process. Unlike the non-steroidal anti-inflammatory drugs (NSAIDs), they do not produce immediate relief of symptoms but take 4–6 months to produce a full response. Examples of this drug group include GOLD, PENICILLAMINE, CHLOROQUINE and METHOTREXATE.

dyspepsia. Indigestion.

elixir. Clear, flavoured liquid preparation of drug frequently containing alcohol and sweetening and colouring agents.

embolus. Mobile blood clot which travels through the bloodstream until it wedges in a blood vessel and blocks the blood supply to the part of the body supplied by that vessel.

embrocation. A liquid formulation for external application on, or rubbing into, a diseased or painful joint or muscle.

emetic. Induces vomiting.

emollient. Topical softening application.

encephalitis. Inflammation of brain tissue.

encephalopathy. Comprehensive term to describe general abnormality of brain tissue function. May be due to many causes.

endogenous. Produced or found within the body.

endometriosis. 'Islands' of uterine lining cells scattered throughout the other abdominal organs. Symptoms include abdominal pain and heavy menstruation.

enema. Drug formulation for rectal administration.

enteric coating. Surface coating of capsules or tablets designed to resist gastric acid acting on it, so that the drug is not released until reaching the small intestine.

enzyme. A reactive protein which mediates a chemical reaction without itself being altered.

essential oil. Volatile oil derived by distillation from part of a plant.

exogenous. Derived from outside the body.

expectorant. Aids removal of sputum from the lungs and respiratory passages.

febrifuge. A preparation that lowers raised body temperature (fever).

fibrates. Lipid-regulating drugs used in patients at risk of clinical manifestations of coronary artery disease. For most patients they are a second-line treatment after/or in addition to the statins, as they are more effective at lowering triglyceride levels than CHOLESTEROL levels, because of their more serious adverse effect profile. In particular, they may cause muscle dysfunction, including myositis.

fibrinolytic. Dissolves or otherwise destroys the fibrin which is formed when blood clots.

fusion inhibitors. A class of antiviral drugs that work by preventing HIV-1 and HIV-2 from entering human cells. Used in the treatment and prevention of AIDS.

GABA (Gamma-aminobutyric acid). Inhibitory neurotransmitter found in the brain. Reduced activity is associated with epilepsy, hence drugs which enhance GABA effects may be used as anticonvulsants.

G6PD (Glucose 6-phosphate dehydrogenase). An enzyme involved in carbohy-

drate metabolism. Some patients exhibit an inherited deficiency of this enzyme and are thus more susceptible to certain diseases and adverse drug effects.

galactorrhoea. Inappropriate production of breast milk in either sex, not associated with a recent pregnancy.

gel. Jelly-like formulation of medicinal ingredients.

gynaecomastia. Abnormal enlargement of the breasts in men.

haematinic. Involved in the normal development of red blood cells.

haemolysis. Increased breakdown of red blood cells.

haemorrhoids. Piles.

haemostatic. Reduces or stops blood loss.

herbicide. Kills plants.

hirsutism. Increased and extensive hair growth.

HIV-1 and HIV-2 (Human immunodeficiency virus). Viruses of the retrovirus family are transmitted either sexually or by injection when, for example, drugs are injected intravenously using non-sterile needles previously used by infected individuals. HIV-1 is the dominant strain in Western countries whereas HIV-2 was first identified in Western Africa. After the initial infection the patient is asymptomatic for a period of years but may become progressively immunocompromised and develop the acquired immune deficiency syndrome (AIDS). When AIDS was first described in the early 1980s, there were no effective antiviral agents for HIV and treatment was symptomatic using antibiotics and antifungals, for example. As a result of subsequent research, an increasing number of antiviral agents have been developed, starting with ZIDOVUDINE. Currently four classes of anti-HIV drugs are described according to their mode of action: (1) nucleoside reverse transcriptase inhibitors, (2) protease inhibitors, (3) non-nucleoside reverse transcriptase inhibitors, (4) fusion inhibitors. When prescribed in the recommended way, by specialists, these drugs have been shown to improve both quality of life and life expectancy in patients who have developed AIDS, or are showing signs of developing it.

HMG CoA reductase. An enzyme involved in cholesterol synthesis in the liver. Inhibited by the statin group of drugs that are used in the treatment and prophylaxis of atherosclerosis.

hormone. Naturally occurring substance which is secreted by a gland into the bloodstream, whence it is carried to the part of the body on which it acts. Insulin, for example, is secreted by the pancreas and acts at sites all over the body.

HRT. Hormone replacement therapy for relief of menopausal/postmenopausal symptoms. Uses small doses of the hormones used for contraception.

hyperaldosteronism. Excessive secretion of the salt-retaining hormone ALDOSTERONE.

hypercalcaemia. Raised serum calcium above normal levels.

hyperglycaemia. Raised blood glucose above normal levels.

hyperkalaemia. Raised serum potassium above normal levels.

hyperlipidaemia. High concentrations of lipids (fats) in the blood, measured as cholesterol and triglycerides. May be inherited, acquired (dietary), or a mixture of both. Untreated hyperlipidaemias are associated with atherosclerotic disease, leading to heart attacks, strokes and poor blood supply to the legs and other parts of the body. Treatment consists of reduction of dietary fat intake, plus lipid-lowering drugs, if necessary.

hypernatraemia. Raised serum sodium above normal levels.

hyperthyroidism. Abnormal increase in thyroid function.

hypnotic. Facilitates sleep.

hypocalcaemia. Reduced serum calcium below normal levels.

hypoglycaemia. Reduced blood glucose below normal levels.

hypokalaemia. Reduced serum potassium below normal levels.

hyponatraemia. Reduced serum sodium below normal levels.

hypotensive. Lowers blood pressure.

hypothyroidism. Abnormal decrease in thyroid function.

immunosuppressant. Tends to suppress the immune response. This effect may be used to suppress some cancers or rejection of transplanted organs, but it makes the body more susceptible to infections.

infusion. Administration of a drug by continuous intravenous drip/injection.

insecticide. Kills insects.

insomnia. Lack of, or inability to, sleep.

isomer. One of two or more molecules having the same number and kind of atoms but differing in the arrangement or configuration of the atoms. Optical isomers are compounds whose structures are mirror images of each other. Isomers may differ in the order in which atoms are joined together, or in the position of atoms or groups of atoms in the molecule.

When a drug exists in more than one isomer, one isomer may have all or most of the pharmacological activity. Recent trends in drug development include the introduction of specific isomers rather than the normal racemic mixtures.

keratolytic. Removes dry scaly skin.

laxative. Relieves constipation.

leukotrienes. Potent inflammatory mediators that play an important role in asthma. When released from eosinophils and mast cells in the inflammatory response, they cause smooth muscle contraction, increased vascular permeability and increased mucus production, all of which adversely affect the breathing.

linctus. Viscous liquid preparation of drug containing sugar or alternative sweetening agent.

liniment. A liquid formulation for external application on, or rubbing into, a diseased or painful joint or muscle.

lotion. Wet dressing used to cleanse and cool inflamed skin lesions.

lozenge. Tablet, originally diamond-shaped, of flavoured medication to be dissolved in the mouth.

melaena. Black stools due to passage of altered blood from haemorrhage.

meningitis. Inflammation of the meninges, the covering of the brain.

minipill. *See* Progestogen-only pill (POP).

miotic. Constricts the pupil of the eye.

mucolytic. Liquifies mucus within the respiratory system.

myalgia. Pain in muscles.

mydriatic. Dilates the pupil of the eye.

narcotic analgesic. Pain-relieving drug of the opium group. Liable to have addictive properties.

nephritis. Inflammation of kidney tissue.

nephrotoxic. Causes damage to the kidneys.

neurokinins. Neurotransmitters that have a key role in the regulation of depression and emesis.

neuropathy. Comprehensive term to describe general abnormality of function of a peripheral nerve, which may be due to many causes.

neurotransmitter. Biochemical substance which acts in the transmission of nerve impulses.

neutrophil. One of the families of white blood cells which is involved in combating bacterial infection.

non-nucleoside reverse transcriptase inhibitors. A class of structurally diverse antiviral drugs which block reverse transcriptase, an enzyme that HIV-1 needs to make more copies of itself. Unlike the nucleoside reverse transcriptase inhibitors, they have no activity against HIV-2. Used in the treatment and prevention of AIDS.

nucleoside reverse transcriptase inhibitors. Antiviral drugs with a chemical structure similar to the chemicals that make up DNA and RNA. They prevent replication of HIV-1 and HIV-2 by blocking the reverse transcriptase enzyme which is essential for replication. Used in the treatment and prevention of AIDS.

oedema. Swelling and congestion of tissues due to accumulation of fluid derived from the blood plasma.

ototoxic. Causes damage to nerves involved in hearing.

parasympatholytic. Antagonizes the action of ACETYLCHOLINE. *See* ANTI-CHOLINERGIC.

parasympathomimetic. Has actions similar to the parasympathetic chemical transmitter in the nervous system ACETYLCHOLINE.

parenteral. Administered by a route other than via the gastro-intestinal tract. Usually refers to intradermal, subcutaneous, intramuscular or intravenous injection.

pastille. A sweetened medicinal formulation with a round flat shape, to be dissolved in the mouth.

peptide. A chain of amino acids.

pessary. Solid-dose drug formulation similar to suppository but placed in the vagina. Usually used for local actions in the vagina but systemic absorption of the drug may occur.

pesticide. Kills pests. This term includes a wide range of compounds (e.g. rodenticides which kill rats and small mammals, insecticides, herbicides). Only a few of these chemicals also have applications as drugs.

pharmaceutical aid. An ingredient used to produce a convenient formulation of a drug for administration by a particular route.

pharmacodynamics. Study of the actions of drugs in living systems.

pharmacokinetics. Study of the fate of drugs in the body. Includes absorption, distribution, metabolism and excretion.

phenothiazine. Drug with a chemical structure similar to CHLORPROMAZINE.

phosphodiesterase. Enzyme, the inhibition of which leads to effects similar to beta-adrenoceptor stimulation.

photophobia. Intolerance to light.

placebo. Inactive substance or preparation used in controlled studies to evaluate the effectiveness of a medicinal substance. In some instances, a placebo may be prescribed to satisfy the patient's desire for medicine. In other instances, a supposedly 'active' drug may be prescribed but the benefits seen relate not to this action but to the 'placebo' effect.

plasma. The cell-free fluid component of the blood.

plasmin. An enzyme which acts on fibrin in small clots in blood vessels with the result that the clot dissolves and disintegrates.

pneumonitis. Inflammation of the tissues of the lung.

polypeptide. A complex molecule made up of peptides.

polysaccharide. A complex sugar molecule.

prodrug. A chemical that is converted into an active drug within the body.

Progestogen-only pill (POP). Oral contraceptive containing only progestogen hormone, as compared to the combined oral contraceptives (COCs) which contain both an oestrogen and a progestogen. Although effective as contraceptives, POPs are less reliable than COCs and are used mainly for those women who cannot tolerate the latter. May cause irregular vaginal bleeding.

prokinetic. Facilitates movement throughout the gastro-intestinal tract by increasing contractions of the gut wall.

prophylactic. Tends to prevent a condition rather than treat it when established.

prostaglandins. A group of very active substances found throughout the body with a large number of actions including effects on the uterus, airways and blood vessels.

protease inhibitors. Antiviral drugs that prevent replication of the HIV virus by blocking the protease enzyme that is essential for this process. See the definition of HIV-1 and HIV-2. Used in the treatment and prevention of AIDS.

protein. A complex molecule made up of polypeptides.

pruritis. Persistent itching.

psychosis. Major disturbance in mental function, with abnormalities in thought processes often accompanied by hallucinations.

purgative. Facilitates evacuation of the bowels.

purine nucleoside. A chemical related to the basic protein structure of which chromosomes are constructed.

quinolones. An expanding group of antibiotics. The initial drugs e.g. NALIDIXIC ACID, CINOXACIN and NORFLOXACIN are used to treat urinary infections. More recent drugs e.g. CIPROFLOXACIN and LEVOFLOXACIN have a broader spectrum of activity and have wider uses including respiratory infections. May cause convulsions and should be used with caution in patients with epilepsy. Rare cases of severe tendonitis have been described, notably in elderly patients on corticosteroid therapy.

receptor. Site on cell surfaces which reacts to drugs or endogenous substance to produce the observed effect.

retinitis. Inflammation of the retina, the layer of nerve cells at the back of the eye which senses light impulses and mediates vision.

retrobulbar neuritis. Inflammation of the optic nerve between the brain and eye.

rhinitis. Inflammation of the nasal passages.

rub. A formulation for topical application.

rubefacient. Causes reddening of the skin.

sclerosing agent. Produces an inflammatory reaction and fibrosis, leading to closure of blood vessels.

sedative. Reduces arousal.

sinus rhythm. The normal regular heart rhythm.

spermicides. A number of different substances used in spermicidal contraceptives and administered topically into the vagina as jelly, cream, foaming tablet, pessary, aerosol or film. Appear to act by reducing surface tension in the sperm cell surface and allowing osmotic imbalance to destroy the cell. Relatively ineffective contraceptives, they should be used in conjunction with a barrier contraceptive (e.g. the cap), unless the couple concerned accept the risk of pregnancy.

statins. A group of orally active inhibitors of the enzyme HMG CoA reductase which reduce CHOLESTEROL synthesis in the liver. Used long term to reduce blood CHOLESTEROL concentrations when diet and exercise are not sufficient. They are beneficial in preventing the complications of atherosclerosis, e.g. myocardial infarction and stroke. Used both for primary prevention in 'at-risk' patients and for secondary prevention, i.e. to reduce the risk of recurrence of myocardial infarctions and strokes. May cause headaches, gastro-intestinal upsets, altered liver function and allergy. Muscle symptoms, including myalgia, myositis and myopathy, occur rarely, notably in patients with a history of liver disease and where multiple lipid-lowering drugs have been used. In extreme cases, rhabdomyolysis and resultant renal failure have occurred. Recently there has been a move to license statins for non-prescription use, starting with SIMVASTATIN.

sulphonylureas. A group of drugs which act on pancreatic, insulin-secreting cells to augment insulin secretion. Used as oral antidiabetic treatment where the pancreas is still capable of secreting useful amounts of insulin, i.e. in late onset/ type 2 diabetes. May cause hypoglycaemia, and this is more likely with the longer acting drugs and in elderly patients.

suppository. Solid-dose, elongated, cone-shaped drug formulation for insertion into the rectum for local treatment (e.g. for haemorrhoids) or for drug absorption (e.g. antiemetic). Has a fatty base which melts at body temperature.

sustained-release formulation. Product specifically designed to release the active drug more slowly and over a prolonged period. Used to increase the interval between doses and prevent toxicity from high drug concentrations achieved in the body when there is rapid absorption.

sympathomimetic. Has actions similar to the chemical transmitters of sympathetic nervous system (ADRENALINE and NORADRENALINE).

tachycardia. Rapid heart rate.

tachyphylaxis. Occurs when repeated doses of the drug produce progressively smaller effects (or else progressively bigger doses are required).

tardive dyskinesia. A neurological syndrome associated with long-term use of dopamine receptor blocking antipsychotic drugs such as phenothiazines, and characterized by involuntary movements.

teratogenic. May produce congenital malformation if given during the first three months of pregnancy.

thiazides. A group of related compounds (e.g. BENDROFLUMETHIAZIDE), with diuretic effects. They act at the distal convoluted tubule of the kidney to reduce reabsorption of salt and water. Moderately potent, but less so than the 'loop diuretics' (e.g. FUROSEMIDE). Active by mouth within one to two hours and a duration of 12–24 hours. May cause hypokalaemia, hyperglycaemia, and hyperuricaemia. Caution in patients with diabetes mellitus and gout. Used in hypertension where they act partly by reducing the peripheral vascular resistance. May cause impotence.

thrombolytic. Breaks down clots in the vascular system.

thrombophlebitis. Formation of clot in an inflamed vein.

thrombus. Blood clot.

tolerance. Has the same meaning as tachyphylaxis (see above).

topical. Applied externally at the site where the drug action is needed (e.g. for treatment of skin rashes or eye infections).

toxoid. A preparation of a bacterial toxin that has its toxic properties removed but has retained its ability to stimulate the body's immunity to it by the production of antibodies.

tranquillizer. *See* antipsychotics.

vaccine. Preparation of live attenuated or dead microorganisms used to induce immunity.

vasoconstrictor. Causes constriction of blood vessels.

vasodilator. Causes dilatation of blood vessels.

vitamin. Chemical essential in small amounts for maintenance of normal growth and health. Must be obtained from external sources, usually dietary. Inadequate intake leads to deficiency diseases.

PART I

Approved Names

A

Abacavir. Antiretroviral enzyme inhibitor used in combination with other drugs to prevent viral replication in HIV infection. May cause gastro-intestinal upset, lethargy, fever, headache and loss of appetite. Severe and even fatal hypersensitivity reactions have occurred and if these are detected further use of the drug is precluded.

Abciximab. Monoclonal antibody which binds to receptors on the walls of blood vessels and thus blocks the formation of a blood platelet clot. Used in non-invasive heart surgery (angioplasty) to reduce the risk of blood clots forming after the operation and reduce the risk of myocardial infarct in patients with unstable angina. May cause bleeding complications and should not be used in any patient with a previous history of such problems.

Acamprosate. Analogue of the neurotransmitter GABA. Used to aid abstinence in chronic alcoholism, where it acts on GABA receptors to reduce craving for alcohol. May cause gastro-intestinal disturbance, skin reactions and fluctuations in libido.

Acarbose. Saccharide that inhibits the digestive enzyme alpha-glucosidase which breaks dietary carbohydrate down to monosaccharides. This leads to a reduction in blood glucose level. Indicated in patients with non-insulin-dependent diabetes who are inadequately controlled by diet alone, or in combination with other oral drug treatment. Adverse effects include flatulence and diarrhoea.

Acebutolol. Beta-adrenoceptor blocking drug, with limited cardioselectivity. Uses, side effects etc. as for PROPRANOLOL.

Aceclofenac. Non-steroidal anti-inflammatory analgesic with actions, uses and adverse effects similar to DICLOFENAC.

Acemetacin. Non-steroid anti-inflammatory/analgesic used in treatment of rheumatoid arthritis, osteoarthritis and postoperative pain and inflammation. Adverse effects include gastro-intestinal symptoms, headache, dizziness, oedema, chest pain, pruritus, blood dyscrasias, tinnitus and blurred vision.

Acenocoumarol. Anticoagulant, with actions, interactions and adverse effects similar to WARFARIN.

Acetaminophen. USA: *see* PARACETAMOL.

Acetazolamide. Weak diuretic. Also used in glaucoma to reduce intraocular pressure, and as an anticonvulsant. Acts by inhibiting carbonic anhydrase and so reduces hydrogen ions available for exchange with sodium ions. May cause drowsiness, mental confusion and paraesthesia.

Acetomenaphthone. *See* VITAMIN K.

Acetylcholine. Neurotransmitter, particularly in parasympathetic system. Peripheral effects include miosis, paralysis of accommodation, increased glandular secretions, contraction of smooth muscle in gastro-intestinal, respiratory and urogenital systems, slowing of heart and vasodilatation. These effects blocked by ATROPINE SULPHATE. Used by ocular irrigation to produce rapid dilation of the pupil during eye surgery.

Acetylcysteine. Mucolytic. Administered by mouth or by inhalation from a nebulizer. Liquefies mucus and aids expectoration in diseases where mucus is troublesome (e.g. chronic bronchitis). May cause bronchospasm, haemoptysis. nausea and vomiting. Used also in lubricant eye drops and intravenously in the treatment of PARACETA-MOL overdosage where it prevents liver damage by restoring or acting as a substitute for depleted liver glutathione stores. In this use may also cause rash, nausea, vomiting and transient bronchospasm.

Acetylsalicylic acid (Aspirin). Antiinflammatory, antipyretic analgesic. Inhibits prostaglandin synthesis, reduces stickiness of blood platelets. Used to reduce risk of stroke and heart attacks. May cause gastric erosion, haemorrhage and hypersensitivity reactions. Tinnitus and hyperventilation leading to respiratory and cardiovascular failure in overdose. Interacts with oral anticoagulants and sulphonylureas. Forced alkaline diuresis may be used to speed elimination in overdosage.

Aciclovir. Antiviral agent used orally, topically and intravenously to treat herpes simplex and varicella zoster infections. Should not be used when patient is dehydrated as may cause rise in blood urea and creatinine.

Acipimox. Reduces raised blood lipids by inhibiting the release of fatty acids from fat tissue. Related chemically to NICOTINIC ACID. Adverse reactions include flushing and headache.

Acitretin. The major metabolite of ETRETI-NATE with similar actions, adverse reactions and contraindications. Patients are advised to avoid alcohol because of increased risk of effects on the foetus.

Aclarubicin. Cytotoxic antibiotic used in treatment of leukaemia. Adverse effects include bone marrow suppression, phlebitis and cardiotoxicity. Related to DAUNORUBICIN but may act by a different mechanism and appears to cause less cardiotoxicity.

Acrivastine. Antihistamine for treatment of allergies and hay fever. It is fast acting and has a short duration of action. It seldom causes drowsiness.

Actinomycin D. Cytotoxic antibiotic used in neoplastic disease. Adverse effects include bone marrow depression.

Activated charcoal. Charcoal is a strong adsorbent. 'Activated' indicates simply that the charcoal meets certain standards in adsorbance tests. Used by mouth in cases of acute poisoning in single doses to reduce absorption of many drugs or other toxins. For a small number of drugs, will enhance excretion if given in multiple doses. May cause nausea and vomiting. Would adsorb oral antidotes and therefore should not be used if these are given. Subsequent black stools should not be mistaken for melaena. Also used in some dressings to adsorb odour and fluid from wounds.

Adalimumab (r). Anticytokine. Human, monoclonal, TNF-α antibody. Has been shown to modulate the inflammatory process and improve quality of life in patients with severe rheumatoid arthritis, who do not respond to, or cannot tolerate, disease-modifying anti-rheumatoid drugs (DMARDs). Given by injection at two-week intervals. Similar to ETANERCEPT and INFLIXIMAB and like them it may cause a wide range of adverse reactions including impaired response to infections. Since some of these reactions relate to the production of antibodies against the drugs, it is hoped that the use of a fully human drug structure in adalimumab will reduce the incidence of such reactions. All anticytokines are recently introduced and are being closely monitored for safety.

Adapalene. VITAMIN A analogue with actions and adverse effects similar to TRETINOIN. Used in topical treatment of severe acne.

Adefovir (r). Oral antiviral used to treat chronic hepatitis B in patients with active liver disease. May cause weakness, gastro-intestinal symptoms, headache and impaired renal function.

Adenosine. Endogenous purine nucleoside which acts on specific receptors in heart muscle and coronary arteries to reduce heart rate. Given by intravenous injection to assist in diagnosis of certain fast heart rhythms and to convert some fast rhythms back to normal 'sinus' rhythm. May cause facial flushing, sweating, burning sensations, chest pain, palpitations, heart block, shortness of breath, headaches and blurred vision.

Adenosine monophosphoric acid (AMP). Source of high-energy phosphate bonds for tissue metabolism. Suggested for use in cardiovascular disease and rheumatism but efficacy unproven.

Adenosine triphosphoric acid (ATP). Source of high-energy phosphate bonds for tissue metabolism. Suggested for use in cardiovascular disease and rheumatism but efficacy unproven.

Adrenaline. Sympathomimetic amine, alpha- and beta-adrenoceptor agonist. Produces vasoconstriction with rise in blood pressure, cardioacceleration and bronchodilation. Used in acute allergic reactions, as peripheral vasoconstrictor, in narrow-angle glaucoma and in cardiac arrest. Toxicity includes hypertension, pulmonary oedema and cardiac arrhythmias.

Agar. Purgative. Increases faecal bulk by same mechanism as METHYLCELLULOSE but less effective.

Alclofenac. Anti-inflammatory analgesic with actions similar to IBUPROFEN.

Alclometasone. Topical corticosteroid for treatment of eczema and other non-infective inflammatory conditions. Actions and adverse effects similar to HYDROCORTISONE.

Aldesleukin. Growth factor produced by recombinant techniques, involved in regu-

lation of normal growth and differentiation of cells involved in immune mechanisms. Used in treatment of renal cancer which has spread throughout the body. Given intravenously, it produces many unwanted effects including fever, rigor, weight gain and hypotension.

Aldosterone. Naturally occurring adrenal (mineralocorticoid) steroid hormone. Acts mainly on salt and water metabolism by increasing salt retention in the kidney; has no useful anti-inflammatory activity. Used only in replacement therapy for adrenal insufficiency.

Alemtuzumab (r). Monoclonal antibody that targets lymphocytes and stimulates cell death. Used by intravenous infusion in treatment of chronic lymphocytic leukaemia when first-line treatments fail. May cause pain at the injection site, fever, anorexia, fluid retention and impairment of function of other body systems including liver and heart.

Alendronic acid. A biphosphonate with actions on remodelling of bone similar to ETIDRONATE. For prevention and treatment of postmenopausal osteoporosis and corticosteroid-induced osteoporosis in women. Also used for prevention of bone loss in men and women at risk of osteoporosis from other causes, e.g. inability to exercise regularly. May cause abdominal pain, gastro-intestinal disturbances, skin rashes, heachaches and bone marrow suppression. Should be swallowed with water and the patient is advised to avoid lying down for 30 minutes, to avoid irritation to the oesophagus.

Alexitol sodium. Complex of sodium poly (hydroxyaluminium) carbonate and hexitol. An antacid with uses and adverse effects similar to ALUMINIUM HYDROXIDE.

Alfacalcidol (1α-Hydroxyvitamin D$_3$). Rapidly converted in the liver to dihydroxyvitamin D$_3$ – the metabolite of VITAMIN D with the most marked effect on calcium and phosphate balance. Used in

Alfentanil

treatment of renal bone disease, hypoparathyroidism, rickets and osteomalacia
when these are resistant to VITAMIN D
itself. May cause hypercalcaemia with risk
of metastatic calcification and renal failure.
Hypercalcaemia treated by stopping the
drug and administration of fluids plus
potent diuretics (e.g. FUROSEMIDE).

Alfentanil (c). Narcotic analgesic, with
actions and uses similar to FENTANYL and
MORPHINE. Has a rapid onset of action, but its
duration of action is less than other narcotic
analgesics. Used as an adjunct to anaesthesia during short surgical procedures.

Alfuzosin. Alpha$_1$ antagonist used for
symptomatic relief in benign prostatic
hypertrophy. Does not reduce or delay
growth of the prostate but reduces urethral
tone and resistance and bladder resistance
thus relieving the more distressing symptoms. May cause dizziness, headache,
gastro-intestinal disturbance, tachycardia,
flushing and itching.

Alginates. Extracts from algae used as
tablet binders and disintegrants, and in
highly adsorbant wound dressings which
aid the removal of exudates. Also used in
antacids where the alginates form a 'raft'
which floats on the surface of the stomach
acid and protects the oesophageal mucosa
in cases of acid reflux.

Alimemazine. Phenothiazine similar to
CHLORPROMAZINE. Used for antiemetic,
sedative and antipruritic effects. Adverse
effects, etc. as for CHLORPROMAZINE.

Allantoin. Used in creams and lotions to
stimulate wound healing.

Allergen extract vaccines. Extracts prepared from common allergens (e.g. grass,
bee venom) for hyposensitization of hyper-
sensitive individuals. Used as graded doses
starting from the lowest. Injected subcutaneously. Avoid in pregnancy, febrile conditions and acute asthma. May cause
allergic reactions.

Allopurinol. Reduces formation of uric
acid from purine precursors by inhibiting
the enzyme xanthine oxidase. Used in
primary and secondary gout.

Allylestrenol. Hormone with actions
similar to PROGESTERONE.

Almasilate. Polymer of aluminium magnesium silicate. Similar antacid properties
to ALUMINIUM HYDROXIDE and MAGNESIUM
TRISILICATE.

Almotriptan. Oral 5-HYDROXYTRYPTAMINE
agonist similar to SUMATRIPTAN. Used to
relieve migraine attacks. Acts by causing
selective constriction of cranial blood
vessels to relieve the throbbing headache
associated with migraine. May cause
dizziness, nausea, vomiting and tiredness. There may be rebound headaches.
Contraindicated if there is a history of
heart disease or other vascular disease.

Aloes. Derived from species of aloe. Used
as purgative, producing motion 6–12 hours
after ingestion. Causes griping. Colours
urine red. May cause nephritis in large
doses.

Aloin. Extract of aloes: see ALOES.

Aloxiprin. Complex of ALUMINIUM
ANTACIDS and ACETYLSALICYLIC ACID,
yielding these agents after breakdown in
the gastro-intestinal tract.

Alprenolol. Beta-adrenoceptor blocking
drug with partial agonist activity (intrinsic
sympathomimetic activity). Uses, side
effects, etc. as for PROPRANOLOL.

Alprostadil. Naturally occurring prostaglandin which increases penile blood
flow by direct relaxation of arterial
smooth muscle and inhibition of throm-
boxane. Used by intracavernous (intrapenile) injection in treatment of erectile
dysfunction. Adverse effects include
burning sensation and pain in the penis.
May also cause a fall in blood pressure,

6

cardiac arrhythmias, dizziness and headaches.

Alteplase. A synthetic plasminogen activator/fibrinolytic agent given intravenously after a myocardial infarct to dissolve thrombi in the coronary artery. Unlike STREPTOKINASE and UROKINASE it acts on plasminogen in the clot rather than in the systemic circulation and is not immunogenic. May cause localized bleeding, intracerebral haemorrhage, nausea and vomiting.

Altretamine. Cytotoxic used in treatment of ovarian cancer and other solid-dose tumours. May cause bone marrow suppression and gastro-intestinal disturbance.

Alum (Potassium aluminium sulphate). Used as solid to stop bleeding; in powder for application to umbilical cord. Precipitates proteins and is a powerful astringent.

Aluminium antacids. Range of aluminium salts, used alone or complexed with other compounds. Neutralize gastric acid in treatment of peptic ulceration. Large doses cause constipation which may be prevented by combination with MAGNESIUM ANTACIDS. May reduce absorption of other drugs (e.g. TETRACYCLINE).

Aluminium carbonate. Nonsystemic (nonabsorbable) antacid. Used in treatment of peptic ulceration where it produces longer neutralization of acid than SODIUM BICARBONATE. Also used in prevention of urinary phosphate stones. May cause constipation. Reduces absorption of TETRACYCLINE given at same time.

Aluminium chloride. Astringent. Precipitates proteins when applied to skin resulting in hardening and reduced secretions. Used to prevent excessive sweating (hyperhidrosis).

Aluminium chlorohydrate. Used topically in antiperspirant preparations. Thought to act by reducing release of sweat by forming a plug using cell proteins which block the sweat duct. May cause redness or irritation.

Aluminium glycinate. See ALUMINIUM ANTACIDS.

Aluminium hydroxide. Nonsystemic (nonabsorbable) antacid. Neutralizes gastric acid and binds phosphate ions in the gut. Used to treat peptic ulceration by reducing gastric acidity and also to increase phosphate excretion when phosphate retention is associated with stone formation (e.g. renal stones). Large doses cause constipation which may be prevented by combination with MAGNESIUM ANTACIDS.

Alverine. Antispasmodic drug used in gut colic; related to PAPAVERINE.

Amantadine. Antiviral agent for prophylaxis against influenza. Antiparkinsonian drug used in mild cases. Adverse effects include dry mouth, visual disturbances, confusion, hallucinations and ankle oedema.

Amethocaine. See TETRACAINE.

Amfetamine (c). A central nervous system stimulant with sympathomimetic effects. Acts by releasing NORADRENALINE from peripheral nerve endings to cause increases in heart rate and blood pressure, and by releasing NORADRENALINE and DOPAMINE centrally to produce a state ranging from increased alertness to increased, and even psychotic, excitation. In the past amfetamine and similar drugs were used to treat a variety of psychiatric disorders and obesity. The evidence for benefit from such uses was limited and the potential for adverse effects, misuses and dependency was large. Amfetamine is no longer prescribed, but derivatives such as DEXAMFETAMINE have limited use as specialist treatments for narcolepsy and attention deficit hyperactivity disorder (ADHD).

Amifostine. Cytoprotective used to reduce the adverse effects of anticancer drugs. It is a prodrug activated by an enzyme which is present in large amounts only where there is a good blood supply. Acts by combining with, and deactivating, the anticancer drug at nontumour sites, but is less active in most tumours since the blood supply is usually relatively reduced, thus allowing the anticancer drug to exert its effect. Adverse effects include nausea, vomiting, dizziness and low blood pressure.

Amikacin. Antimicrobial with actions and uses similar to GENTAMICIN.

Amiloride. Potassium-sparing diuretic. Acts by inhibiting exchange of sodium for potassium in the distal tubule of the kidney. Relatively weak diuretic used when there is particular danger of potassium loss (e.g. fluid overload due to liver failure). Often combined with a thiazide (e.g. BEN-DROFLUMETHIAZIDE) or FUROSEMIDE. Danger of excessive potassium retention. May cause nausea, vomiting and diarrhoea.

Aminacrine. See AMINOACRIDINE.

Amino acids. Dietary components. Breakdown products of proteins. Some may be synthesized in the body, others (the 'essential' amino acids) cannot, and must be taken in at least minimum amounts for normal health.

Aminoacridine. Skin disinfectant.

Aminobenzoic acid. Member of the vitamin B complex found in some compound vitamin preparations. Used as a lotion to protect the skin from ultraviolet radiation.

Aminoglutethimide. Has inhibitory actions on adrenal cortex. May be used to suppress adrenal activity in hyperadrenalism, particularly when due to adrenal carcinoma. Also used to reduce oedema caused by hyperaldosteronism and in sex hormone-dependent prostatic and breast carcinoma. Adverse effects include drowsiness, confusion, skin rashes, gastric discomfort, bone marrow suppression, hypothyroidism and virilism.

Aminophylline (Theophylline ethylenediamine). Relaxes smooth muscle, dilates bronchi, increases heart rate and force, and has diuretic action. Used in cardiac and bronchial asthma. Given orally, intravenously or by suppository. Adverse effects include nausea, vomiting, if given orally; vertigo, restlessness, cardiac arrhythmias, if given intravenously.

5-Aminosalicylic acid. See MESALAZINE.

Amiodarone. Cardiac antiarrhythmic. Adverse effects include hepatitis, disturbances of thyroid function, corneal deposits, nerve damage, skin photosensitivity, sleep disturbance and a metallic taste.

Amisulpride. Oral antipsychotic which acts by blocking presynaptic (in low doses) and postsynaptic (at high doses) DOPAMINE receptors (D_2 and D_3). It is thus used to control both the negative and positive symptoms of schizophrenia. May cause agitation, gastro-intestinal disorders, weight gain and movement disorders.

Amitriptyline. Antidepressant. Actions and adverse effects similar to IMIPRAMINE. Also has sedative and anxiolytic properties.

Amlodipine. Antianginal/antihypertensive vasodilator, with actions, uses and adverse effects similar to NIFEDIPINE. Long duration of action allows once daily dosage.

Ammonium chloride. Acidifying agent. Also used as expectorant and diuretic.

Amobarbital (c). Barbiturate hypnotic/sedative. General depressant action on CNS. Used in treatment of insomnia and anxiety. Frequently has a 'hangover' effect with impairment of mental and physical performance. Tolerance and addiction may occur, with insomnia, delirium and convulsions on withdrawal. Metabolized by liver and therefore used with caution in liver disease. Induces its own metabolism and that of some other drugs with danger of adverse drug interaction. Coma with respiratory depression in overdosage. No antidote; treated by supportive measures.

Amorolfine. Antifungal agent similar to TERBINAFINE, but marketed as a lacquer for treatment of fungal infections of the nails. May cause pruritus.

Amoxapine. Tricyclic antidepressant which inhibits reuptake of NORADRENALINE and SEROTONIN in neurones. Adverse effects and precautions as for AMITRIPTYLINE. Said to have a more rapid onset of antidepressant effects and to be one of the less sedative tricyclics.

Amoxicillin. Similar to AMPICILLIN but better absorbed.

Amoxycillin. *See* AMOXICILLIN.

Amphetamine. *See* AMFETAMINE.

Amphotericin. Antifungal. Used topically for skin infections or by intravenous injection for severe generalized fungal infections. Topically it may produce irritation of skin. Systemic side effects are often severe, including headache, vomiting, fever, joint pains, convulsions and kidney damage.

Ampicillin. Penicillin antibiotic with broader spectrum of activity than BENZYLPENICILLIN; active against typhoid fever. Adverse effects as for BENZYLPENICILLIN. Rash common if given to patients with infectious mononucleosis (i.e. glandular fever).

Amprenavir. Antiviral protease inhibitor. Inihibits HIV maturation/proliferation. Used for treatment of HIV infections in combination with other antiviral agents. May cause gastro-intestinal disturbance, liver dysfunction, bone marrow suppression, fatigue and muscle disorders, metabolic disorders and skin rashes.

Amsacrine. Cytotoxic drug with actions, indications and adverse effects similar to DOXORUBICIN.

Amyl nitrite (m). Vasodilator with actions similar to GLYCERYL TRINITRATE but with more rapid onset of action and shorter duration of effect. Abused in the belief that it expands creativity, appreciation of music and sexual experience. Not used to treat angina because adverse effects are accentuated and beneficial actions are too short-lived. Used as an immediate antidote to cyanide poisoning to induce formation of methaemoglobin which combines with cyanide to form nontoxic cyanmethaemoglobin.

Amylobarbitone. *See* AMOBARBITAL.

Amylocaine. Local anaesthetic with actions similar to LIDOCAINE.

Anagrelide (r). Enzyme inhibitor with specific effects on the enzymes involved in formation of blood platelets. Used to treat primary or essential thrombocythaemia, a myeloproliferative disorder, in order to reduce the risk of vascular thrombosis. Less likely to cause global bone marrow suppression than earlier treatments i.e. CHLORAMBUCIL, BUSULPHAN and INTERFERON ALFA. May cause anaemia, headache, gastrointestinal disturbance and fluid retention.

Anakinra (r). Interleukin-1 receptor antagonist that suppresses the inflammatory process in rheumatoid arthritis. Used by injection in combination with METHOTREXATE when the response to that drug is inadequate. May cause injection site reactions, headache and impaired response to infections.

Anastrozole. Anti-oestrogen, acts by inhibition of an enzyme responsible for production of non-ovarian oestrogens. Breast cancer after the menopause is usually oestrogen-dependent and non-ovarian sources are of increased importance. Used, therefore, to treat advanced breast cancer in postmenopausal women. May cause hot flushes, vaginal irritation, hair thinning, gastro-intestinal disturbance, rash and headaches.

9

Ancrod

Ancrod. Anticoagulant enzyme from venom of Malayan pit viper. Given intravenously. May produce allergic reactions.

Anethole. Essential oil with odour of anise. Used as a carminative and expectorant.

Aneurine (Thiamine, Vitamin B_1). Vitamin. Deficiency may cause cardiac failure (wet beri-beri), peripheral neuritis (dry beri-beri) and Wernicke's encephalopathy.

Anistreplase. An acylated complex of human plasminogen with STREPTOKINASE which produces plasmin when injected intravenously and dissolves blood clots. Acylation delays plasmin release. Used after acute myocardial infarction. May produce allergic reactions, treated as for STREPTOKINASE.

Antazoline. Antihistamine with actions and uses similar to PROMETHAZINE.

Anthraquinone glycosides. Derivative of Chinese rhubarb used with SALICYLIC ACID for topical treatment of inflamed and ulcerated conditions in the mouth.

Anti-D immunoglobulin. Human immunoglobulin active against rhesus (Rh_0D) antibodies. Given to rhesus negative mothers prophylactically or after delivery of a rhesus positive child, intended to prevent haemolytic disease of newborn in subsequent pregnancies. May cause anaphylactoid reactions in patients who have antibodies against immunoglobulin A, or who have previously had atypical reactions to blood products.

Antidiuretic hormone. *See* VASOPRESSIN.

Antipyrene. *See* PHENAZONE.

Apomorphine. Stimulates DOPAMINE receptors. Used by injection for treatment of patients with Parkinson's disease resistant to other therapy. Adverse affects similar to those of BROMOCRIPTINE, particularly nausea and vomiting.

Apraclonidine. $Alpha_2$ agonist which reduces secretion of aqueous humour in the anterior chamber of the eye. Used to prevent or reduce intraocular pressure following laser surgery to the eye. May cause lid retraction, blanching of the conjunctiva, dilated pupils and drowsiness.

Aprepitant (r). Oral antiemetic. Neurokinin receptor antagonist, acting peripherally and centrally to block the emetic effects of neurokinin. Used in combination with an antihistamine antiemetic and a corticosteroid to prevent acute and delayed nausea and vomiting associated with cancer chemotherapy. May cause tiredness, constipation or diarrhoea, headaches and hiccups.

Aprotinin. Inhibits enzymes that digest proteins. Used in acute pancreatitis. Adverse effects include allergic reactions.

Arachis oil. Extract of ground nut used for nutrition and for softening both faeces and ear wax.

Arginine. Essential amino acid used in treatment of liver coma and in tests of growth hormone secretion.

Aripiprazole (r). Atypical antipsychotic. Used for the treatment of adult schizophrenia. May cause gastro-intestinal disturbance, insomnia, drowsiness and abnormal movements. In rare instances has caused tachycardia, postural hypotension and seizures. May increase stroke, ischaemic attacks and fatalities in elderly patients. Rarely, may cause hyperglycaemia. May reduce glucose control in patients with diabetes or risk factors for diabetes.

Arsenic trioxide (r). Intravenous treatment for acute leukaemia that has relapsed or not responded to standard chemotherapy. May cause metabolic and cardiac disturbances.

Artemether (r). Antimalarial used in combination with LUMEFANTRINE for the treatment of acute, uncomplicated malaria, particularly if there is resistance to older drugs. Contraindicated if the patient is taking other drugs which influence liver metabolism of drugs. May cause headache, dizziness, abdominal pain and anorexia.

Ascorbic acid. *See* VITAMIN C.

Aspirin. *See* ACETYLSALICYLIC ACID.

Astemizole. Antihistamine. Withdrawn because of the risk of serious cardiac arrhythmias.

Atazanavir (r). Antiviral protease inhibitor. Inhibits HIV maturation and proliferation. Used in combination with other antivirals to slow or halt HIV infection. May cause gastro-intestinal disturbances, liver dysfunction, bone marrow suppression, fatigue and muscle disorders, metabolic disorders and skin rashes.

Atenolol. Beta-adrenoceptor blocking drug with limited cardioselectivity. Uses, side effects, etc. as for PROPRANOLOL.

Atomoxetine (r). CNS stimulant used for attention deficit hyperactivity disoder (ADHD). May cause anorexia, gastrointestinal upset, palpitations, increased blood pressure, insomnia and tremors. In some patients may increase the risk of suicidal thoughts, hostility and emotional lability.

Atorvastatin. Statin. Enzyme inhibitor with actions, uses, precautions and adverse effects similar to SIMVASTATIN.

Atosiban. OXYTOCIN receptor antagonist used as an intravenous infusion to suppress uterine contractions and thus delay premature birth. May cause nausea, vomiting, headache, flushing, tachycardia, hypotension and hyperglycaemia, but incidence of adverse effects is less than with beta-agonists such as SALBUTAMOL. Not used before 24 weeks or after 33 weeks duration of the pregnancy, or if there is evidence of severe illness in the foetus or the mother.

Atovaquone. Antiprotozoal. Acts to block nucleic acid synthesis and thus cell growth in certain parasites. Active against the malarial parasite *Pneumocystis carnii*. Used to treat malaria resistant to first-line drugs and to treat *Pneumocystis carnii* pneumonia, a common infective complication in advanced AIDS. May cause rash, nausea, vomiting, diarrhoea, headache, fever and insomnia.

Atracurium. Nondepolarizing skeletal muscle relaxant with uses and adverse effects similar to TUBOCURARINE.

Atropine. *See* ATROPINE SULPHATE.

Atropine methonitrate. Anticholinergic with actions, uses and adverse effects similar to ATROPINE SULPHATE, but has less effect upon CNS and is sometimes considered less toxic.

Atropine sulphate. Parasympatholytic derivative of belladonna plants (e.g. deadly nightshade). Blocks peripheral autonomic cholinergic nerve junctions. Causes dilatation of pupils, paralysis of ocular accommodation, tachycardia, reduced gut motility, decreased secretions and CNS stimulation. Used intravenously in treatment of bradycardia and anticholinesterase poisoning (e.g. due to organophosphorus insecticides), intramuscularly as part of pre-operative medication, and topically in the eye for optical refraction in children. For parkinsonism and peptic ulceration it has largely been replaced by other anticholinergics. May cause dry mouth, blurred vision, glaucoma and retention of urine. In overdosage, there is tachycardia, fever, flushed skin, dehydration and excitement. Anticholinesterase (e.g. NEOSTIGMINE) may be used as antidote.

Attapulgite. Form of magnesium aluminium silicate used as adsorbent agent in treatment of acute poisoning, in diarrhoea and in topical deodorant preparations.

Auranofin. Orally active gold compound for treatment of rheumatoid arthritis.

Aurothiomalate sodium

Actions, uses and adverse effects similar to AUROTHIOMALATE SODIUM.

Aurothiomalate sodium. Preparation of gold for intramuscular injection in treatment of active rheumatoid arthritis. Adverse effects include allergic reactions such as rashes, blood dyscrasias, jaundice, kidney dysfunction, peripheral neuritis and encephalitis.

Azapropazone. Non-steroid anti-inflammatory/analgesic used in arthritic conditions. Adverse effects include gastro-intestinal disturbances, allergic rashes and photosensitivity. Contraindicated in patients with a history of peptic ulceration.

Azatadine. Antihistamine with actions, uses and adverse effects similar to PROMETHAZINE.

Azathioprine. Derivative of MERCAPTOPURINE, used primarily as immunosuppressant agent in patients receiving organ transplants. Adverse effects include bone marrow depression.

Azelaic acid. Antibacterial, anti-inflammatory agent used topically for acne. Prevents growth of the bacteria involved in the development of acne lesions, and reduces the inflammatory response of the white blood cells. Also reduces proliferation of skin cells in the lesions. May cause local skin irritation and photosensitivity.

Azelastine. Antihistamine (H_1) nasal spray used for symptomatic relief of allergic rhinitis. By this route the drug does not cause sedation although nasal irritation and taste disturbance may occur.

Azithromycin. Bactericidal antibiotic with spectrum of activity and adverse effects similar to ERYTHROMYCIN, but requires only once daily administration.

Azlocillin. Broad-spectrum antibiotic, with actions and adverse effects similar to CARBENICILLIN.

Aztreonam. Bactericidal antibiotic for injection. May be used cautiously in patients allergic to PENICILLINS and cephalosporins. Adverse effects include rashes, diarrhoea and vomiting.

B

Bacampicillin. Prodrug antibiotic. Readily absorbed from gastro-intestinal tract and rapidly metabolized to the active drug AMPICILLIN, whose actions, uses and adverse effects it shares.

Bacitracin. Peptide antibiotic active mainly on Gram-positive cocci. Nephrotoxic on systemic administration. Only used topically for skin infections.

Baclofen. Used in treatment of skeletal muscle spasticity. Adverse effects include nausea and sedation.

Balsalazide. Prodrug combines MESALAZINE (5-aminosalicylic acid) with an inert carrier. Passes unchanged to the colon where bacterial enzymes release MESALAZINE. Used by mouth in the treatment of ulcerative colitis. May cause headaches and abdominal pain.

Bambuterol. Bronchodilator, prodrug for TERBUTALINE which improves its availability and prolongs its action. Uses and adverse effects similar to TERBUTALINE.

Becaplermin. Genetically engineered growth factor which stimulates the cellular mechanisms associated with wound healing. Used by application to diabetic leg ulcers to promote formation of new tissue and then improve healing. May be associated with redness and pain. Should not be used if there is underlying infection of the bones (osteomyelitis) or malignancy.

Beclometasone. Potent synthetic CORTICOS-TEROID. Used by inhalation for treatment of asthma and for the prophylactic treatment of asthma and chronic obstructive pulmonary disease (COPD). May cause paroxysmal bronchospasm and oral candidiasis but systemic absorption from inhaled corticosteroids is low and systemic adverse effects are infrequent, except when the highest doses are used for a prolonged time.

Beclomethasone. See BECLOMETASONE.

Belladonna extract. Plant extract containing ATROPINE SULPHATE and having similar actions, uses and adverse effects.

Bendrofluazide. See BENDROFLUMETHI-AZIDE.

Bendroflumethiazide. Thiazide diuretic used in the treatment of fluid overload and in control of high blood pressure. Acts by reducing sodium reabsorption in the kidney. Less potent than FUROSEMIDE and MERSALYL but has longer action. It is effective orally. May cause excessive loss of potassium in urine and increase in blood uric acid or glucose. Consequently can produce symptoms of hypokalaemia, gout or diabetes. May produce impotence.

Benorilate. Analgesic/anti-inflammatory combination that breaks down in the body into ACETYLSALICYLIC ACID and PARACETA-MOL, and has the actions of each.

Benorylate. See BENORILATE.

Benoxinate. See OXYBUPROCAINE.

Benperidol. Tranquillizer, with actions, uses, etc. similar to HALOPERIDOL.

Benserazide. Dopamine decarboxylase inhibitor used with LEVODOPA in fixed dose combinations as CO-BENELDOPA. Prevents peripheral breakdown of LEVODOPA, allowing reduced dosage and decreased side effects.

Bentonite. Native colloidal hydrated aluminium silicate used as an adsorbent in

Benzalkanium

treatment of poisoning, and as a pharmaceutical aid in preparation of drug formulations.

Benzalkonium. Topical disinfectant used in creams, lozenges and irrigating solutions.

Benzathine penicillin. Long-acting form of BENZYLPENICILLIN, with similar actions and adverse effects.

Benzatropine. Antispasmodic parasympatholytic used in parkinsonism. Similar to TRIHEXYPHENIDYL, but more potent and can be given by intramuscular injection. Particularly useful in treating drug-induced parkinsonism.

Benzethonium. Similar to BENZALKONIUM.

Benzhexol. See TRIHEXYPHENIDYL.

Benzocaine. Weak local anaesthetic similar to LIDOCAINE. Used in proprietary preparations for sore throats.

Benzoctamine. Anxiolytic. Actions, uses and adverse effects similar to DIAZEPAM.

Benzoic acid. Used topically for mild fungus infections of skin.

Benzoin. Plant resin extract used as inhalation to reduce catarrh in upper respiratory tract and as topical skin preparation to reduce or prevent dryness and fissures.

Benzoylmetronidazole. Antibacterial, formulated as suspension for those unable to swallow tablets. Otherwise identical to METRONIDAZOLE.

Benzoyl peroxide. Antiseptic/keratolytic. Powder used in dusting powders and in creams and lotions in treatment of burns, skin ulcers and acne.

Benzthiazide. Diuretic, with actions similar to CHLOROTHIAZIDE.

Benztropine. See BENZATROPINE.

Benzydamine. Analgesic with antiinflammatory and antipyretic properties similar to ACETYLSALICYLIC ACID. Used topically as cream for musculoskeletal pains and as a mouthwash for sore throat. Overdosage by mouth has caused agitation, anxiety, hallucinations and convulsions.

Benzyl benzoate. Used as insect repellent, in treatment of scabies, and as antipruritic. May cause allergic rashes.

Benzyl nicotinate. Vasodilator related to NICOTINIC ACID.

Benzylpenicillin. Bactericidal antibiotic (*see* PENICILLINS). Unstable at acid pH, poorly active by mouth. Given parenterally. Active against most Gram-positive and some Gram-negative organisms. Inactivated by penicillinase. Adverse effects include hypersensitivity reactions, both immediate and delayed, and encephalopathy with convulsions if given intrathecally or in massive doses.

Beractant. A synthetic surfactant used to treat lung damage (respiratory distress syndrome) in preterm infants. Similar to COLFOSCERIL.

Betahistine. Vasodilator with actions similar to HISTAMINE. Used in Ménière's disease to reduce episodes of dizziness.

Betamethasone. Potent synthetic CORTICOSTEROID similar to DEXAMETHASONE.

Betaxolol. Beta-adrenoceptor blocking drug with cardioselectivity. Used as an antihypertensive, and as eye drops for glaucoma. Adverse effects and precautions as for PROPRANOLOL.

Betazole. Related to HISTAMINE, with similar actions and uses.

Bethanechol. Parasympathomimetic drug, with actions of ACETYLCHOLINE.

14

Bisoprolol

Bethanidine. *See* BETANIDINE.

Bevacizumab (r). Intravenous antineoplastic used in combination with other chemotherapy to treat metastatic colorectal cancer. May cause gastro-intestinal bleeding and perforation and impaired wound healing.

Bexarotene (r). Oral cytotoxic used to treat skin lesions associated with advanced lymphoma. May cause raised blood lipids, hypothyroidism and headache.

Bezafibrate. Fibrate, lipid-regulating drug. Acts by reducing CHOLESTEROL synthesis and increasing the breakdown of lipids. Used to treat hyperlipidaemias not responding to diet alone. More effective at reducing triglyceride levels than CHOLESTEROL levels. Fibrates are generally used as second-line treatment in patients who do not tolerate or fully respond to statins, which are the drugs of choice for reducing CHOLESTEROL levels. May cause gastrointestinal disturbances, headache, rash, drowsiness and muscle disease, notably myositis.

Bicalutamide. Antiandrogen used in the treatment of cancer of the prostate. May cause hot flushes, itching, breast enlargement/tenderness and angina.

Bile salts. Extracted from animal bile. Used to stimulate bile flow without increasing its bile salts and pigment contents (e.g. after biliary operations). Included in some compound preparations for treatment of biliary insufficiency, but of doubtful efficacy.

Bimatoprost (r). Prostaglandin analogue (a prostamide) thought to regulate ocular pressure by a natural mechanism. Used as eye drops to reduce pressure in glaucoma when beta-blocker drugs are contraindicated or inadequate. May cause reddening of the eyes, itching and growth of eyelashes and darkening of the eyelids.

Biotin (Vitamin H). Found in liver, kidney, yeast, eggs and milk. Until recently there was no known clinical deficiency state. Induced deficiency caused dermatitis, lassitude, anorexia and parasthesiae. It is now known that several extremely rare inborn metabolic disorders present with similar symptoms and respond to biotin.

Bisacodyl. Purgative that acts by stimulating sensory nerve endings in wall of large bowel. Available for oral and rectal use. Suppositories may cause mild burning sensation in the rectum.

Bismuth aluminate. *See* BISMUTH ANTACIDS.

Bismuth antacids. Insoluble bismuth salts have weak antacid properties and are claimed to protect the stomach. Largely superseded by more effective antacids. Prolonged, excessive use may allow sufficient absorption to cause toxicity with kidney damage, liver damage and CNS effects.

Bismuth carbonate. *See* BISMUTH ANTACIDS.

Bismuth chelate. *See* TRI-POTASSIUM DICITRATO BISMUTHATE.

Bismuth oxide. *See* BISMUTH ANTACIDS.

Bismuth salicylate. Bismuth salt administered by mouth for protective effect on stomach and bowels. Converted to bismuth and SODIUM SALICYLATE in small intestine. Used as symptomatic treatment for indigestion, nausea and diarrhoea.

Bismuth subgallate. Insoluble powder used for eczema and as suppositories for haemorrhoids.

Bismuth subnitrate. *See* BISMUTH ANTACIDS.

Bisoprolol (r). Cardioselective beta-adrenoceptor blocking drug. Used in the

15

treatment of hypertension and angina. Actions and adverse effects similar to ATENOLOL.

Bivalirudin (r). Anticoagulant, short-acting thrombin inhibitor. Used by intravenous infusion in patients undergoing percutaneous coronary intervention (PCI) procedures, as treatment for coronary artery disease. May cause allergic reactions, including anaphylaxis and bleeding episodes.

Bleomycin. Cytotoxic antibiotic used to treat lymphomas and solid tumours. Toxic effects include lung fibrosis and skin pigmentation.

Boric acid. Weak anti-infective powder used in dusting powders, lotions and ointments.

Bortezomib (r). Cytotoxic. Protease inhibitor used intravenously in multiple myeloma when other, longer established therapies have failed to stop progress of the disease. May cause peripheral neuropathy, gastro-intestinal disorders, fever and fatigue.

Bosentan (r). Receptor antagonist that blocks the constrictor effects of endothelin, the hormone that increases resistance in blood vessels resulting in cardiovascular disorders. Bosentan has proved effective in reducing pulmonary vascular hypertension and may have a role in treating heart failure from all causes. It may cause a fall in systemic blood pressure and should not be used if there is pre-existing hypotension. Other adverse effects include palpitations, flushing, oedema and hepatic impairment.

Botulinum A toxin-haemagglutinin complex. Neurotoxin derived from the bacterium *Clostridium botulinum*. Binds to endings of nerves which supply muscles, to prevent the release of ACETYLCHOLINE, so producing weakness or paralysis of those muscles, from which recovery occurs after 2–3 months. Used by local injection to treat patients with troublesome spasm of the eyelids, strabismus (squint) and twitching of muscles around the mouth. Effects seen within 2–5 days of injection. Unwanted effects include bruising around the eye, double vision, drooping eyelid and weakness of facial muscles. Also used to relieve spasticity in the feet in children with cerebral palsy and upper limb spasticity in stroke patients. Unwanted effects include leg pain, weakness and urinary incontinence.

Bran. Purgative, nonirritant. Byproduct of milling of wheat. Contains indigestible cellulose which increases intestinal bulk. Crude bran is unpalatable; processed bran is pleasant cereal. Large doses needed for effect. Danger of bowel obstruction if pre-existing bowel narrowing.

Bretylium. Adrenergic neurone blocking drug with actions similar to GUANETHIDINE. Used mainly in cardiac arrhythmias. Side effects have limited its use as antihypertensive.

Brimonidine. Selective alpha-adrenoceptor blocking agent used topically in the treatment of glaucoma. Less likely to produce systemic CNS or cardiac effects than some other glaucoma treatments. May cause local irritation, allergic reactions and drowsiness. Acts by reducing formation of aqueous humour and improving drainage.

Brinzolamide. Carbonic anhydrase enzyme inhibitor with actions similar to DORZOLAMIDE. Use topically as eye drops alone or in addition to beta-blocker eye drops as treatment for open-angle glaucoma. May caused blurred vision, headache, ocular discomfort and bitter taste.

Bromazepam (m). Benzodiazepine anxiolytic, with actions and adverse effects similar to DIAZEPAM.

Bromides. CNS depressants, now largely superseded by safer drugs.

Bromocriptine. Stimulates DOPAMINE receptors. Used in treatment of acromegaly, for inhibition or suppression of lactation, and in conditions due to excessive prolactin secretion, including some cases of infertility and in some patients with Parkinson's disease. Adverse effects include nausea, hypotension and cold extremities.

Brompheniramine. Antihistamine, with actions similar to PROMETHAZINE.

Bronopol. Antibacterial preservative used in topical preparations.

Buclizine. Antihistamine/antiemetic drug with actions similar to PROMETHAZINE.

Budesonide. Synthetic CORTICOSTEROID similar to BECLOMETASONE. Used by inhalation for treatment of asthma and for the prophylactic treatment of asthma and chronic obstructive pulmonary disease (COPD). May cause paroxysmal bronchospasm and oral candidiasis but systemic absorption from inhaled corticosteroids is low and systemic adverse effects are infrequent, except when the highest doses are used for a prolonged time. Also applied intranasally for allergic rhinitis, and topically for psoriasis and eczema and systemically in a controlled-release form for Crohn's disease.

Bumetanide. Potent diuretic, with actions and uses similar to FUROSEMIDE. Adverse effects similar to BENDROFLUMETHIAZIDE.

Bupivacaine. Local anaesthetic similar to LIDOCAINE, but produces longer anaesthesia.

Buprenorphine (c). Narcotic analgesic with antagonist properties for injection or as sublingual tablets or transdermal patches (r). Actions, uses and adverse effects similar to PENTAZOCINE.

Bupropion. Oral, sustained-release aid to smoking cessation. Thought to act on dopaminergic/noradrenergic pathways which are associated with nicotine addiction. Used alone or in combination with NICOTINE patches. Taken 5–8 days before complete cessation of smoking is attempted. Full course of treatment is 8–9 weeks. May cause insomnia, headache, dry mouth, altered taste, gastro-intestinal disturbance and rashes. Contraindicated in patients with history of seizure, eating disorders, liver failure, known CNS tumour, or abrupt withdrawal of alcohol or benzodiazepines.

Buserelin. Hormone. Analogue of gonadotrophin-releasing hormone that suppresses androgen production by testes. Used in treatment of carcinoma of the prostate and endometriosis. May cause hot flushes, nasal irritation and loss of libido.

Buspirone. Anxiolytic used in short-term relief of the symptoms of anxiety. Acts by different (but, as yet, undefined) mechanisms to the benzodiazepines. Does not have muscle relaxant or anticonvulsant effects. Takes longer to have an effect than the benzodiazepines, but appears to cause less sedation and is less likely to lead to dependence. May cause headaches and dizziness.

Busulfan. Cytotoxic drug given orally or intravenously (r) used in neoplastic disease, particularly myeloid leukaemia. Adverse effects include skin pigmentation, cataract, pulmonary fibrosis and bone marrow depression.

Busulphan. *See* BUSULFAN.

Butacaine. Local anaesthetic used by injection or by spray on to the mucosa of the nose and throat. Actions and adverse effects similar to LIDOCAINE.

Butetamate. Sympathomimetic amine, with actions similar to EPHEDRINE.

Butobarbital (c). Barbiturate hypnotic essentially like AMOBARBITAL.

Butobarbitone. *See* BUTOBARBITAL.

Butorphanol (d). Analgesic injection, with actions and uses similar to MORPHINE, but has narcotic antagonist activity similar to NALOXONE. May cause sedation, dizziness, nausea, changes in mood and vivid dreams. Has low potential for dependence and addiction, and may precipitate withdrawal symptoms in narcotic addicts. May depress respiration and therefore caution is advised if used in patients with respiratory disease. NALOXONE, but not NALORPHINE or LEVAL-LORPHAN, may be used as antagonist.

Butoxyethyl nicotinate. *See* NICOTINIC ACID.

Butriptyline. Antidepressant, with actions and uses similar to IMIPRAMINE.

Butyl nitrite (m). Vasodilator with actions, adverse effects and abuse potential similar to AMYL NITRITE.

C

Cabergoline. Ergot derivative with DOPAMINE agonist activity. A prolactin antagonist similar to BROMOCRIPTINE but with less risk of cardiac toxicity at recommended doses. Used after pregnancy to suppress unwanted lactation and to facilitate conception when infertility is associated with high prolactin levels. Also used to control symptoms of Parkinson's disease.

Caffeine. Active principle from tea and coffee, used as mild CNS stimulant. Adverse effects include restlessness, excitement and dependence after prolonged excessive ingestion. Claimed to enhance the absorption and thus the effectiveness of ERGOTAMINE in migraine.

Calamine. Zinc carbonate used in dusting powders, creams, lotions, etc.

Calciferol. *See* VITAMIN D.

Calcipotriol. Synthetic analogue of VITAMIN D used topically as treatment for psoriasis. Acts on VITAMIN D receptors in skin cells (keratocytes) to reduce cell proliferation and thus corrects one of the key abnormalities in that condition. Unlike CALCITRIOL (natural vitamin D_3) this drug has little effect on calcium metabolism thus reducing the risk of hypercalcaemia. May cause local irritation.

Calcitonin (salmon). Synthetic hormone which regulates plasma calcium concentrations. Used short term to lower high calcium levels in Paget's disease of bone and metastatic cancer. Also used for pain relief. Adverse effects include gastrointestinal disturbances, skin rashes and dizziness. Anaphylactic reactions have been reported.

Calcitriol (1α,25-Dihydroxycholecalciferol). More potent active metabolite of VITAMIN D. Used intravenously in dialysis patients to treat/prevent hypocalcaemia and renal bone disease and orally to treat postmenopausal osteoporosis.

Calcium carbonate. Nonsystemic (nonabsorbable) antacid. Used in treatment of peptic ulceration where it produces longer neutralization of acid than SODIUM BICARBONATE. Frequent use may cause constipation. Small amounts are absorbed and in some subjects may cause renal stones (i.e. nephrocalcinosis). When formulated as an effervescent tablet, yields CALCIUM CITRATE in the stomach.

Calcium chloride. Used intravenously as a source of calcium ions in treatment of cardiac arrest. Orally, could be used as a dietary supplement, but is very irritant to the gastro-intestinal tract. CALCIUM GLUCONATE or CALCIUM PHOSPHATE are preferred for this purpose.

Calcium citrate. Absorbable calcium salt used as a calcium supplement in deficiency states and in osteoporosis. Adverse effects include gastro-intestinal disturbances, bone pain, thirst, increased urine output, muscle weakness and confusion.

Calcium gluconate. Source of calcium for deficiency states.

Calcium hydrogen phosphate. Source of calcium and phosphate for treatment of dietary insufficiency.

Calcium iodide. Used as an expectorant.

Calcium lactate. *See* CALCIUM GLUCONATE.

19

Calcium laevulinate

Calcium laevulinate. Source of calcium for treatment of dietary insufficiency.

Calcium levofolinate. The active isomer of LEUCOVORIN.

Calcium pantothenate. Source of PANTOTHENIC ACID. Considered a vitamin but no proven deficiency has been discovered. No accepted therapeutic role, but used in some vitamin mixtures.

Calcium phosphate. Source of calcium for treatment of dietary insufficiency.

Calcium polystyrene sulphonate. Ion exchange resin used to treat electrolyte abnormalities by changing absorption or excretion in the gut.

Camphene. *See* CAMPHOR.

Camphor. Used internally as carminative and externally as rubefacient.

Candesartan cilexetil. Prodrug, rapidly absorbed and converted to candesartan angiotensin II receptor antagonist with actions and adverse effects similar to LOSARTAN. Used as an antihypertensive and in treatment of heart failure. Rarely, bone marrow suppression has been reported.

Cannabis (m). Dried extract of the plant *Cannabis sativa*, smoked or taken by mouth for the promotion of mood elevation. The main active principle is tetrahydrocannabinol. Adverse effects include nausea, vomiting, anxiety and psychotic episodes. Tolerance and psychological dependence occur but physical dependence is not a serious problem. Overdose causes exacerbation of the adverse effects and is managed by supportive treatment. Cannabinoids have antiemetic effects. NABILONE is a cannabis derivative used to treat nausea and vomiting from cytotoxic drugs.

Capecitabine (r). Noncytotoxic drug which acts as a precursor for the cytotoxic FLUOROURACIL. Given orally, after absorption it is converted into FLUOROURACIL by enzymes

that are present in colorectal cancer. Used to treat metatstatic tumours. Adverse effects include bone marrow suppression and CNS disturbance but better tolerated than when FLUOROURACIL itself is administered.

Capreomycin. Peptide antibiotic, mainly used in tuberculosis. Adverse effects include ototoxicity and nephrotoxicity.

Capsaicin. Naturally occurring substance found in *Capsicum* (sweet pepper). When applied to the skin it depletes local pain-conducting nerve fibres of pain transmitter substance. Used topically to treat post-herpetic neuralgia (pain persisting after shingles, which is caused by infection with the herpes zoster virus). Claimed to be effective in treating pain after psoralin ultraviolet activation therapy and in erythromelalgia. Should not be applied to broken skin. May cause skin irritation.

Capsicum. Essential oil used internally as carminative and externally as rubefacient.

Captopril. Inhibits angiotensin-converting enzyme (ACE) involved in formation of hormone concerned with maintenance of blood pressure and constriction of blood vessels. Used in treatment of hypertension, kidney disease in diabetic patients, chronic heart failure and in prevention of recurrent myocardial infarction. Adverse effects include hypotension, proteinuria and renal impairment, skin rashes and cough. Bone marrow depression and loss of taste may occur with high doses.

Caraway. Essential oil used as carminative.

Carbachol. Parasympathomimetic, with actions and adverse effects similar to ACETYLCHOLINE, but more prolonged. Used as miotic eye drops in glaucoma and for improvement of postoperative intestinal or bladder muscle tone.

Carbamazepine. Anticonvulsant. Acts by suppressing epileptic discharges in the brain. Used in prevention of epilepsy, in suppression of pain in trigeminal neuralgia (but is not an analgesic) and in mania. May cause drowsiness, blurred vision, dizziness and gastro-intestinal upsets. Skin rashes and adverse effects on the liver and bone marrow are relatively common. Coma with convulsions in overdosage. No antidote; supportive treatment only.

Carbaryl. Anticholinesterase. Used topically as an insecticide (e.g. for lice).

Carbenicillin. PENICILLIN antibiotic, particularly active against Gram-negative bacteria especially *Pseudomonas* and *Proteus*. Adverse effects as for BENZYLPENICILLIN.

Carbenoxolone. Used in treatment of gastric and duodenal ulcers and for mouth ulcers. Has ALDOSTERONE-like actions. Adverse effects include oedema, hypertension, hypokalaemia and muscle pain.

Carbidopa. Dopamine decarboxylase inhibitor used with LEVODOPA in fixed dose combinations as CO-CARELDOPA. Similar actions to BENSERAZIDE.

Carbimazole. Depresses formation of thyroid hormone. Used in treatment of hyperthyroidism. Adverse effects include allergic rashes, nausea, diarrhoea, blood abnormalities and keratitis.

Carbinoxamine. Antihistamine, with actions similar to PROMETHAZINE.

Carbocisteine. Mucolytic used to reduce viscosity of sputum.

Carboplatin. Cytotoxic with actions, uses and adverse effects similar to CISPLATIN.

Carboprost. Synthetic prostaglandin used in treatment of postpartum haemorrhage which fails to respond to OXYTOCIN or SYNTOCIN/ERGOMETRINE. Adverse effects include gastro-intestinal disturbances, hyperthermia, flushing, asthma, hypertension, dyspnoea and pulmonary oedema.

Carisoprodol. Used to treat painful muscle spasm.

Carmellose (r). Cellulose derivative employed in artificial tears and as a pharmaceutical aid in drug formulations.

Carmustine. Intravenous cytotoxic, inactivates DNA, RNA and several enzymes. Crosses the blood-brain barrier, thus useful for brain tumours as well as certain other neoplastic diseases. Rapidly degraded from the parent drug to active metabolites. Adverse effects include nausea, vomiting, burning sensation at injection site, renal and hepatic damage, and delayed bone marrow suppression.

Carteolol. Beta-adrenoceptor blocking drug used in prevention of angina. Actions and adverse effects similar to PROPRANOLOL.

Carvedilol. Nonselective beta-adrenoceptor antagonist with alpha-antagonist activity. Used as prophylaxis of stable angina and in treatment of hypertension where its effects are similar to PROPRANOLOL. Also used for chronic cardiac failure. May be used with care for patients with chronic heart failure. Adverse effects include dizziness, headache, gastro-intestinal upset, postural hypotension and pain in extremeties.

Cascara. Purgative from bark of buckthorn tree. Stimulates gut movement via the nerve plexus in the large bowel wall. Produces reddish-brown discolouration of urine and may cause excessive catharsis. Excreted in milk of lactating mothers and may cause diarrhoea in infants. Prolonged use causes black pigmentation in colon (melanosis coli).

Castor oil. Purgative, with action upon small intestine as well as large intestine useful when prompt evacuation is required (e.g. before bowel X-rays). Chronic use not recommended as it causes reduced absorption of nutrients. Also used topically on skin for its emollient effect.

Cefaclor. Cephalosporin antibiotic. Orally active and has wider range of activity than earlier drugs of that group. Actions, uses and adverse effects similar to CEPHALOTHIN.

Cefadroxil

Cefadroxil. Cephalosporin antibiotic similar to CEFALEXIN.

Cefalexin. Cephalosporin antibiotic, with similar activity and adverse effects to CEPHALOTHIN, but well absorbed by mouth.

Cefamandole. Newer cephalosporin antibiotic for injection. Has wider range of antibacterial activity than earlier drugs of this group. Actions, uses and adverse effects similar to CEPHALOTHIN.

Cefazolin. Cephalosporin antibiotic similar to CEFALEXIN.

Cefixime. Cephalosporin antibiotic with wide range of activity. Adverse effects include gastro-intestinal disturbances, headache, dizziness and skin reactions.

Cefotaxime. Broad-spectrum cephalosporin antibiotic for injection, with actions, uses and adverse effects similar to CEPHALOTHIN.

Cefoxitin. Cephamycin antibiotic for injection. Related to the cephalosporins with similar actions, uses and adverse effects, but may have broader spectrum of activity.

Cefpirome. Broad-spectrum cephalosporin antibiotic which is active against beta-lactamase producing bacteria. Uses and adverse effects similar to other cephalosporin antibiotics.

Cefpodoxime proxetil. Cephalosporin antibiotic, administered orally as its proxetil ester, which is hydrolysed in the gut wall to produce the active drug. Has a broad spectrum of antibacterial activity. Adverse effects include gastro-intestinal and allergic reactions.

Cefradine. Cephalosporin antibiotic similar to CEFALEXIN.

Ceftazidime. Cephalosporin antibiotic used orally and by injection. Has wider range of antibacterial activity than earlier drugs of this group. Adverse effects similar to CEPHALOTHIN.

Ceftibuten. Orally active cephalosporin antibiotic. Adverse reactions include gastro-intestinal disturbance, headache and rash.

Ceftizoxime. Cephalosporin antibiotic for injection. Has range of antibacterial activity similar to CEFTAZIDIME. Adverse effects similar to CEPHALOTHIN.

Ceftriaxone. Broad-spectrum cephalosporin antibiotic for injection, with actions, uses and adverse effects similar to CEPHALOTHIN.

Cefuroxime. Cephalosporin antibiotic used orally and by injection. Has wider range of antibacterial activity than earlier drugs in this group. Actions, uses and adverse effects similar to CEPHALOTHIN.

Celecoxib. Non-steroidal anti-inflammatory analgesic with selective inhibition of the cyclo-oxygenase enzyme-2 (COX-2). Thus it reduces prostaglandin production at the sites of inflammation without affecting the protective effects of COX-1 prostaglandins on the gastro-intestinal tract. Used for symptomatic relief of pain in osteoarthritis and rheumatoid arthritis. Gastro-intestinal effects are reduced but not eliminated. May also cause dizziness, fluid retention, hypertension, headache and itching. Should be used with caution in patients with renal, cardiac or hepatic impairment, and renal function should be monitored. Contraindicated in moderate or severe congestive heart failure.

Celiprolol. Cardioselective beta-adrenoceptor blocking drug with actions and adverse effects similar to ATENOLOL/ACEBUTOLOL. Used to treat hypertension.

Cephalexin. See CEFALEXIN.

Cephalothin. Cephalosporin antibiotic, particularly useful against penicillinase-producing *Staphylococcus aureus*. Must be given parenterally. Adverse effects mainly hypersensitivity reactions.

Cephamandole. See CEFAMANDOLE.

Cephazolin. *See* CEFAZOLIN.

Cephradine. *See* CEFRADINE.

Ceratonia. Powder prepared from the endosperm of the locust bean tree (*Ceratonia siliqua*). Used as a mucilage to thicken feeds for children with diarrhoea.

Cerivastatin. Enzyme inhibitor active in reducing cholesterol synthesis with actions and uses similar to SIMVASTATIN. Adverse effects include headache, rhinitis, cough, influenza-like symptoms, arthralgia, myalgia, back pain, abdominal pain and insomnia. Withdrawn following reports of rhabdomyolysis associated with its use, particularly in combination with GEMFIBROZIL.

Certoparin. Anticoagulant, low molecular heparin similar to ENOXAPARIN.

Cetalkonium. Topical disinfectant.

Cetirizine. Antihistamine used for hay fever and allergic skin conditions. It is rapidly absorbed and has a long duration of action suitable for once-daily dosing. It is related to HYDROXYZINE, but produces less sedation and only mild side effects, including headache, dizziness agitation, dry mouth and gastro-intestinal upset.

Cetomacrogol. Emulsifying wax used in formulating oil-in-water emulsions.

Cetostearyl alcohol. Mixture of solid alcohols used for emulsifying properties in oil-in-water formulations including preparations for protection of dry skin.

Cetrimide. Topical disinfectant used in many skin preparations.

Cetrorelix. Synthetic luteinizing hormone (LH) releasing hormone (LHRH) antagonist used to suppress premature LH release in patients undergoing controlled ovarian stimulation for assisted conception. May cause local reactions at injection site, nausea and headaches.

Cetuximab (r). Cytotoxic. Monoclonal antibody targeted at the cell growth mechanisms in colorectal cancer. Used intravenously to treat metastatic disease when established treatments, including IRINOTECAN, have failed. May cause hypersensitivity reactions, including skin reactions, fever and bronchospasm.

Cetyl alcohol. Used in manufacture of ointments and creams.

Cetylpyridinium. Topical disinfectant used in skin and mouth preparations.

Chamomile oil. An ESSENTIAL OIL used to treat early stages of skin inflammation, e.g. nappy rash, cracked nipples. Contact sensitivity has been described.

Charcoal. *See* ACTIVATED CHARCOAL.

Chenodeoxycholic acid. Naturally occurring bile acid which prevents formation and aids dissolution of gall stones.

Chloral betaine. *See* CLORAL BETAINE.

Chloral hydrate. Hypnotic. Available only as a liquid. Converted by liver to trichloroethanol which causes generalized CNS depression. Used for insomnia, especially in children and the elderly. Relatively 'safe'. Addiction is rare. Coma in overdosage. No antidote; treated by supportive measures.

Chlorambucil. Cytotoxic drug related to CHLORMETHINE. Used in neoplastic conditions of lymphoid tissues. Adverse effects include bone marrow depression.

Chloramphenicol. Broad-spectrum bacteriostatic antibiotic, which should be reserved for treatment of typhoid fever and life-threatening infections. Adverse effects include aplastic anaemia. Produces 'grey baby syndrome' in neonates and premature babies.

Chlorbutol. *See* CHLOROBUTANOL.

Chlorcyclizine

Chlorcyclizine. Antihistamine, with similar actions and adverse effects to PRO-METHAZINE. Used mainly as an antiemetic.

Chlordiazepoxide (m). Benzodiazepine anxiolytic similar to DIAZEPAM but less hypnotic and less anticonvulsant activity. Used in treatment of anxiety.

Chlorexolone. Diuretic, with actions, uses and adverse effects similar to BENDROFLUMETHIAZIDE.

Chlorhexidine. Topical disinfectant used in skin preparations, urethral catheterization, cytoscopy, and as preservative in eye drops.

Chlormethiazole. *See* CLOMETHIAZOLE.

Chlormezanone. Anxiolytic, muscle relaxant. Sometimes used as a hypnotic. Actions similar to MEPROBAMATE. Adverse effects include drowsiness, dizziness, headache, skin rashes and jaundice.

Chlorobutanol. Antibacterial and antifungal preservative for topical applications.

Chlorocresol. Disinfectant used in sterilizing solutions and as a preservative in creams.

Chlorofluoromethane. Aerosol propellant for drugs administered by inhalation. Also used as a spray for muscle pain where it produces local anaesthesia due to intense coldness.

Chlorophenoxyethanol. Topical antibacterial.

Chloropyramine. Antihistamine similar to PROMETHAZINE.

Chloroquine. Antimalarial agent, which has also been used in rheumatoid arthritis. Adverse effects include skin pigmentation, alopecia, neuropathy, and corneal and retinal damage.

Chlorothiazide. Thiazide diuretic similar to BENDROFLUMETHIAZIDE.

Chloroxylenol. Topical disinfectant used chiefly on skin.

Chlorphenamine. Antihistamine, with actions, uses and adverse effects similar to PROMETHAZINE.

Chlorphenesin. Topical antibacterial/antifungal agent.

Chlorpheniramine. *See* CHLORPHENAMINE.

Chlorphentermine (c). Anorectic, sympathomimetic amine. Actions and adverse effects similar to DIETHYLPROPION.

Chlorpromazine. Phenothiazine tranquillizer. Causes selective depression of the brain structures responsible for control of behaviour and wakefulness. Has anticholinergic alpha-adrenergic blocking and dopaminergic effects amongst other pharmacological effects. Used in psychotic disorders, particularly schizophrenia and agitated depression; in terminal illness to enhance analgesia; to control nausea and vomiting; and for hiccups. Adverse effects include postural hypotension, dry mouth, blurred vision, involuntary movements, cholestatic jaundice, photosensitivity and deposits in lens and cornea. Used only with caution in liver disease and epilepsy (may precipitate convulsions). In overdosage causes coma, involuntary movements, convulsions, hypotension and arrhythmias. No antidote; supportive treatment only.

Chlorpropamide. Long-acting oral antidiabetic drug that stimulates pancreatic insulin release in maturity-onset diabetes mellitus. Adverse effects include hypoglycaemia, particularly in the elderly, allergic reactions, jaundice, and flushing with alcohol. Action may be potentiated by salicylates and sulphonamides. No longer recommended because it has the highest incidence of adverse reactions in this class of drugs. Sometimes used in diabetes insipidus where it is thought to increase the response of the kidney to any remaining natural antidiuretic hormone.

Chlorprothixene. Phenothiazine tranquillizer essentially similar to CHLORPROMAZINE.

Chlorquinaldol. Topical antibacterial/antifungal similar to HYDROXYQUINOLINE. Used in skin infections.

Chlortalidone. Diuretic essentially similar to BENDROFLUMETHIAZIDE.

Chlortetracycline. Bacteriostatic antibiotic, with actions, adverse effects and interactions similar to TETRACYCLINE.

Chlorthalidone. *See* CHLORTALIDONE.

Cholecalciferol. *See* COLECALCIFEROL.

Cholesterol. Natural fatty constituent of all animal cells and a precursor of steroids. Used topically in creams for soothing and water-absorbing properties.

Cholestyramine. *See* COLESTYRAMINE.

Choline magnesium trisalicylate. A mixture of CHOLINE SALICYLATE and magnesium salicylate with actions, uses and adverse effects similar to ACETYLSALICYLIC ACID.

Choline salicylate. Similar actions to ACETYLSALICYLIC ACID.

Choline theophyllinate. Oral preparation of THEOPHYLLINE, with actions similar to AMINOPHYLLINE. Main use is in chronic bronchitis.

Chorionic gonadotrophin. Hormone produced in the placenta. Used in treatment of anovulatory infertility and failure of development of the testes or ovaries. May cause fluid retention and therefore used with caution if there is evidence of cardiac or renal failure.

Chymotrypsin. Animal pancreatic enzyme used to reduce soft tissue inflammation, particularly associated with trauma. Adverse effects include allergic reactions.

Ciclesonide (r). Potent synthetic corticosteroid prodrug used by inhalation in prophylaxis of asthma. Broken down by lung enzymes to form an active metabolite. It has similar effects and adverse effects to BECLOMETASONE.

Ciclosporin. Potent immunosuppressant antibiotic used to prevent rejection after organ and tissue transplantation. Also used to treat severe rheumatoid arthritis, severe psoriasis unresponsive to conventional treatment and severe atopic dermatitis when other treatments fail. Adverse effects include impairment of liver and renal function.

Cidofovir. Antiviral agent active against cytomegalovirus, which may be a cause of serious infection in immunocompromised patients, especially those with AIDS.

Cilastatin. Structurally similar to the antibiotic IMIPENEM, but has no antibacterial activity. Given with IMIPENEM it reduces the metabolism of the latter and prolongs its effectiveness. For adverse effects *see* IMIPENEM.

Cilazapril. Prodrug ACE inhibitor metabolized to the active drug cilazaprilat. Used to treat hypertension. Actions and adverse effects similar to CAPTOPRIL.

Cilostazol (r). Antiplatelet-vasodilator thought to act via mechanisms that modify intracellular calcium. Used to prevent blood clots and improve blood flow in patients with exercise-related painful impairment of blood flow to the legs and feet (intermittent claudication). Adverse effects include headache, angina, fluid retention and increased risk of bleeding.

Cimetidine. Selectively blocks histamine receptors mediating gastric acid secretion. Used in peptic ulceration and gastric hyperacidity, oesophageal reflux and prophylaxis of gastro-intestinal bleeding in seriously ill patients. Adverse effects include diarrhoea, dizziness, rash and breast enlargement in males. Danger of

Cinacalcet

CNS depression and confusional states in renal failure, the elderly or seriously ill patients. Increases effects of some other drugs including WARFARIN and PHENYTOIN by reducing their metabolism and excretion.

Cinacalcet (r). Lowers active parathyroid hormone levels by increasing the sensitivity of the parathyroid gland to calcium. Used to treat parathyroid hormone overactivity in patients with end-stage renal disease or on dialysis, and in parathyroid carcinoma. May cause nausea, vomiting, anorexia, dizziness and reduced blood calcium levels.

Cinchocaine. Local anaesthetic with actions similar to LIDOCAINE.

Cinnarizine. Antihistamine similar to PROMETHAZINE, chiefly used in treatment of vertigo and vomiting.

Cinoxacin. Antibacterial for urinary infections. Actions and adverse effects similar to NALIDIXIC ACID.

Ciprofibrate. Lipid-lowering drug. Acts by reducing cholesterol synthesis and increasing breakdown of lipids. Used to treat hyperlipidaemias not responding to treatment with diet alone. May cause headache, dizziness, drowsiness, rash, muscle pains and gastro-intestinal disturbance.

Ciprofloxacin. Broad-spectrum antibiotic used in a wide range of infections, notably urinary and respiratory, where the organisms are resistant to PENICILLINS and cephalosporins. Also used topically for conjunctivitis. Causes bacterial death whether or not the bacteria are growing. Adverse effects include rashes, gastro-intestinal disturbance, headaches, dizziness, tiredness, tendon damage and, if injected, pain at the injection site. Structure similar to NALIDIXIC ACID.

Cisapride. A prokinetic agent related to METOCLOPRAMIDE which facilitates movement throughout the gastro-intestinal tract. Used to treat symptoms and lesions of gastro-oesophageal reflux and relieve symptoms of delayed gastric emptying. May cause abdominal cramps, diarrhoea, hypersensitivity reactions, convulsions, impaired liver function and serious cardiac arrhythmias. Suspended because cardiac reactions have resulted in fatalities.

Cisatracurium. Nondepolarizing muscle relaxant with an intermediate duration of action. Used in surgery and intensive care. Mechanism of action similar to TUBOCURARINE, but without significant adverse effects on blood pressure.

Cisplatin. Cytotoxic platinum compound used in treatment of metastatic testicular and ovarian tumours, mesothelioma and non-small cell lung cancer. May cause renal damage, ototoxicity, bone marrow suppression, nausea, vomiting and allergic reactions.

Citalopram. Antidepressant. Selective serotonin reuptake inhibitor. Used to treat depressive illness and panic disorders. Less sedating and fewer effects upon the heart than the tricyclic antidepressants but may still cause palpitations and low blood pressure. Other unwanted effects include gastro-intestinal disturbances and a wide range of neuropsychiatric symptoms. Similar symptoms may also occur if the treatment is suddenly stopped or withdrawn too quickly.

Cladribine. Cytotoxic with specific effects in hairy cell leukaemia. Adverse effects include bone marrow suppression, renal and neurotoxicity. May also cause gastrointestinal disturbance and painful reactions at injection sites.

Clarithromycin. Bactericidal antibiotic with spectrum of activity similar to ERYTHROMYCIN, but requires only twice daily administration and unwanted gastrointestinal effects appear to be less frequent.

Clavulanic acid. Inhibits the enzyme penicillinase which inactivates PENICILLIN antibiotics. Used with AMOXICILLIN to increase its spectrum of activity. Rare side effects include severe liver toxicity.

Clemastine. Antihistamine, with actions and uses similar to PROMETHAZINE, but with less sedative effects.

Clindamycin. Antibacterial for staphylococcal bone and joint infections, with limited use because of serious side effects including antibiotic-associated colitis.

Clioquinol. Used in treatment of gut amoebiasis and to protect against gut infections, used topically for skin infections. Prolonged large oral doses may produce neuropathy.

Clobazam (m). Benzodiazepine anxiolytic with actions, uses and adverse effects similar to DIAZEPAM. May also be used for long-term anticonvulsant therapy, similar to CLONAZEPAM.

Clobetasol. Topical CORTICOSTEROID for psoriasis and eczema.

Clobetasone. Topical CORTICOSTEROID for psoriasis and eczema.

Clodantoin. Topical antifungal agent.

Clofazimine. Antileprotic/anti-inflammatory, used for control of reactions occurring with DAPSONE treatment. Adverse effects include skin pigmentation, red urine and diarrhoea.

Clomethiazole. Sedative/hypnotic/anticonvulsant. Depressant action on CNS. Used for sedation or hypnosis in agitated or confused patients especially the elderly. Also for treatment of acute withdrawal symptoms in alcoholics and drug addicts and control of sustained epileptic fits (status epilepticus). May cause tingling in nose and sneezing. Effects potentiated by CHLORPROMAZINE, HALOPERIDOL and related drugs. Coma with respiratory depression in overdosage. No antidote. Symptomatic treatment is adequate.

Cloral betaine

Clomifene. Sex hormone used in infertility due to failure of ovulation. Acts both on the pituitary gonadotrophic hormones and on the ovary permitting ovulation. Should not be used in liver failure or if patient has ovarian cysts. Danger of multiple births, especially at higher doses.

Clomiphene. See CLOMIFENE.

Clomipramine. Antidepressant drug, with actions and uses similar to IMIPRAMINE.

Clomocycline. Bacteriostatic antibiotic, with actions, adverse effects and interactions similar to TETRACYCLINE.

Clonazepam (m). Benzodiazepine anticonvulsant similar to DIAZEPAM but has greater anticonvulsant activity. Used intravenously for control of status epilepticus, orally for prevention of all types of epilepsy.

Clonidine. Reduces sympathetic activity by central action, and reduces vascular reactivity. Used in hypertension and in migraine. Antihypertensive effect blocked by tricyclic antidepressants. Adverse effects include sedation, depression, dryness of mouth and fluid retention. Rapid withdrawal may be associated with 'rebound hypertension'.

Clopamide. Diuretic essentially similar to BENDROFLUMETHIAZIDE.

Clopidogrel. Antiplatelet drug that irreversibly alters platelet binding to fibrin and thus reduces aggregation for the duration of the life of the affected platelets. Used in patients with a history of atherosclerosis to prevent further ischaemic strokes or myocardial infarcts and in established peripheral vascular disease to reduce tissue damage and eventual gangrene. May cause bleeding episodes, skin rashes and gastrointestinal disturbance.

Cloral betaine. Complex of CHLORAL HYDRATE and trimethyl glycine. Rapidly broken down in the body to yield CHLORAL HYDRATE.

27

Clorazepate

Clorazepate. Anxiolytic, with actions, uses and adverse effects similar to DIAZEPAM. Long-acting and has sedative effects, so is best given at night. Metabolized to desmethyldiazepam, an active metabolite of DIAZEPAM.

Clorexolone. Diuretic essentially similar to BENDROFLUMETHIAZIDE.

Clorprenaline. Bronchodilator similar to EPHEDRINE.

Clotrimazole. Antifungal agent used topically for skin infections with *Candida*.

Cloxacillin. Penicillinase-resistant PENICILLIN with actions and adverse effects similar to BENZYLPENICILLIN. Use restricted to treatment of penicillinase-producing *Staphylococcus aureus* infections.

Clozapine. Antipsychotic/tranquillizer, used in treatment-resistant schizophrenia. Actions and adverse effects similar to CHLORPROMAZINE but with fewer dopamine antagonist effects and reduced tendency to involuntary movements. Has been associated with bone marrow depression and is used only if haematological monitoring is arranged.

Coal tar. Keratolytic used in topical preparations for eczema and psoriasis.

Co-amilofruse. Contains AMILORIDE and FUROSEMIDE in a fixed ratio.

Co-amilozide. Contains AMILORIDE and HYDROCHLOROTHIAZIDE in a fixed ratio.

Co-amoxiclav. Contains AMOXICILLIN and CLAVULANIC ACID in a fixed ratio. May cause liver injury.

Co-beneldopa. Contains BENSERAZIDE and LEVODOPA in a fixed ratio.

Cobalt edetate. *See* DICOBALT EDETATE.

Cobalt tetracemate. *See* DICOBALT EDETATE.

Cocaine (c). Local anaesthetic and sympathomimetic amine. Stabilizes nerve cell membranes to prevent impulse transmission. Little used except topically in eye or respiratory passages. Frequent use may cause corneal ulceration. Stimulates CNS with euphoria and consequent risk of addiction. Chronic misuse leads to delusions, hallucinations and paranoia.

Co-careldopa. Contains CARBIDOPA and LEVODOPA in a fixed ratio.

Co-codamol. Contains CODEINE and PARACETAMOL in a fixed ratio.

Co-codaprin. Contains CODEINE and ACETYLSALICYLIC ACID in a fixed ratio.

Co-danthramer. Contains DANTRON and POLOXAMER in a fixed ratio.

Co-danthrusate. Contains DANTRON and DOCUSATE SODIUM in a fixed ratio.

Codeine (m). Weak narcotic analgesic. (c) when formulated for injection. Used for somatic (deep) pain often combined with ACETYLSALICYLIC ACID or PARACETAMOL. Also causes constipation and suppresses the cough reflex. May therefore be used as an antidiarrhoeal and in cough mixtures. Addiction unusual. Coma with respiratory depression in overdosage. NALOXONE is antidote.

Co-dergocrine. Mixture of dihydroergocornine, dihydroergocristine and dihydroergocryptine, ergot derivatives that are alpha-adrenoceptor blockers and vasdilators. Used in elderly patients with mild to moderate dementia. Adverse effects include nausea, headache, nasal congestion; dizziness and postural hypotension in patients with hypertension.

Cod-liver oil. Oil obtained from fresh cod liver. Used as a source of VITAMINS A and D.

Co-dydramol. Contains DIHYDROCODEINE and PARACETAMOL in a fixed ratio.

Co-fluampicil. Contains FLUCLOXACILLIN and AMPICILLIN in a fixed ratio.

Co-flumactone. Contains HYDROFLUME-THIAZIDE and SPIRONOLACTONE in a fixed ratio.

Colaspase. *See* L-ASPARAGINASE.

Colchicine. Used for relief of pain in acute gout. Adverse effects include nausea, vomiting, colicky pain and diarrhoea.

Colecalciferol. Naturally occurring form of VITAMIN D.

Colestipol. Ion exchange resin which lowers plasma cholesterol levels through binding with bile acids in the intestinal lumen. Used as an adjunct to diet in treatment of high cholesterol levels. May cause constipation. Must be taken mixed with water or may cause oesophageal damage.

Colestyramine. Resin that binds bile salts in gut. Used in pruritus associated with jaundice and to reduce blood cholesterol. Adverse effects include nausea, diarrhoea and constipation.

Colfosceril. A synthetic surfactant used to treat lung damage (respiratory distress syndrome) in preterm infants.

Colistin. A polymyxin antibiotic active against Gram-negative bacteria. Not absorbed by mouth but effective topically (e.g. within gut or on skin or eyes). Can also be given by intramuscular injection but injections may be painful and associated with neurological symptoms. Rarely, may cause skin sensitivity.

Collagen. Purified bovine collagen injection used as a bulking injection in the peri-urethral area to reduce stress incontinence at the bladder neck. The additional bulk reduces the urethral luminal space allowing effective contraction of the urethral muscle. Adverse effects include urinary infections, urinary retention and discomfort or bleeding at the site of the injections.

Compound gentian infusion. Bitter extract from the dried root of *Gentiana lutea*. Used to stimulate gastric acid secretion and thus to stimulate appetite.

Co-phenotrope. Contains DIPHENOXYLATE and ATROPINE SULPHATE in a fixed ratio.

Copper acetate. Used topically for its astringent properties.

Copper sulphate. Used as an emetic, together with iron in treatment of anaemia, and as astringent in topical preparations. Large doses may cause copper poisoning. Syrup of IPECACUANHA is generally considered a safer emetic.

Co-prenozide. Contains OXPRENOLOL and CYCLOPENTHIAZIDE in a fixed ratio.

Co-proxamol. Contains DEXTROPROPOXY-PHENE and PARACETAMOL in a fixed ratio. There is no evidence for increased benefit from this combined formulation and clear evidence of danger from overdose, especially if taken with alcohol. For these reasons, in January 2005, the CHM announced a phased withdrawal of all co-proxamol-containing products. This allows 6–12 months for all patients currently being treated with the drug to be assessed and their treatment changed as appropriate.

Corticosteroids. General term to include natural and synthetic steroids, with actions similar to HYDROCORTISONE, which is produced in the adrenal cortex. They possess anti-inflammatory and salt-retaining properties. Adverse effects include oedema, hypertension, diabetes, bone thinning with fractures, muscle wasting, infections and psychosis.

Corticotrophin. *See* CORTICOTROPIN.

Corticotropin. Pituitary hormone that controls functions of adrenal cortex.

Cortisone

Cortisone. Naturally occurring adrenal (glucocorticoid) steroid hormone. Has effects upon fat, protein and carbohydrate metabolism, and possesses marked anti-inflammatory activity. Used for replacement therapy in adrenal insufficiency, anti-inflammatory activity in a wide range of conditions, and immunosuppression after organ transplantation or in certain leukaemias. Adverse effects include retention of salt and water, fulminating infections, osteoporosis, peptic ulceration, muscle wasting, hypertension, diabetes mellitus, weight gain, moon face, cataracts and psychiatric disturbance. On withdrawal of large doses after long periods of treatment there may be failure of the natural adrenal hormone secretion.

Co-simalcite. Contains activated DIMETICONE and HYDROTALCITE in a fixed ratio.

Co-tenidone. Contains ATENOLOL and CHLORTALIDONE in a fixed ratio.

Co-trimazine. Antibacterial. Combination of SULFADIAZINE and TRIMETHOPRIM. Actions and adverse effects similar to CO-TRIMOXAZOLE but SULFADIAZINE is metabolized less than SULFAMETHOXAZOLE resulting in higher drug concentrations in kidneys and urine. Used for urinary tract infections.

Co-trimoxazole. Antimicrobial. Combination of SULFAMETHOXAZOLE and TRIMETHOPRIM. Broad antibacterial spectrum, active against typhoid fever. Adverse effects include rashes and blood dyscrasias.

Co-zidocapt. Contains CAPTOPRIL and HYDROCHLOROTHIAZIDE in a fixed ratio.

Cresol. Antiseptic. Used as disinfectant or preservative and also as an inhalant for relief of congestion in bronchitis, asthma and the common cold. If ingested in concentrated solutions, there may be local corrosion, depression of the CNS and damage to the liver and kidneys.

Crotamiton. Topical treatment for scabies.

Cyanocobalamin. Largely replaced by HYDROXOCOBALAMIN.

Cyclizine. Antihistamine, with actions similar to PROMETHAZINE. Main use as antiemetic.

Cyclobarbital (c). Barbiturate hypnotic, with actions, uses and adverse effects similar to AMOBARBITAL.

Cyclopenthiazide. Thiazide diuretic similar to BENDROFLUMETHIAZIDE.

Cyclopentolate. Anticholinergic, with actions and adverse effects similar to ATROPINE SULPHATE but with more rapid onset and shorter duration. Used as eye drops to dilate the pupil and to assist optical refraction.

Cyclophosphamide. Cytotoxic used in wide variety of neoplastic diseases. Activated by metabolism in the liver and excreted mainly in the urine. Adverse effects include baldness, cystitis, and renal and bone marrow toxicity.

Cycloserine. Antibiotic used in tuberculosis and in *Escherichia coli* and *Proteus* infections. Adverse effects include ataxia, drowsiness and convulsions.

Cyclosporin. *See* CICLOSPORIN.

Cyproheptadine. Antihistamine similar to PROMETHAZINE. Stimulates appetite.

Cyproterone. Hormone with antiandrogenic and some progestogenic activity used in the treatment of prostatic carcinoma. Has also been used in sexual disorders in the male, acne and hirsutism. May cause gynaecomastia, galactorrhoea, sedation, mood changes, altered hair pattern, skin rashes, weight gain, headache, anaemia, liver toxicity and fluctuations in blood pressure. Also avoided in liver disease, thromboembolic disorders, diabetes and immature youths.

Cysteamine. *See* MERCAPTAMINE.

30

Cytosine arabinoside

Cysteine. Amino acid containing sulphur.

Cytarabine (Cytosine arabinoside). Antiviral agent used systemically for herpes encephalitis. Cytotoxic, used in treatment of leukaemia and Hodgkin's disease. Adverse effects include bone marrow depression.

Cytosine arabinoside. *See* CYTARABINE.

D

Dacarbazine. Cytotoxic. May cause bone marrow suppression.

Daclizumab (r). Recombinant, humanized monoclonal antibody specific for the T-cell activating site that becomes active in transplant rejection. Used intravenously to prevent rejection of kidney transplants. No evidence for associated increased risk of infections or other illnesses associated with immunosuppression.

Dactinomycin. *See* ACTINOMYCIN D.

Dakin's solution. Contains calcium hypochlorite, SODIUM BICARBONATE, BORIC ACID. Used as wound disinfectant.

Dalfopristin. Antibiotic derived from *Streptomyces pristinaespiralis.* Used in combination with QUINUPRISTIN, another antibiotic from the same source. This combination acts synergistically against Gram-positive organisms. Used by injection only when specifically indicated in order to reduce the potential for development of bacterial resistance. Adverse reactions include injection site pain, headache, itching and joint pain.

Danaparoid sodium. Low molecular weight heparinoid used for prevention of deep vein thrombosis. Actions, adverse effects and precautions similar to HEPARIN.

Danazol. Used in endocrine disturbances where pituitary control of gonad hormone production is required.

Danthron. *See* DANTRON.

Dantrolene. Used in control of skeletal muscle spasticity. Adverse effects include sedation, weakness and diarrhoea.

Dantron. Purgative, with actions etc. similar to CASCARA. Use limited to elderly or terminally ill patients because of some incidence of tumour formation in animals at high doses and reports of genotoxicity.

Dapsone. Sulphone drug used in treatment of leprosy and dermatitis herpetiformis. Adverse effects include allergic dermatitis, nausea, vomiting, tachycardia, haemolytic anaemia and liver damage.

Daptomycin (r). Antibiotic for intravenous infusion. Used for complicated skin and soft tissue infections which are caused by Gram-positive bacteria. Destroys Gram-positive bacteria by binding with cell membranes, but is inactive against Gram-negative organisms. In mixed infections it should be co-administered with another, appropriate antibiotic. May cause headaches, gastro-intestinal disturbance, injection site reactions, fungal infections, muscle pain and myositis. Muscle damage can be detected early by monitoring plasma enzymes.

Darbepoetin alfa (r). Recombinant human erythropoetin. Stimulates red blood cell/ haemoglobin production. Used to treat anaemia associated with chronic renal failure and in some specified adult cancer patients. Administered intravenously or subcutaneously as corrective and maintenance therapy. May cause headache, hypertension and thrombosis and pain at injection site. Isolated cases of pure red cell aplasia have been reported.

Daunomycin. *See* DAUNORUBICIN.

Daunorubicin (Rubidomycin, Daunomycin). Cytotoxic antibiotic used in neoplastic disease. Adverse effects include cardiotoxicity and bone marrow depression.

Debrisoquine. Adrenergic neurone blocking drug used in hypertension. Adverse effects as for GUANETHIDINE. Discontinued in 2003.

Deferiprone. Oral iron chelator used to treat transfusional iron overload, e.g. thalassaemia major. May cause gastrointestinal upsets, rashes, joint pains, kidney and liver dysfunction and bone marrow suppression.

Deglycyrrhizinized liquorice. Mild anti-inflammatory agent. Used in treatment of peptic ulcer. Adverse effects include oedema and hypertension.

Dehydrocholic acid. Used to stimulate secretion of bile flow without increasing its content of bile solids (e.g. after surgery of biliary tract).

Demecarium. Anticholinesterase used by instillation into eye in glaucoma. Actions those of ACETYLCHOLINE.

Demeclocycline. Bacteriostatic antibiotic with actions, adverse effects and interactions similar to TETRACYCLINE.

Deoxyribonuclease. Animal pancreatic enzyme used to resolve clots and exudates associated with trauma and inflammation.

Deptropine. Antihistamine similar to PROMETHAZINE.

Dequalinium. Topical antibacterial/antifungal used in oral infections.

Deserpidine. *See* RESERPINE.

Desferrioxamine. Binds with iron. Used orally and parenterally in treatment of acute iron poisoning and in conditions associated with excessive iron storage in tissues, where it increases urinary iron excretion. Adverse effects include allergic reactions.

Desipramine. Antidepressant. Active metabolite of IMIPRAMINE, whose actions and adverse effects it shares.

Desirudin. Recombinant hirudin genetically engineered from yeast. Hirudin is a natural anticoagulant found in leeches that acts by different mechanisms to heparin. Administered by subcutaneous injection in prevention of deep vein thrombosis following hip or knee replacement surgery. May cause bleeding, wound secretions and haematomas. Fever, insomnia and high potassium levels may also occur.

Desloratadine. Nonsedating, second generation antihistamine. The active metabolite of LORATIDINE, it does not block potassium channels in cardiac cells and thus is thought unlikely to cause the cardiac arrhythmias associated with the parent compound. Used in the treatment of seasonal affective rhinitis (hay fever).

Desmopressin. Synthetic analogue of VASOPRESSIN. Longer acting and causes less vasconstriction. Active by mouth and by nasal absorption. Used to counteract high volumes of urine production in diabetes insipidus and to reduce night-time urine volume in nocturnal enuresis. May cause fluid retention and therefore careful dose titration is required. Other adverse effects include headache, nausea and abdominal pain. The nasal spray may cause nasal congestion, rhinitis and local bleeding.

Desogestrel (r). Sex hormone, with actions and adverse effects similar to PROGESTERONE. Used for oral contraception in combination with an oestrogenic hormone or as a progestogen-only pill (POP).

Desonide

Desonide. Topical corticosteroid for psoriasis and eczema.

Desoximetasone. CORTICOSTEROID for topical skin use. Actions and adverse effects similar to DEXAMETHASONE.

Desoxymethasone. *See* DESOXIMETASONE.

Dexamethasone. Potent synthetic CORTICOSTEROID with actions, etc. similar to CORTISONE. Anti-inflammatory activity is much increased in potency, with no increase in salt and water-retaining activity.

Dexamfetamine (c). CNS stimulant amfetamine with uses limited to the specialist care of narcolepsy and attention deficit hyperactivity disorder (ADHD). May cause a wide range of adverse effects including anorexia, insomnia, excitability, tremor, headache and convulsions. In the longer term may lead to tolerance, dependency and abuse.

Dexamphetamine. Former BAN for DEXAMFETAMINE. *See* AMFETAMINE.

Dexfenfluramine. Dextro-isomer of FENFLURAMINE. More active serotonin agonist than the laevo-isomer and thus has greater effect in reducing obesity than the d-l (dextro-laevo) mixture FENFLURAMINE. Claimed to have a greater effect in reducing obesity but with lower incidence of adverse effects. Has been associated with cardiac valve anomalies in some asymptomatic patients.

Dexibuprofen (r). The active isomer of IBUPROFEN. It has similar actions and adverse effects to IBUPROFEN and is licensed for the relief of mild to moderate pain and inflammation associated with osteoarthritis and other musculoskeletal diseases.

Dexketoprofen. The active analgesic dextro-isomer of KETOPROFEN. The laevo-isomer has no analgesic effect but is thought to contribute to the adverse effects. Thus the dextro-isomer is an effective treatment for arthritis with a potential to reduce adverse effects.

Dextranomer. Spherical beads of dextran for surface application to skin wounds. Takes up fluid exudate by capillary action and aids removal of bacteria and tissue debris, thus improving wound healing.

Dextrans. Polysaccharides used intravenously instead of blood or plasma to maintain blood volume and assist capillary flow. Used also as a lubricant in drops for dry eyes. Adverse effects include allergic reactions.

Dextromethorphan. Cough suppressant. Adverse effects include slight psychic dependence and abuse.

Dextromoramide (c). Narcotic analgesic essentially similar to MORPHINE but more reliable when taken by mouth. Useful in the management of severe chronic pain in terminal disease.

Dextropropoxyphene (c) (m). Weak narcotic analgesic with potency less than CODEINE. Used in moderate pain, commonly with PARACETAMOL when the latter drug is not fully effective. In normal doses, causes less nausea, vomiting and constipation than codeine. Coma with depressed respiration in overdosage. NALOXONE is antagonist.

Dextrose. Carbohydrate used orally or intravenously as a source of calories in cases of undernutrition. Readily absorbed from the gastro-intestinal tract. Metabolized by energy-producing pathways or stored in the liver as glycogen. Concentrated solutions by mouth may cause nausea and vomiting, intravenously may cause thrombophlebitis.

Diamorphine (Heroin) (c). Narcotic analgesic similar to MORPHINE. Less likely to cause nausea, vomiting, constipation and hypotension, but greater euphoriant action makes it more addicting and liable to greater abuse.

Diamthazole. Topical antifungal agent. Adverse effects include convulsions if absorbed.

Diazepam (m). Benzodiazepine minor tranquillizer (anxiolytic)/hypnotic with anticonvulsant properties. Acts centrally on the limbic system. Used in treatment of anxiety and as a hypnotic. Useful also in reduction of muscle tone in spasticity and as an anticonvulsant given intravenously for status epilepticus. May cause ataxia, nystagmus and sedation. May impair psychomotor performance. Caution required if driving or operating machinery. Coma in overdosage but little respiratory depression. Supportive treatment is usually adequate. May cause dependence, even in therapeutic doses.

Diazoxide. Used to reduce blood pressure in severe hypertension and to increase blood sugar level in hypoglycaemia. Adverse effects include excessive hair growth, nausea, vomiting, oedema, diabetes and hypotension.

Dibromopropamidine. See DIBROMPROPAMIDINE.

Dibrompropamidine. Topical antibacterial/antifungal.

Dichloralphenazone. Hypnotic. Combination of CHLORAL HYDRATE and PHENAZONE. Converted back to parent compounds by the liver. Used for insomnia especially in children and the elderly. Relatively 'safe'. Addiction is rare, but rashes and blood disorders may be caused by PHENAZONE. Withdrawn.

Dichlorofluoromethane. See CHLOROFLUOROMETHANE.

Dichlorophen. Used in treatment of tapeworms. Adverse effects include nausea, vomiting, and bowel colic.

Diclofenamide. Used in treatment of respiratory failure from chronic bronchitis and in glaucoma. Adverse effects include electrolyte imbalance.

Diclofenac. Non-steroid anti-inflammatory/analgesic/antipyretic used in treatment of rheumatoid arthritis and osteoarthritis. Adverse effects include gastro-intestinal upsets, headache and dizziness.

Dicobalt edetate (Cobalt edetate, Cobalt tetracemate). Antidote for cyanide poisoning. Binds with cyanide and prevents its effects upon cell metabolism.

Dicophane. Insecticide used as dusting powder and lotion for fleas and lice. Very toxic if absorbed.

Dicyclomine. See DICYCLOVERINE.

Dicycloverine. Parasympatholytic used in spasm of gastro-intestinal and urinary tracts and to reduce gastric acid in peptic ulceration. Actions, etc. similar to ATROPINE but weaker.

Didanosine. Antiviral drug which prevents replication of the human immunodeficiency virus (HIV) involved in AIDS. Adverse reactions include headache, rash, gastro-intestinal upset, pancreatitis and peripheral neuropathy. More rarely, anorexia, metabolic disorders, alopecia, anaphylaxis, blood dycrasias, liver failure and changes to the optic nerve or retina.

Dienestrol. Synthetic female sex hormone used for menopausal symptoms and for suppressing lactation. Adverse effects include nausea, vaginal bleeding and oedema.

Dienoestrol. See DIENESTROL.

Diethylamine salicylate. Rubefacient with actions similar to SALICYLIC ACID.

Diethylcarbamazine. Used in filariasis. Adverse effects include anorexia, nausea, vomiting and encephalopathy. Allergic reactions may accompany release of foreign proteins on death of the worms.

Diethylpropion (c). Anorectic/sympathomimetic amine. Actions those of AMFETA-

Diethylstilbestrol

MINE but less central stimulation and abuse potential.

Diethylstilbestrol. Sex hormone, with actions, uses and adverse effects similar to ESTRADIOL.

Diflucortolone. CORTICOSTEROID for topical use in inflammatory skin conditions. Actions and adverse effects similar to CORTISONE.

Diflunisal. Analgesic related to ACETYL-SALICYLIC ACID, but with longer duration of action and no effects on blood platelet function. May cause gastro-intestinal symptoms including ulceration and bleeding, although less common than with ACETYLSALICYLIC ACID. Should not be used if there is a history of hypersensitivity to ACETYLSALICYLIC ACID.

Digitalis. Crude foxglove extract, with same actions, etc. as DIGOXIN but content of active drug is less reliable.

Digitoxin. Foxglove derivative, with similar actions, etc. to DIGOXIN.

Digoxin. Foxglove derivative. Increases force of contraction of heart and slows heart rate, thus making cardiac function more efficient. Used in heart failure and certain abnormal heart rhythms. Influenced by serum potassium levels and by kidney function. In therapeutic overdose, causes vomiting, abdominal pain, diarrhoea, impaired colour vision, slow heart rate and abnormal heart rhythms.

Digoxin-specific antibody. Fragment (F(ab)) of sheep antibody specific for DIGOXIN and related cardiac drugs. Used to reverse DIGOXIN toxicity by the antibody/antigen reaction which removes the drug and prevents its effects at tissue sites. Given intravenously in a dose determined by the DIGOXIN dose taken. The antibody/antigen complexes are excreted in the urine.

Dihydrocodeine. Mild narcotic analgesic similar to CODEINE, but more potent in relief of pain and more likely to cause

constipation. (c) when formulated for injection.

Dihydroergotamine. For migraine. Drops, tablets, nasal spray or intramuscular injection. Used both for prevention and for symptomatic treatment. Has vasoconstrictor effects similar to ERGOTAMINE but milder and with much reduced tendency to hypertension or effects on the uterus. No evidence of ergotism on prolonged or excessive use.

Dihydrotachysterol. Closely related to VITAMIN D and has similar actions. Used in treatment of rickets and osteomalacia resistant to VITAMIN D. Also used in treatment of osteodystrophy due to chronic renal failure and in hypoparathyroidism. Contraindicated in hypercalcaemia, where it may cause ectopic calcification and renal failure.

Di-iodohydroxyquinoline. Used orally for amoebiasis and topically as skin antiseptic.

Diloxanide. Used in the treatment of intestinal amoebiasis, usually in combination with other drugs. Adverse effects include flatulence, vomiting and pruritus.

Diltiazem. For treatment and prevention of angina and mild to moderate hypertension. Blocks calcium entry into heart muscle and prevents the heart from 'overworking' during exercise. Contraindicated in patients with slow heart rates and poor conduction of cardiac impulse. Adverse effects may include heart block, ankle swelling, nausea, rash and headache.

Dimenhydrinate. Antihistamine/antiemetic with actions similar to PROMETHAZINE.

Dimercaprol. Binds to heavy metals. Used parenterally in treatment of heavy metal poisoning to increase urinary metal excretion. Adverse effects include nausea, vomiting and hypertension.

Dimethicone. *See* DIMETICONE.

Dimethyl sulfoxide. Used as a solvent in pharmaceutical manufacture. Used alone to reduce inflammation, for example, in the bladder.

Dimethyl sulphoxide. *See* DIMETHYL SULFOXIDE.

Dimeticone. Used in protective creams and in antacid preparations. Consists of finely divided silicone polymers. In the gut reduces surface tension of small gas bubbles. This allows them to coalesce into larger pockets of gas which are more easily expelled. Also formulated as a lotion for treatment of head lice which are killed by dimeticone's effect on their ability to maintain water balance.

Dinoprost (Prostaglandin $F_2\alpha$). Used for induction of abortion.

Dinoprostone (Prostaglandin E_2). Used for induction of abortion and of labour. Prostaglandins are produced in the ovary and uterus with rising concentrations in blood and amniotic fluid at term and during labour. A sustained-release pessary formulation may be used to produce gradual effects. Adverse effects include protracted, painful uterine contractions. Contraindicated if there has been previous uterine surgery or complications of pregnancy.

Dioctyl sodium sulphosuccinate. *See* DOCUSATE SODIUM.

Diphenhydramine. Antihistamine drug, with actions similar to PROMETHAZINE.

Diphenoxylate (c) (m). Reduces gut motility. Used in control of diarrhoea. Related to MORPHINE; adverse effects include drowsiness, euphoria, respiratory depression, coma and dependence.

Diphenylpyraline. Antihistamine similar to PROMETHAZINE.

Dipipanone (c). Narcotic analgesic essentially similar to METHADONE.

Dipivefrine. Prodrug, metabolized to ADRENALINE after absorption. Used as eye drops for chronic open-angle glaucoma where the prodrug passes through the cornea more readily than ADRENALINE. May cause transitory stinging of the eyes.

Diprophylline. Bronchodilator, with actions similar to AMINOPHYLLINE.

Dipyridamole. Used in treatment of angina. Reduces platelet stickiness. Adverse effects include flushing, headache and hypotension.

Disopyramide. Used in abnormal heart rhythms. Adverse effects include dry mouth, blurred vision and urinary hesitancy.

Distigmine. Anticholinesterase: *see* NEOSTIGMINE.

Disulfiram. Blocks alcohol metabolism at stage of acetaldehyde. Produces nausea, vomiting, severe headache, chest pain, dyspnoea, hypotension and collapse if taken before alcohol. Used in treatment of alcoholism. Other adverse effects include impotence, neuropathy and interference with anticoagulant activity of WARFARIN.

Dithranol. Used topically in psoriasis and other chronic skin conditions where it is thought to act by reducing the rate of skin cell formation. Adverse effects include staining of clothes and severe irritation to the eyes and skin.

Dobutamine. Synthetic beta-adrenoceptor agonist chemically similar to ISOPRENALINE. Stimulates cardiac beta-adrenoceptors directly causing an increase in cardiac output with less increase in cardiac rate than with ISOPRENALINE. Used as infusion in treatment of shock. Unlike DOPAMINE does not cause constriction of peripheral blood vessels and rise in blood pressure but lacks the favourable effect of the latter on renal blood flow. May cause cardiac arrhythmias, but less frequently than with ISOPRENALINE.

Docetaxel. Cytotoxic. A semi-synthetic derivative of a natural substance (taxoid)

Docusate sodium

found in the Pacific yew tree. Most active against rapidly growing tumours, it is used in locally advanced or metastatic breast cancer and in hormone refractory metastatic prostate carcinoma, in combination with corticosteroids. Adverse effects include bone marrow suppression, bleeding, rashes and a wide range of systemic effects.

Docusate sodium. Laxative. Promotes water penetration into faeces with softening and increased rate of transit along large bowel. Should not be given together with mineral oil laxatives (e.g. LIQUID PARAFFIN) as these may enhance absorption of the oil.

Domiphen. Topical disinfectant used in skin and mouth preparations.

Domperidone. Antiemetic, with DOPAMINE antagonist actions similar to METOCLO-PRAMIDE. Used to control nausea and vomiting due to cancer chemotherapy. Adverse effects include drowsiness, involuntary movements and cardiac dysrhythmias.

Donepezil. Central acetylcholinesterase inhibitor used to improve cognitive function in mild to moderate cases of Alzheimer's dementia. Brain acetylcholine, which is involved in memory storage and retrieval, is deficient in this condition. Inhibition of acetylcholinesterase reduces breakdown of acetylcholine and thus increases levels. May cause nausea, vomiting, dizziness, insomnia, fatigue, muscle cramps. Rarely seizures, extrapyramidal symptoms, heart block, bradycardia and liver dysfunction. Peripheral anticholinesterase effects are low but caution is needed in cases with known bladder outflow obstruction, gastric ulceration and asthma. Diagnosis and treatment must be undertaken in a specialist clinic. Long-term benefits remain uncertain and care is needed in case there are interactions with other drugs.

Dopamine. Naturally occurring precursor of NORADRENALINE that possesses sympatho-mimetic properties in its own right. Used intravenously in treatment of shock where it increases cardiac output with less risk of arrhythmias than ISOPRENALINE. Unlike DOBUTAMINE or ISOPRENALINE has a vasodilator action on blood vessels to kidneys and may help to improve kidney function. Larger doses may cause peripheral vasoconstriction with a rise in pressure (*see* DOBUTAMINE).

Dopexamine. Beta-adrenoreceptor agonist which increases cardiac output and increases blood flow to peripheral blood vessels and blood vessels in the kidney. Unlike DOPAMINE it does not produce vasoconstriction at high doses. May produce nausea, vomiting and tachycardia at high doses.

Dornase alfa. Synthetic (recombinant) enzyme that breaks down the DNA content of purulent sputum. Used by inhalation in cystic fibrosis to assist in clearing sputum from the lungs. Adverse effects include pharyngitis/laryngitis and skin rash.

Dorzolamide. Carbonic anhydrase enzyme inhibitor with actions similar to ACETA-ZOLAMIDE but with better ocular penetration when used topically. Used as eye drops for treatment of open-angle glaucoma, alone or in conjunction with a topical beta-adrenoceptor blocking drug. Adverse effects include a bitter taste, conjunctivitis, blurred vision and headache.

Dosulepin. Tricyclic antidepressant, with actions, uses, etc. similar to IMIPRAMINE. Also has mild tranquillizing action, which may be useful in agitated depression. May cause extrapyramidal adverse effects.

Dothiepin. *See* DOSULEPIN.

Doxapram. CNS stimulant used to stimulate respiration. Adverse effects include convulsions and abnormal heart rhythms.

Doxazosin. Long-acting antihypertensive with alpha-adrenoceptor blocking effects. May also be used to reduce symptoms of urinary obstruction caused by benign prostatic hypertrophy. Adverse effects include dizziness, vertigo, headache, fatigue, asthenia, oedema and, rarely, incontinence. Similar in action to PRAZOSIN.

Doxepin. Tricyclic antidepressant, with actions, uses, etc. similar to IMIPRAMINE. Also has mild tranquillizing effect which may relieve anxiety associated with depression. Also has potent inhibitory effects on peripheral histamine receptors H_1 and H_2. This action is used topically in a cream as treatment for the pruritis (itching) associated with eczema. May cause local irritation, dry mouth and drowsiness.

Doxorubicin (r). Cytotoxic antibiotic used in neoplastic disease. Adverse effects include bone marrow depression, cardiotoxicity, and gastro-intestinal disturbances.

Doxycycline. Bacteriostatic antibiotic, with actions, adverse effects and interactions similar to TETRACYCLINE. Unlike other tetracyclines, is not excreted by kidneys. Therefore used where renal impairment is a complication. The capsule formulation is apt to stick to the oesophageal mucosa where it dissolves and causes mucosal damage due to high acidity. A soluble formulation is available.

Doxylamine. Antihistamine similar to PROMETHAZINE.

Drospirenone (r). Synthetic progesterone used as an oral contraceptive with an oestrogen. It may help to reduce fluid retention, acne and seborrhoeic skin changes, which are sometimes associated with other combined products. Also used for hormone replacement therapy and subject to intensive monitoring when used for this indication.

Drostanolone (m). Anabolic steroid given by intramuscular injection. Adverse effects as for TESTOSTERONE.

Duloxetine (r). Antidepressant. Like VENLEFAXINE acts by inhibiting reuptake of SEROTONIN and NORADRENALINE. Used to treat major depressive episodes. May cause gastro-intestinal upset, weight loss, drowsiness and impaired sexual function. Also licensed to treat moderate to severe stress incontinence in women, where it is thought to act by increasing SEROTONIN and NORADRENALINE levels in the nerves which control muscle tone in the urethral sphincter. Used orally, in combination with pelvic floor muscle training.

Dutasteride. Enzyme inhibitor used to treat benign prostatic hyperplasia. Actions and adverse effects similar to FINASTERIDE.

D-Xylose. Sugar similar to glucose. Readily absorbed from the normal small intestine but has low rate of metabolism with consequent excretion of approximately 30 per cent unchanged in the urine. Used as a test for intestinal malabsorption since lower absorption results in lower levels in the urine. May cause diarrhoea, nausea and abdominal discomfort.

Dydrogesterone. Actions similar to PROGESTERONE, but does not inhibit ovulation and does not have contraceptive effect.

Dyflos. Organophosphorus, long-acting anticholinesterase, with actions, etc. similar to PHYSOSTIGMINE.

39

E

Econazole. Antifungal agent, with actions, uses and adverse effects similar to MICONAZOLE.

Ecothiopate. Anticholinesterase similar to DYFLOS.

Edrophonium. Short-acting anticholinesterase, with actions similar to PHYSOSTIGMINE. Used in diagnosis of myasthenia gravis.

Efalizumab (r). Monoclonal antibody injection which inhibits the immunological cascade found in active psoriasis. Used when other systemic therapies such as CICLOSPORIN and METHOTREXATE have failed or are contraindicated. May cause flu-like symptoms and exacerbation of symptoms of psoriasis, including arthritis. Contraindicated if there is any history of malignancy or tuberculosis.

Efavirenz. Antiviral. Non-nucleoside reverse transcriptase inhibitor used in combination with other antiviral drugs in HIV-1-positive patients with evidence of immunodeficiency.The antiviral activity is very specific and HIV-2 is not sensitive to this drug. May cause skin rashes, impaired concentration, dizziness and psychosis, also gastro-intestinal upset and headache. May cause interactions with other drugs that are metabolized in the liver.

Eflornithine (r). Enzyme inhibitor which is active against a key enzyme involved in hair growth. Does not remove hairs but reduces the number present and makes those that remain less visible. Used topically for the treatment of facial hirsutism in women. May cause skin reactions,

including itching, tingling, redness and acne.

Eformoterol. *See* FORMOTEROL.

Egg phosphatide. *See* LECITHINS.

Eletriptan (r). Oral 5-hydroxytryptophan receptor antagonist with actions and adverse effects similar to SUMATRIPTAN.

Embramine. Antihistamine similar to PROMETHAZINE.

Emedastine. Histamine H_1 receptor antagonist used topically to reduce eye symptoms in hay fever (seasonal allergic conjunctivitis). May cause topical dryness, skin reactions, headache or rhinitis.

Emetine. Anti-amoebic agent given by subcutaneous injection. Adverse effects include nausea, vomiting, hypotension and cardiac arrhythmias.

Emtricitabine (r). Oral antiviral. Nucleoside reverse transcriptase inhibitor used in combination with other antiviral treatments in HIV-1-positive patients with evidence of immunodeficiency. May cause jaundice, gastro-intestinal upset, headache and tiredness.

Enalapril. Antihypertensive, with actions, uses and adverse effects similar to CAPTOPRIL.

Enflurane. Inhalation anaesthetic similar to HALOTHANE.

Enfuvirtide (r). Antiviral for subcutaneous injection. A fusion inhibitor that acts by preventing the AIDS virus, HIV-1, from fusing with the immunocompetent cells and thus destroying them. Used in combination with other antiviral treatments in HIV-1-positive patients with evidence of immunodeficiency. May cause injection site reactions and a wide range of symptoms related to the gastro-intestinal and nervous systems.

Enoxaparin. A low molecular weight HEPARIN prepared by fractionating naturally occurring HEPARIN. Has increased effect against thrombus (clot) formation but with less tendency to haemorrhagic adverse effects. *See* HEPARIN.

Enoximone. Increases cardiac output by increasing stroke volume and reducing venous pressure without significant increase in heart rate. Used intravenously in heart failure refractory to other drugs. May cause hypotension, headache and insomnia. Gastro-intestinal symptoms, fever and urinary retention may also occur.

Entacapone. Inhibitor of the enzyme catecholamine-o-methyltransferase (COMT). Used in treatment of the on–off syndrome of patients treated for parkinsonism with LEVODOPA and a dopa decarboxylase inhibitor. COMT is the main enzyme metabolizing LEVODOPA in such patients and the loss of control (off symptoms) is due to low levels of LEVODOPA. May exacerbate the adverse symptoms from LEVODOPA.

Ephedrine (m). Sympathomimetic amine with alpha- and beta-adrenoceptor effects. Bronchodilator used in bronchial asthma. Also as mydriatic and nasal decongestant. Adverse effects include tachycardia, anxiety and insomnia.

Epinastine (r). Antihistamine with selective action for the H$_1$ receptor, which is activated in seasonal allergic conjunctivitis (hay fever). Used as eye drops to relieve symptoms. Is absorbed from the eye into the blood but does not cross the blood/brain barrier so is nonsedating. May cause a burning sensation when instilled in the eye.

Epinephrine. rINN for ADRENALINE.

Epirubicin. Cytotoxic antibiotic with uses, actions and adverse effects similar to DOXORUBICIN.

Eplerenone (r). ALDOSTERONE antagonist with actions similar to SPIRONOLACTONE. Has less affinity for androgen or progesterone receptors and thus causes fewer adverse effects. Not used as a diuretic but as an addition to standard therapy for left ventricular heart failure after recent myocardial infarction. May cause excessive potassium retention, nausea, diarrhoea and low blood pressure.

Epoetin alfa. A synthetic preparation of human erythropoietin hormone, normally produced by the kidneys, which increases red blood cell production. Used to treat anaemia in patients with chronic renal failure on dialysis, where the kidney is no longer able to produce sufficient hormone, and anaemia caused by chemotherapy with platinum-containing compounds. Adverse effects include raised blood pressure, thrombosis at injection sites, influenza-like symptoms, convulsions and skin reactions. Very rarely pure red cell aplasia has been reported.

Epoetin beta. Hormone preparation similar to EPOETIN ALFA.

Epoprostenol (Prostacyclin) (r). Endogenously produced prostaglandin with potent vasodilator properties. Inhibits platelet aggregation. Administered by continuous intravenous infusion because of its short duration of action. Used to preserve platelet function during cardiac bypass procedures and charcoal haemoperfusion. May be used as an anticoagulant alternative to HEPARIN in renal dialysis. Adverse effects include headache, flushing, hypotension and increased bleeding.

Eprosartan. Antihypertensive. Selective angiotensin II antagonist with actions, uses and adverse effects similar to LOSARTAN. Not metabolized by the enzyme system

Epsom salts

that gives susceptibility to drug interactions. May thus be safer at the same drug concentrations.

Epsom salts. *See* MAGNESIUM SULPHATE.

Eptifibatide. Prevents platelet aggregation. Used intravenously in conjunction with ASPIRIN and unfractionated heparin to prevent myocardial infarction in patients with unstable angina or other evidence of threatened infarction. May cause bleeding at any vulnerable site, therefore contraindicated if there is a recent history of haemorrhagic stroke or other bleeding. Use with care if there is a history of peptic ulceration or recent surgery.

Ergocalciferol. Form of VITAMIN D obtained from fungi and yeasts.

Ergometrine. Derivative of ergot – a fungus which grows on rye. Causes contraction of uterine muscle. Used in obstetrics after delivery of the baby to prevent or reduce maternal haemorrhage. Adverse effects as for ERGOTAMINE.

Ergotamine. Ergot derivative similar to ERGOMETRINE but with vasoconstricting and alpha-adrenoceptor blocking activity. Used in treatment of migraine by oral, intramuscular, sublingual, aerosol or suppository routes. Adverse effects include nausea, vomiting, headache, convulsions and cold extremities. Rarely, may cause myocardial infarct in patients with no known history of coronary heart disease.

Erlotinib. Oral antineoplastic used to treat advanced non-small cell lung cancer when other treatments have failed. May cause gastro-intestinal disturbance, rash and shortness of breath due to damage to the alveolar cells.

Ertapenem (r). Intravenous broad-spectrum antibiotic which acts by inhibiting bacterial cell wall synthesis. Used to treat intra-abdominal infections, community-acquired pneumonia and acute gynaecological infections. Similar to IMIPENEM.

Adverse effects include diarrhoea, nausea, vomiting, headache, pain at the injection site, rash and itching and, less commonly, CNS disturbances.

Erythromycin. Bactericidal antibiotic, with spectrum of activity similar to BEN-ZYLPENICILLIN, plus some strains of *Haemophilus influenzae* and mycoplasmas. Adverse effects include diarrhoea and liver damage with jaundice. Used systemically for a wide range of infections, especially in penicillin-sensitive individuals. Also used topically for treatment of mild to moderate acne.

Escitalopram. Antidepressant: the active isomer of CITALOPRAM with which it shares both actions and adverse effects.

Eserine. *See* PHYSOSTIGMINE.

Esomeprazole. Proton pump inhibitor, the S-isomer of OMEPRAZOLE. Has the same actions, uses and adverse effects as OMEPRAZOLE but undergoes less rapid (first pass) metabolism and has potential to be more effective due to increased bioavailability.

Essential oils. Volatile, odorous mixtures of plant origin with a mild irritant effect on skin and mucous membranes. Used as carminatives for the gastro-intestinal tract (induce feelings of warmth and salivation), or as counterirritants on the skin (cause warmth and smarting). Also widely used as flavours and in 'traditional' medicines.

Estradiol. Naturally occurring sex hormone (OESTROGEN). Controls development and function of female sex organs, working in conjunction with PROGESTERONE. Could be used for menstrual disorders, OESTROGEN deficiency, oral contraception and suppression of certain neoplastic disease, but mainly superseded by related compounds. Also used for prevention of osteoporosis. May cause withdrawal bleeding, breast development in the male, salt and water retention, nausea and vomiting, stimulation of tumours and arterial and venous thrombosis. Use avoided in patients with known risks of these effects.

Estramustine phosphate. Cytotoxic drug used in neoplastic disease. Adverse effects include lower abdominal burning sensation and bone marrow depression.

Estriol. Sex hormone (OESTROGEN) similar to ESTRADIOL, but more active by mouth. Used mainly for menopausal disorders.

Estrone. Sex hormone (OESTROGEN) similar to ESTRADIOL. Used mainly for menopausal disorders.

Etacrynic acid. Potent diuretic. Action and uses similar to FUROSEMIDE. Adverse effects similar to BENDROFLUMETHIAZIDE. May also cause transient deafness.

Etamivan. Respiratory stimulant essentially similar to NIKETHAMIDE. May be used in respiratory depression of the newborn.

Etamsylate. Haemostatic agent used to control surgical and menstrual blood loss.

Etanercept (r). Anticytokine. Recombinant human tumour necrosis factor alpha (TNF-α). Acts by neutralizing TNF-α mediated cell responses in joint (synovial tissues) and possibly by modulating further stages in the inflammatory process of arthritis. Used subcutaneously to treat active rheumatoid arthritis and juvenile chronic arthritis that have not responded to disease-modifying agents such as METHO-TREXATE, severe active ankylosing spondylitis and severe plaque psoriasis. Adverse effects include injection site reactions and vulnerability to infections, allergic reactions and blood disorders. May cause cardiovascular and CNS effects.

Ethacrynic acid. See ETACRYNIC ACID.

Ethambutol. Antituberculous drug. Well tolerated but high doses toxic to optic nerve, producing central or periaxial retrobulbar neuritis.

Ethamsylate. See ETAMSYLATE.

Ethanolamine. Sclerosing agent used in the injection treatment of varicose veins. Contraindicated if there is thrombophlebitis. May cause hypersensitivity allergic reactions.

Ethinylestradiol. Synthetic female sex hormone with similar actions and adverse effects to DIENESTROL. Combined with progestational drug in some oral contraceptives and in treatment of acne and hirsutism.

Ethinyloestradiol. See ETHINYLESTRADIOL.

Ethionamide. Antituberculous agent. High incidence of adverse effects, mainly on gastro-intestinal tract.

Ethisterone. Similar actions and adverse effects to PROGESTERONE.

Ethoheptazine. Analgesic for mild to moderate pain. Adverse effects include nausea and drowsiness.

Ethomoxane. Alpha-adrenoceptor blocking drug similar to PHENTOLAMINE.

Ethosuximide. Anticonvulsant. Suppresses epileptic discharges in the brain. Used in treatment of petit mal (absence seizures) but not for major epilepsy. May cause nausea and vomiting, drowsiness or excitation, photophobia, and Parkinson-like symptoms. Coma with respiratory depression in overdosage. No antidote. Supportive treatment only.

Ethotoin. Anticonvulsant essentially similar to PHENYTOIN but less toxic and less effective.

Ethyl biscoumacetate. Anticoagulant drug, with actions similar to WARFARIN.

Ethylene diamine. Pharmaceutical aid used in manufacture of AMINOPHYLLINE, and of some creams for topical application. Can produce allergic dermatitis by both topical and systemic administration.

Ethyl nicotinate

Ethyl nicotinate. Topical vasodilator. *See* NICOTINIC ACID.

Ethylestrenol (m). Anabolic steroid. Adverse effects as for TESTOSTERONE.

Ethyl salicylate. Similar to METHYL SALICYLATE.

Ethynodiol. *See* ETYNODIOL.

Etidronate. A biphosphonate which influences bone structure and strength by increasing bone mass and reducing bone reabsorption. Used to treat osteoporosis and Paget's disease of bone (osteitis deformans), but less likely to cause oesophageal irritation. Adverse effects similar to ALENDRONATE but less likely to cause oesophageal irritation.

Etodolac. Non-steroid anti-inflammatory/analgesic, with actions and uses similar to IBUPROFEN. Adverse effects include gastrointestinal intolerance, but claimed to produce less gastric bleeding than other drugs in this group.

Etomidate. Used by injection for induction of anaesthesia. May cause pain on injection, hypotension and involuntary movements.

Etoposide. Cytotoxic drug used in treatment of malignant disease. Adverse effects include nausea, vomiting and bone marrow depression.

Etoricoxib (r). Non-steroidal anti-inflammatory analgesic with selective inhibition of the cyclo-oxygenase enzyme-2 (COX-2). Thus it reduces prostaglandin production at the sites of inflammation without affecting the protective effects of COX-1 prostaglandins on the gastro-intestinal tract. Used for symptomatic relief of pain in osteoarthritis and rheumatoid arthritis. Gastro-intestinal effects are reduced but not eliminated. May also cause dizziness, fluid retention, hypertension, headache and itching. Should be used with caution in patients with renal, cardiac or hepatic impairment, and renal function should be monitored. Contraindicated in moderate or severe congestive heart failure.

Etosalamide. Analgesic, with similar actions and adverse effects to SALICYLAMIDE.

Etretinate. Synthetic derivative of retinoic acid (VITAMIN A) used in treatment of severe intractable psoriasis and some other serious disorders of skin growth. Adverse effects include teratogenic actions, dryness of mouth and other mucous membranes, exfoliation of the skin, hair loss, and disorders of liver function and blood fats. Acute overdosage produces severe headache, nausea, vomiting and drowsiness, requiring immediate withdrawal of the drug and nonspecific supportive treatment. Contraindicated in pregnancy.

Etynodiol. Similar actions and adverse effects to PROGESTERONE. Combined with oestrogenic agent in some oral contraceptives.

Eucalyptus. Essential oil used internally to relieve catarrh and externally as rubefacient.

Eucatropine. Parasympatholytic mydriatic similar to HOMATROPINE.

Exemestane. Hormone antagonist/aromatase inhibitor effective against hormone-dependent breast cancer. Used in treatment of metastatic breast cancer in post-menopausal women in whom anti-oestrogen therapy has failed. May cause hot flushes, sweating, gastro-intestinal upset, tiredness, headache and depression.

Ezetimibe (r). Acts in the small intestine to inhibit absorption of cholesterol. Used to lower body cholesterol levels usually in conjunction with a statin. May cause headache, abdominal pain and diarrhoea. Rare cases of myopathy and rhabdomyolysis have been reported.

F

Factor VIIa. Activated Factor VII used intravenously to treat bleeding problems in patients with haemophilia type A or B. May cause skin reactions, gastro-intestinal disturbance and malaise. There is a danger of excessive clotting in patients with advanced atherosclerosis, crush injuries and septicaemia. May also cause angina, cardiac arrhythmia and hypotension.

Factor VIII. Blood clotting factor that is deficient in haemophilia and von Willebrand's disease. Used intravenously to stop episodes of uncontrollable bleeding.

Factor IX concentrate. HIV-free clotting factor purified and concentrated from human blood plasma. May cause headache, fever, flushing, vomiting and thromboembolic episodes.

Famciclovir. Antiviral agent used orally to treat herpes zoster infections, shingles and genital herpes. It is a prodrug, which is rapidly metabolized to its active metabolite PENCICLOVIR in the liver. Should only be used with caution in patients with renal impairment. Adverse effects include headache and nausea.

Famotidine. Gastric histamine receptor blocker, with actions and uses similar to CIMETIDINE, but longer duration of action. May cause tiredness, headache, dizziness, constipation, diarrhoea, anorexia and other minor gastro-intestinal symptoms.

Felbinac. Non-steroid anti-inflammatory/analgesic derived from FENBUFEN, for topical application after soft-tissue injury. It acts locally and has minimal systemic effects. It may cause mild local erythema, dermatitis and pruritus. It is contraindicated in hypersensitivity to ACETYLSALICYLIC ACID.

Felodipine. Calcium antagonist with actions and adverse effects similar to NIFEDIPINE. Used to treat hypertension and angina.

Felypressin. Vasoconstrictor polypeptide used in some local anaesthetic preparations. Less likely than sympathomimetic vasoconstrictors to cause cardiac arrhythmias, and does not interact with antidepressant drugs.

Fenbufen. Non-steroid anti-inflammatory/analgesic, with action and uses similar to IBUPROFEN. Has long duration of action and needs only twice-daily dosage. Adverse effects include gastro-intestinal intolerance, skin rashes, dizziness and headaches. Contraindicated in hypersensitivity to ACETYLSALICYLIC ACID.

Fenclofenac. Anti-inflammatory/analgesic, with actions, uses and adverse effects similar to IBUPROFEN.

Fenfluramine. Anti-obesity, with central anorectic and peripheral metabolic effects. Claimed to be effective in autism. May produce diarrhoea, sedation and sleep disturbance. Contraindicated in patients taking monoamine oxidase inhibitors. Has been associated with cardiac valve abnormalities in some asymptomatic patients.

Fennel. Essential oil used as carminative.

Fenofibrate. Fibrate, lipid-regulating drug. Acts by reducing CHOLESTEROL synthesis and increasing the breakdown of lipids. Used to treat hyperlipidaemias not responding to diet alone. More effective at

Fenoprofen

reducing triglyceride levels than CHOLES-TEROL levels. Fibrates are generally used as second-line treatment in patients who do not tolerate or fully respond to statins, which are the drugs of choice for reducing CHOLESTEROL levels. May cause gastrointestinal disturbances, headache, rash, drowsiness and muscle disease, notably myositis.

Fenoprofen. Anti-inflammatory/analgesic, with similar actions and uses to INDO-METACIN.

Fenoterol. Actions and adverse effects similar to SALBUTAMOL.

Fentanyl (c). Narcotic analgesic, with actions and uses similar to MORPHINE. More potent analgesic and respiratory depressant, but shorter action. May be administered transdermally from patches.

Fenticonazole. Antifungal used topically as pessaries for vulvovaginal candiasis. Actions and effectiveness similar to MICONAZOLE and CLOTRIMAZOLE. Used as a single dose or on three consecutive nights. May cause local irritation.

Ferric ammonium citrate. Actions and adverse effects similar to FERROUS SULPHATE.

Ferric chloride. Iron salt included in some 'tonics' or treatments for iron deficiency. Actions and adverse effects similar to FERROUS SULPHATE.

Ferric hydroxide. Iron salt, with actions similar to FERROUS SULPHATE.

Ferrous fumarate. Actions and adverse effects similar to FERROUS SULPHATE.

Ferrous gluconate. Actions and adverse effects similar to FERROUS SULPHATE.

Ferrous glycine sulphate. *See* FERROUS SULPHATE.

Ferrous succinate. Actions and adverse effects similar to FERROUS SULPHATE.

Ferrous sulphate. Used as a source of iron to replenish body iron stores in iron deficiency anaemia. Adverse effects include black faeces, abdominal pain, constipation and diarrhoea. Liquid formulations can stain teeth black.

Fexofenadine. Nonsedative antihistamine used in treatment of hay fever (seasonal allergic rhinitis). Has actions and adverse effects similar to TERFENADINE and ASTEMI-ZOLE, but appears to lack cardiac effects.

Filgrastim. Human growth factor which stimulates production of white blood cells within the bone marrow. Made by recombinant DNA technology. Used to enhance white blood cell production in patients whose bone marrow function is depressed by cytotoxic treatment. Adverse effects include muscle pain and painful micturition.

Finasteride. Enzyme inhibitor which blocks the formation of the male sex hormone dihydrotestosterone from testosterone. The former is active in promoting benign growth of the prostate gland in older men, whilst the latter maintains male sexual characteristics. Used in the treatment of benign prostatic hypertrophy. Finasteride reduces the size of the gland without causing feminizing side effects. Should not be used to treat cancer of the prostate, as it may cause impotence and decreased libido.

Flavoxate. Antispasmodic used in bladder disorders. Adverse effects include headache and dry mouth.

Flecainide. Antiarrhythmic, with actions and adverse effects similar to LIDOCAINE but active by mouth. Used to treat and prevent life-threatening, irregular cardiac rhythms.

Flosequinan. Direct-acting vasodilator with effects upon arterioles and veins. Used in treatment of cardiac failure when it reduces the stress on the heart, both from venous inflow and resistance to arterial outflow. Acts by relaxing muscles in the blood vessel walls. May cause headaches, dizziness, palpitations, low blood pressure, joint pains, rashes and photosensitivity. Withdrawn due to evidence of increasing risk of hospitalization and mortality of patients with congestive heart failure.

Fluclorolone. Topical CORTICOSTEROID used in psoriasis and eczema.

Flucloxacillin. Antibiotic. Similar properties to CLOXACILLIN, but better absorbed.

Fluconazole. Antifungal agent used to treat vaginal and oral fungal infections. Adverse effects include nausea, headache and abdominal discomfort.

Flucytosine. Antifungal agent active orally against systemic *Candida* infections. Adverse effects include bone marrow depression.

Fludarabine. Cytotoxic used in treatment of chronic lymphocytic leukaemia where it may achieve complete or partial remission. Adverse effects include bone marrow suppression, fever and infection.

Fludrocortisone. Potent salt-retaining CORTICOSTEROID used in adrenal insufficiency. Adverse effects include oedema, hypertension and electrolyte imbalance.

Fludroxycortide. Topical CORTICOSTEROID used in psoriasis and eczema.

Flufenamic acid. Anti-inflammatory/analgesic essentially similar to MEFENAMIC ACID.

Flumazenil. Benzodiazepine antagonist which completely or partially reverses the central sedative effects. Used to reverse benzodiazepine effects after short diagnostic and therapeutic procedures. Its use in the reversal of benzodiazepine overdose is not yet established, and it is not licensed for this purpose. Adverse effects may include withdrawal symptoms and convul-

sions in patients dependent on benzodiazepines.

Flumetasone. Topical CORTICOSTEROID used in psoriasis and eczema.

Flumethasone. *See* FLUMETASONE.

Flunisolide. Potent synthetic CORTICOSTEROID similar to DEXAMETHASONE. Used by nasal spray for treatment of allergic rhinitis.

Flunitrazepam (c). Benzodiazepine hypnotic/anxiolytic with actions, uses and adverse effects similar to NITRAZEPAM. Recommended only for short-term treatment of insomnia.

Fluocinolone. Topical CORTICOSTEROID used in psoriasis and eczema.

Fluocinonide. Topical CORTICOSTEROID used in psoriasis and eczema.

Fluocortolone. Topical CORTICOSTEROID used in psoriasis and eczema.

Fluorescein. Staining agent used for detection of damage to the cornea and as a test of pancreatic function.

Fluorometholone. Potent synthetic CORTICOSTEROID, similar to DEXAMETHASONE.

Fluorouracil. Cytotoxic, used in the treatment of metastatic cancer of the colon, breast cancer and other solid tumours. May be used topically for some skin lesions including genital warts. Adverse effects include bone marrow suppression and CNS disturbances.

Fluoxetine (m). Antidepressant which acts by blocking reuptake of SEROTONIN into nerve cells. It has a lower incidence of noradrenergic and cholinergic side effects than tricyclic antidepressants (e.g. IMIPRAMINE) and is less likely to cause sedation and cardiac side effects. It also seems to be safer in overdose. May cause nausea, headache, insomnia, dizziness, asthenia, rash, convulsions, hypomania and mania.

Flupenthixol

Flupenthixol. *See* FLUPENTIXOL.

Flupentixol. Antipsychotic, with anti-depressant and anxiolytic actions but little sedative effects. Used in depressive and anxiety states associated with inertia and apathy. Adverse effects include restlessness, insomnia, hypotension and extrapyramidal disturbances. Not recommended for children or excitable patients or in advanced cardiac, renal or hepatic disease.

Fluphenazine. Phenothiazine tranquillizer similar to CHLORPROMAZINE, but longer acting. Used in treatment of psychoses, confusion and agitation. Oral treatment required only once a day. Available as a 'depot' intramuscular injection which is active for 10–28 days. Adverse effects similar to CHLORPROMAZINE but more frequently causes involuntary movements.

Fluprednidene. Topical CORTICOSTEROID used in psoriasis and eczema.

Flurandrenolone. *See* FLUDROXYCORTIDE.

Flurazepam (m). Benzodiazepine tranquillizer/hypnotic. Used in the treatment of insomnia. Essentially similar to NITRAZEPAM.

Flurbiprofen. Anti-inflammatory/analgesic, with actions, uses and adverse effects similar to IBUPROFEN. Used in inflammatory joint diseases and as eye drops to prevent trauma-induced pupil constriction during eye surgery.

Fluspirilene. Tranquillizer used in schizophrenia. Adverse effects include involuntary movements and low blood pressure.

Flutamide. Antiandrogen used to block effects of male sex hormones on growth of cancer of the prostate gland. May cause gynaecomastia, breast tenderness and milk production, also gastro-intestinal disturbances and insomnia.

Fluticasone. Potent synthetic CORTICO-STEROID similar to BECLOMETASONE. Used by inhalation for treatment of asthma and for the prophylactic treatment of asthma and chronic obstructive pulmonary disease (COPD). Formulated as nasal drops and nasal spray for allergic rhinitis. May cause paroxysmal bronchospasm and oral can-didiasis but systemic absorption from inhaled corticosteroids is low and systemic adverse effects are infrequent, except when the highest doses are used for a prolonged time.

Fluvastatin. Statin. Enzyme inhibitor with actions, uses, precautions and adverse effects similar to SIMVASTATIN.

Fluvoxamine. Antidepressant. Acts by blocking reuptake of SEROTONIN into nerve cells. Does not have anticholinergic effects and thus is less likely to cause cardiac side effects than tricyclic antidepressants (e.g. IMIPRAMINE). May cause nausea, constipation, weight loss, drowsiness, anxiety and tremor. Should not be used with THEO-PHYLLINE or AMINOPHYLLINE because it may affect their metabolism and precipitate toxic effects such as nausea, headache, vomiting and agitation.

Folic acid. Used in folate-deficient megaloblastic anaemias of pregnancy, malnutrition and malabsorption states. May precipitate neuropathy in untreated HYDROXOCOBALAMIN deficiency.

Folinic acid. Used as an antidote to antifolate cytotoxic agents and in the treatment of megaloblastic anaemias, other than due to VITAMIN B_{12} (HYDROXOCOBALAMIN) deficiency.

Fomepizole. A specific antidote for ethylene glycol poisoning. It inhibits the enzyme responsible for the metabolism of ethylene glycol to its toxic metabolites.

Fomivirsen. Antiviral agent specific for cytomegalovirus (CMV) infections. Used by intraocular (intravitreal) injection to delay progress of CMV retinitis in AIDS patients. May cause blurring of vision, local swelling, pain and inflammation.

Conjunctival and retinal haemorrhage may occur.

Fondaparinux (r). Antithrombotic. Acts by selective inhibition of coagulation Factor X. Used as an alternative to low molecular weight HEPARIN for the prevention of venous thromboembolism in orthopaedic surgery. Also for treatment of deep vein thrombosis and pulmonary embolism. Adverse effects include bleeding, bruising anaemia and reduced blood platelets. May cause fluid retention and abnormal liver function tests.

Formaldehyde. As a solution used topically for treatment of warts.

Formestane. Inhibits enzyme involved in production of oestrogen, leading to prolonged suppression of oestrogen secretion in the ovaries and adrenal glands. Used to treat advanced oestrogen-dependent breast cancer. May cause hot flushes, vaginal bleeding, joint pains, fluid retention and gastro-intestinal disturbance.

Formoterol. Long-acting selective beta-adrenoceptor agonist. Used by inhalation for maintenance therapy in asthma, particularly when night-time or exercise-induced symptoms are a problem. Adverse effects similar to SALBUTAMOL. Should only be used in addition to inhaled or oral steroids and should not replace them.

Fosamprenavir (r). Prodrug of the antiviral protease inhibitor AMPRENAVIR. Similar actions to AMPRENAVIR but shows reduced incidence of adverse effects, notably gastro-intestinal disturbances and rash. Used in combination with RITONAVIR and other antivirals to slow or halt HIV-1 infections.

Foscarnet. Antiviral drug which inhibits the replication of both human immunodeficiency viruses (HIV) involved in AIDS and the herpes viruses. Adverse effects include impaired renal function, hypocalcaemia, hypoglycaemia, epileptic seizures, decrease in haemoglobin con-

centration, headache, nausea, vomiting and rash.

Fosfomycin. Bactericidal antibiotic that acts by inhibiting bacterial cell wall synthesis. It has a broad spectrum of activity and rapidly achieves high urinary concentrations after oral administration. It is used for prophylaxis and treatment of urinary tract infections. Adverse effects include rashes and gastro-intestinal disturbances.

Fosinopril. Antihypertensive with similar actions to CAPTOPRIL also used to treat congestive heart failure. Adverse effects include dizziness, cough, gastro-intestinal disturbances, palpitations, chest pain, rash, musculoskeletal pain, fatigue and taste disturbances.

Fosphenytoin. Inactive prodrug converted rapidly in the liver to the active anticonvulsant PHENYTOIN. Highly water-soluble, so intravenous or intramuscular injection does not cause painful irritant effects associated with injection of PHENYTOIN in propylene glycol and alcohol solution. Used for emergency control of seizures. Systemic adverse effects similar to PHENYTOIN.

Framycetin. Antibiotic derivative of NEOMYCIN used topically for skin infections and by mouth for gastroenteritis and bowel sterilization.

Frangula. Mild purgative, with actions, etc. similar to CASCARA.

Frovatriptan. 5-HYDROXYTRYPTAMINE agonist used in the treatment of acute migraine headache. Actions and adverse effects similar to SUMATRIPTAN but of longer duration (due to longer half-life).

Frusemide. See FUROSEMIDE.

Fuller's earth. Adsorbent. Used in poisoning due to the weedkiller Paraquat, which it binds strongly. Administered orally or directly into stomach via nasogastric tube. May be given with MAGNESIUM SULPHATE to

Fulvestrant

promote diarrhoea and thus attempt to empty the gut of Paraquat.

Fulvestrant (r). Cytotoxic. Hormone antagonist similar to TAMOXIFEN. Used by intramuscular injection in treatment of breast cancer. May cause hot flushes, headaches, gastro-intestinal upset, rashes and injection site reactions.

Furazolidone. Poorly absorbed antibacterial drug used in bacterial diarrhoea and gastroenteritis. Adverse effects include nausea, vomiting, rashes, haemolysis in predisposed patients and flushing with alcohol.

Furosemide. Potent diuretic which causes greater reduction in sodium reabsorption by the kidney than occurs with the thiazide diuretics (*see* BENDROFLUMETHIAZIDE). Rapid onset of action when given orally or intravenously. Used in emergency treatment of fluid overload, especially pulmonary oedema and in cases resistant to thiazides. May also be used as antihypertensive. Adverse effects similar to BENDROFLUMETHIAZIDE.

Fusafungine. Antibiotic administered by aerosol for infections of upper respiratory tract.

Fusidic acid. Steroid antibiotic used for infections by PENICILLIN-resistant *Staphylococci*. Adverse effects include nausea and vomiting.

G

Gabapentin. Anticonvulsant. Structurally similar to the neurotransmitter GABA but mode of action uncertain. Used as an adjunct to other anticonvulsant therapy. Adverse effects include drowsiness, dizziness, headache, tremor, nausea and vomiting. Also used to treat pain resulting from damage to nerve tissue such as neuralgia.

Galantamine. Reversible central acetylcholinesterase inhibitor used to improve cognitive function in mild to moderate Alzheimer's dementia. Brain ACETYL-CHOLINE is involved in memory storage and retrieval and is deficient in this condition. Inhibition of acetylcholinesterase reduces breakdown of ACETYLCHOLINE and thus increases levels. May cause gastrointestinal disturbance, tiredness, dizziness and confusion; less commonly insomnia, tremor, severe bradycardia and convulsions. Long-term benefits remain uncertain and care is needed in case there are interactions with other drugs. Diagnosis and treatment must be undertaken from a specialist clinic.

Gallamine. Skeletal muscle relaxant used during surgical procedures under general anaesthesia. Has action similar to TUBOCU-RARINE.

Gamma-benzene hexachloride. Applied topically for treatment of lice, scabies and other infestations. Adverse effects include convulsions if ingested.

Gamolenic acid. Essential fatty acid derived from the evening primrose plant for systemic treatment of atopic eczema. May cause nausea, diarrhoea and headache and cyclical or noncyclical breast pain. Appears to reduce breast pain by reducing sensitivity to cyclical hormone changes. The product licence has been withdrawn by the CHM because there is inadequate evidence of efficacy.

Ganciclovir. Antiviral agent for cytomegalovirus infections, such as retinitis and pneumonitis, in immunocompromised patients, including those suffering from AIDS. It prevents the virus from replicating and stops the progression of the infection, but it is not a cure and if the treatment is stopped the virus may begin to replicate again. May cause fever, rashes, depression and impairment of liver and kidney function. May be given prophylactically to kidney or liver transplant patients to prevent cytomegalovirus disease from developing.

Ganirelix. Gonadotropin-releasing hormone antagonist. Used by injection or intranasally to reduce luteinizing hormone surges in women undergoing in vitro fertilization. May cause pain at injection site, headaches and vaginal bleeding.

Gefarnate. Used for treatment of peptic ulcer. May cause skin rashes.

Gelatin. Protein used as a nutrient in the preparation of some oral medicines and suppositories, and in a sponge-like form as a haemostatic.

Gemcitabine. Cytotoxic used as palliative treatment for non-small cell lung cancer (the major form of that disease in the UK) and breast cancer. Adverse effects include bone marrow suppression, nausea, vomiting, fever and muscle pains.

Gemeprost. Synthetic prostaglandin which acts on the uterus to prepare it for delivery of

Gemfibrozil

the foetus. Used as a pessary to prepare the uterus for surgical termination of pregnancy.

Gemfibrozil. Fibrate, lipid-regulating drug. Acts by reducing CHOLESTEROL synthesis and increasing the breakdown of lipids. Used to treat hyperlipidaemias not responding to diet alone. More effective at reducing triglyceride levels than CHOLESTEROL levels. Fibrates are generally used as second-line treatment in patients who do not tolerate or fully respond to statins, which are the drugs of choice for reducing CHOLESTEROL levels. May cause gastro-intestinal disturbances, headache, rash, drowsiness and muscle disease, notably myositis.

Gentamicin. Bactericidal aminoglycoside antibiotic injection with spectrum similar to NEOMYCIN, but specially active against *Pseudomonas aeruginosa.* Adverse effects include ototoxicity and nephrotoxicity, particularly in renal failure. Potentiates neuromuscular blockade.

Gestodene. Sex hormone, with actions, uses and adverse effects similar to NORGESTREL. Combined with oestrogenic agent as an oral contraceptive.

Gestonorone. Hormone with similar actions to PROGESTERONE.

Gestrinone. A synthetic steroid for treatment of endometriosis. Has anti-oestrogenic and androgenic activity which reduces the size of the endometrial tissue fragments and leads to their regression. May cause temporary suppression of normal menstruation. Adverse effects include acne, fluid retention, nervousness, depression, voice changes and increased hair growth.

Gestronol. *See* GESTONORONE.

Glatiramer. Immunomodulator used as a 'disease-modifying drug' to reduce the frequency of relapse in ambulatory patients suffering from relapsing, remitting multiple sclerosis. Administered by weekly subcutaneous injection. May cause pain at injection site and post-injection reactions including nausea, hypertension, palpitations and shortness of breath. May also cause joint pains, rash and tissue swelling.

Glauber's salts. *See* SODIUM SULPHATE.

Glibenclamide. Long-acting oral antidiabetic drug, that stimulates pancreatic insulin release in maturity-onset diabetes mellitus. Adverse effects include hypoglycaemia, particularly in the elderly, allergic reactions, jaundice and flushing with alcohol. Action may be potentiated by salicylates and sulphonamides.

Gliclazide. Short-acting oral antidiabetic drug, with actions, uses and adverse effects similar to GLIBENCLAMIDE, but excreted more rapidly and thus shorter acting. Recommended when there is greater danger of hypoglycaemia (e.g. in the elderly).

Glimepiride. Long-acting oral antidiabetic drug with actions, uses and adverse effects similar to GLIBENCLAMIDE.

Glipizide. Long-acting oral antidiabetic drug, with actions and uses similar to GLIBENCLAMIDE.

Gliquidone. Short-acting oral antidiabetic drug, with actions, uses and adverse effects similar to GLIBENCLAMIDE, but excreted more rapidly and thus shorter acting. Recommended when there is greater danger of hypoglycaemia (e.g. in the elderly).

Glucagon. Polypeptide hormone produced by alpha-cells of pancreas. Causes increase in blood sugar, release of several other hormones, and increases force of cardiac contraction. Used in tests of carbohydrate metabolism and in treatment of heart failure. May cause nausea and vomiting but cardiac arrhythmias are said not to occur.

Glucose. Source of carbohydrate nutrition. Administered by mouth or intravenously as a dietary supplement. Also used acutely to reverse hypoglycaemic attacks associated with diabetes melitus.

Glutaraldehyde. As a solution used to treat warts.

Gluten. Constituent of wheat starch responsible for bowel disorders in gluten-sensitive individuals. These conditions respond to treatment with a gluten-free diet.

Glycerin. Carbohydrate used as a sweetening agent in some mixtures and pastilles and as high-calorie source in intravenous feeds. Used topically in skin preparations for water retaining and softening properties. In suppositories or enemas, it promotes bowel peristalsis and evacuation.

Glycerin suppositories. Local lubricant purgative.

Glycerol. *See* GLYCERIN.

Glycerophosphates. Used widely in 'tonic' preparations as a source of phosphorus.

Glyceryl trinitrate. Vasodilator for symptomatic or prophylactic treatment of angina pectoris. Administered as sublingual tablets or oral spray for rapid absorption at onset of symptoms or applied as gel to skin for sustained absorption in prophylaxis. May also be used intravenously to treat cardiac failure, during hypotensive surgery or during cardiac surgery to prevent myocardial infarction. Adverse effects include headache, dizziness and flushing. Also formulated as an ointment to relieve pain associated with anal fissures. Applications to skin may cause local allergic reactions. Loses potency if not stored away from light and under cool conditions.

Glycine. Amino acid used with antacids in gastric hyperacidity, and with ASPIRIN to reduce its gastric irritation.

Glycol salicylate. Rubefacient. Essentially similar to SALICYLIC ACID.

Glycopyrronium. Anticholinergic similar to ATROPINE, used in peptic ulcer, gastric hyperacidity and to reduce excessive sweating.

Gold salts. Anti-inflammatory agent, apparently specific for rheumatoid arthritis. Mechanism of action unknown. Given by mouth or as a course of intramuscular injections. Toxic reactions are common including stomatitis, dermatitis, nausea, vomiting and diarrhoea. May cause hepatitis, nephritis and bone marrow depression. Not given if evidence of pre-existing liver or kidney disease.

Gonadorelin. Hormone produced in the hypothalamus of the brain which stimulates the ovarian hormones luteinizing hormone (LH) and follicle-stimulating hormone (FSH). Used as pulsatile subcutaneous or intravenous injection for treatment of amenorrhoea and infertility due to ovarian hormone deficiency. May cause gastro-intestinal symptoms, skin rashes and abdominal pain.

Gonadotrophin. Pituitary hormone that stimulates gonadal activity. Used in infertility and delayed puberty.

Goserelin. Hormone, analogue of gonadotrophin-releasing hormone. Used for depot administration in abdominal wall to treat cancer of the prostate gland, endometriosis and breast cancer. Acts by reducing production of male sex hormones. May cause hot flushes, loss of libido, breast development, bruising at injection site and transient increase in bone pain.

Gramicidin. Antibiotic used by local application to skin, wounds, burns and nose and mouth infections. Toxic if ingested or injected.

Granisetron. Potent antiemetic with actions similar to ONDANSETRON.

Griseofulvin. Antifungal active both topically and systemically. Used to treat infections of skin, nails and hair. May cause gastro-intestinal disturbances, headaches, tiredness and rashes.

Guaifenesin. Used to reduce sputum viscosity.

Guaiphenesin

Guaiphenesin. *See* GUAIFENESIN.

Guanethidine. Adrenergic neurone blocking drug. Used in hypertension. Eye drops used in glaucoma and hyperthyroid eye signs. Adverse effects include postural hypotension, nasal stuffiness, diarrhoea, fluid retention and impotence. Action antagonized by tricyclic antidepressants and sympathomimetics (e.g. when used as nasal decongestants in 'cold cures').

Guanochlor. Antihypertensive adrenergic neurone blocking drug with actions similar to GUANETHIDINE.

Guanoxan. Antihypertensive adrenergic neurone blocking drug with actions similar to GUANETHIDINE.

Guar flour. *See* GUAR GUM.

Guar gum. Binding agent in tablets, thickening agent in foods. Takes in moisture from the gut and produces feeling of satiety by the bulk thus formed. Used in treatment of obesity and in diabetes mellitus where it may help to stabilize blood glucose levels. Unwanted effects include abdominal bloating, indigestion, diarrhoea and flatus.

H

Haemophilus influenza type b vaccine. Vaccine prepared from the purified polysaccharide of the capsule of the Haemophilus influenza type b virus, conjugated with the tetanus protein (Act-HIB) or diphtheria protein (Hib-TITER) to increase its effectiveness and duration of protection. Recommended for general vaccination programmes in infants over two months of age to reduce incidence of childhood meningitis due to this organism. Local skin redness may occur at the injection site.

Halcinonide. Topical CORTICOSTEROID used in psoriasis and eczema.

Halofantrine. Antimalarial effective in acute treatment of infections resistant to CHLOROQUINE, and other antimalarials. May cause gastro-intestinal disturbances and potentially fatal cardiac arrhythmias. Also a risk of fatal arrhythmias if given together with MEFLOQUINE or other drugs which may induce arrhythmias or electrolyte imbalance. Fatty foods may increase absorption and should therefore be avoided.

Haloperidol. Butyrophenone tranquilliser. Used in treatment of psychosis where it has similar effects to CHLORPROMAZINE but more potent. Has antiemetic action but lacks anticholinergic and alpha-adrenolytic effects. May cause involuntary movements, drowsiness, depression, hypotension, sweating, skin reactions and jaundice. In overdosage, effects and treatment similar to CHLORPROMAZINE.

Halothane. Potent inhalational anaesthetic used for major surgery. Adverse effects include slowing of the heart and fall in blood pressure. May cause liver damage with jaundice in susceptible patients on repeated exposure.

Heparin. Anticoagulant produced in mast cells and obtained from bovine lung. Acts by preventing several reactions in the blood-clotting mechanism. Given by injection only. Used to prevent formation or spread of blood clots as in deep vein thrombosis, pulmonary embolism and unstable coronary artery disease, and to prevent clotting during haemodialysis or haemofiltration. May produce allergic reactions and, on prolonged use, osteoporosis. Heparin-induced haemorrhage may be controlled by PROTAMINE SULPHATE. Low molecular weight heparins are prepared by fractionating naturally occurring HEPARIN. They share some of the properties and actions of standard HEPARIN but have a longer duration of action and are less likely to cause bleeding and other side effects.

Heparinoid. HEPARIN derivative or similar substance with uses and effects similar to HEPARIN.

Hepatitis A vaccine. Vaccine prepared from purified inactivated viral antigens for protection against transmissible viral hepatitis. Used in high-risk groups (e.g. healthcare personnel). Adverse effects include fever, malaise, nausea, loss of appetite and soreness at injection site.

Hepatitis B vaccine. Vaccine prepared from purified inactivated viral antigens for protection against transmissible viral hepatitis. Used in 'at-risk' populations (e.g. healthcare personnel and drug abusers). Adverse effects include fever, joint pains, nausea, tiredness and rashes.

Heroin

Heroin (c). *See* DIAMORPHINE.

Hetastarch. Polysaccharide used intravenously instead of blood or plasma to maintain blood volume.

Hexachlorophane. *See* HEXACHLOROPHENE.

Hexachlorophene. Topical antiseptic used in soaps, creams, lotions, and dusting powders. Adverse effects include allergy, light sensitivity and CNS effects if absorbed or ingested.

Hexamine. *See* METHENAMINE.

Hexetidine. Topical antibacterial/antifungal/antitrichomonas.

Hexobarbital (c). Barbiturate hypnotic essentially like AMOBARBITAL.

Hexylresorcinol. Antiworm. Also used as antiseptic agent for throat infections.

Histamine. Mediator of many body functions including gastric secretion, inflammatory and allergic responses. Produces skin vasodilation. Was used in test of gastric acid production. Adverse effects include headache, hypotension, bronchospasm and diarrhoea.

Homatropine. Parasympatholytic with actions, toxic effects, etc. similar to ATROPINE. Used as a mydriatic because when compared with ATROPINE its action is more rapid, less prolonged and more easily reversed by PHYSOSTIGMINE.

Human menopausal gonadotrophins. Preparation containing human follicle stimulating hormone and luteinizing hormone used to treat infertility due to failure of gonadotrophin stimulation, by stimulating ovulation in women and sperm production in men. Should not be used in other causes of infertility. May cause allergic reactions including skin rashes.

Hyaluronic acid. Animal (rooster) derived hyaluronic acid which has pharmacological and physiological actions in joint (synovial) fluids. Used by intra-articular injection in osteoarthritis of the knee where the concentration of hyaluronic acid is reduced. May cause transient pain, redness and swelling at the injection site.

Hyaluronidase. Enzyme that assists dispersal and absorption of subcutaneous and intramuscular injections. Hastens resorption of blood and fluid in body cavities. Adverse effects include allergic reactions.

Hydralazine. Vasodilator antihypertensive drug. Adverse effects include tachycardia, headache, bone marrow depression, acute rheumatoid syndrome and systemic lupus erythematosus syndrome.

Hydrochlorothiazide. Thiazide diuretic similar to BENDROFLUMETHIAZIDE.

Hydrocortisone. Naturally occurring adrenocorticosteroid hormone with similar actions, etc. to CORTISONE.

Hydroflumethiazide. Thiazide diuretic similar to BENDROFLUMETHIAZIDE.

Hydrogen peroxide. Disinfectant/deodorant. Acts by rapid but short-lived release of oxygen. Used for cleaning wounds. Also helps to detach dead tissue. Other uses include mouthwash, treatment of acne and minor skin infections, and bleaching hair.

Hydromorphone (c). Opioid analgesic with greater potency than MORPHINE but with similar adverse effects. Used by injection in the management of moderate to severe pain.

Hydrotalcite. Antacid used in peptic ulcer and gastric hyperacidity.

Hydrous wool fat. Purified waxy substance obtained from the wool of sheep plus water. Used as a base for ointments. May produce skin sensitization.

Hydroxocobalamin (Vitamin B_{12}). Used for the treatment of pernicious anaemia or specific deficiency states. Parenteral.

Hydroxyapatite. Calcium salt used as a source of calcium and phosphorus in osteoporosis, rickets and osteomalacia.

Hydroxycarbamide. Cytotoxic agent for oral administration. Used mainly in the treatment of chronic myeloid leukaemia and polycythaemia. May cause bone marrow suppression, nausea and skin reactions.

Hydroxychloroquine. Antimalarial agent: *see* CHLOROQUINE.

Hydroxyprogesterone. Hormone that has been used to prevent threatened abortion but no longer recommended for this purpose. Rarely, may cause liver tumours.

Hydroxyquinoline. Topical antibacterial/ antifungal deodorant.

5-Hydroxytryptamine. Neurotransmitter with central and peripheral actions. Thought to be involved in the vascular headache of migraine and to be deficient in some types of depression.

Hydroxyurea. *See* HYDROXYCARBAMIDE.

Hydroxyzine. CNS depressant. Used to relieve tension and anxiety in emotional disturbances but less effective than CHLOR-PROMAZINE and similar tranquillizers in the psychoses. May cause excessive drowsiness, headache, dry mouth, itching and convulsions. Coma in overdosage. No antidote; supportive treatment only.

Hyoscine butylbromide. Parasympatholytic, with peripheral actions similar to ATROPINE SULPHATE but of shorter duration. Used as an antispasmodic similar to PROPANTHELINE but effective only by injection.

Hyoscine hydrobromide. Parasympatholytic, with central and peripheral actions similar to ATROPINE SULPHATE except that it produces central depression and hypnosis rather than stimulation and tends to slow the heart. Used for pre-operative medication where the hypnotic effect makes it preferable to ATROPINE and as an antiemetic for travel sickness. Adverse effects, etc. otherwise as for ATROPINE SULPHATE.

Hyoscine methobromide. Similar to HYOSCINE HYDROBROMIDE.

Hypromellose. Indigestible plant residue similar to METHYLCELLULOSE but used mainly in eye drops as lubricant (e.g. in so-called artificial tears for dry eyes).

I

Ibandronic acid (r). Biphosphonate with actions and uses similar to ETIDRONATE. Also used intravenously to reduce tumour-induced hypercalcaemia. May cause fever, hypocalcaemia, bone pain and bronchospasm.

Ibuprofen. Non-steroid anti-inflammatory/analgesic/antipyretic. Reduces inflammation by inhibition of prostaglandin synthesis, which is part of the inflammatory process. Used in rheumatoid arthritis and other arthritic conditions. Used also as a general purpose mild analgesic and as an antipyretic in febrile conditions of childhood. Also inhibits prostaglandin synthesis in gastric mucosa, thus reducing their protective effect and causing gastric intolerance. Gastro-intestinal symptoms, including blood loss, are less common than with ASPIRIN. Other adverse effects include headache, other CNS symptoms and hypersensitivity reactions.

Ichthammol. Dermatological preparation, with slight antibacterial effects. Used in creams and ointments for chronic skin conditions.

Icodextrin. Nonabsorbable glucose polymer used in ambulatory peritoneal dialysis as treatment of end-stage chronic renal failure. Avoids the weight gain and high glucose/insulin levels associated with dialysis solution based on glucose. May cause abdominal pain, muscle cramps, fluid and electrolyte imbalance.

Idarubicin. Cytotoxic antibiotic with actions, uses and adverse effects similar to DAUNORUBICIN.

Idoxuridine. Antiviral agent used in local treatment of herpes infections.

Ifosfamide. Cytotoxic drug, with uses and adverse effects similar to CYCLOPHOSPHAMIDE.

Iloprost (r). Synthetic analogue of EPOPROSTENOL (PROSTACYCLIN), an endogenous anticoagulant, with the same actions and adverse effects. Used by intermittent inhalation through a nebulizer to improve symptoms and exercise tolerance in patients with advanced pulmonary hypertension. Longer acting than EPOPROSTENOL so does not need to be given continuously. Adverse effects similar to EPOPROSTENOL but may also include persistent coughing.

Imatinib (r). Enzyme inhibitor that reduces proliferation of leukaemic cells. Used orally to treat chronic myeloid leukaemia. May cause headache, nausea, vomiting and bone marrow suppression. Liver and kidney insufficiency occur rarely.

Imidapril. Prodrug for IMIDAPRILAT, a long-acting ACE inhibitor which allows once-daily dosage in treatment of hypertension. Actions, uses and adverse effects similar to other ACE inhibitors, e.g. ENALAPRIL.

Imipenem. Intravenous broad-spectrum antibiotic which acts by inhibiting bacterial cell wall synthesis, similar to PENICILLINS and cephalosporins. Active against many penicillin-resistant strains. Given in combination with CILASTATIN, a structurally similar compound with no antibacterial activity which helps to reduce the metabolism of imipenem and thus to prolong its effectiveness. Adverse effects include nausea, vomiting, diarrhoea, blood dyscrasias and disturbance of renal, hepatic and CNS functions. May cross-react in patients with PENICILLIN hypersensitivity.

Imipramine. Antidepressant, blocks neuronal reuptake of NORADRENALINE, DOPAMINE, and 5-HYDROXYTRYPTAMINE. Adverse effects include anticholinergic actions of dry mouth, blurred vision, precipitation of glaucoma, retention of urine, and constipation; also produces cardiac arrhythmias, potentiates direct sympathomimetic pressor amines and antagonizes action of GUANETHIDINE, BETANIDINE, DEBRISOQUINE and CLONIDINE. Coma, convulsions and cardiac arrhythmias in overdosage. Treatment supportive.

Imiquimod. Immune response modifier that induces the production of INTERFERON ALFA and other cytokines. Used topically in the treatment of genital and anal warts and basal cell carcinoma. May cause local skin reactions.

Immunoglobulin G. Concentrate of antibodies derived from human plasma. Used to convey short-term immunity to some virus infections including hepatitis A, measles and rubella. Used in cases of congenital and acquired immunoglobulin deficiency and after bone marrow transplantation.

Inactivated lactobacilli. Vaccine from bacteria found in the vagina of women suffering from trichomonal infection. The vaccine provokes the immune response to infections including trichomoniasis and thus helps to prevent recurrent infections.

Indapamide. Derivative of FUROSEMIDE, used as antihypertensive in subdiuretic doses. Larger doses have diuretic action and adverse effects similar to BENDROFLUMETHIAZIDE.

Indinavir. Antiviral protease inhibitor which inhibits HIV maturation and proliferation. Used in combination with other antiviral agents to slow or halt HIV infection. May cause gastro-intestinal disturbance, skin reactions, muscle disorders, fatigue, and metabolic disorders.

Indometacin. Non-steroid anti-inflammatory/analgesic, used in treatment of inflammatory joint disease. Adverse effects include headache, vertigo, depression, confusion and gastro-intestinal symptoms including perforation and haemorrhage. No longer used to treat inflammatory joint disease but, when used intravenously, has become the treatment of choice to promote closure of patent ductus arteriosus in neonates, probably by inhibiting an action of prostaglandin. As such, it is used only in intensive care units, where it is possible to monitor closely for the intended effects and possible adverse reactions including haemorrhagic, renal and gastro-intestinal disorders.

Indomethacin. *See* INDOMETACIN.

Indoprofen. Non-steroid anti-inflammatory/analgesic, with actions, uses and adverse effects similar to IBUPROFEN. Recently withdrawn.

Indoramin. Alpha-adrenoceptor blocking drug, used in hypertension, peripheral vascular disease, prophylaxis of migraine and symptomatic relief of urinary symptoms due to prostatic hypertrophy. Acts by relaxation of muscles in blood vessels and in prostate gland. Produces sedation and nasal stuffiness.

Infliximab (r). Anticytokine. Human–mouse monoclonal antibody that inhibits tumour necrosis factor alpha (TNF-α). Acts by binding with TNF-α in the colon and joint tissues to reduce the inflammatory changes which would otherwise be stimulated. Used by intravenous infusion to treat severe active Crohn's disease, ankylosing spondylitis, ulcerative colitis, plaque psoriasis or rheumatoid arthritis that have not responded to other treatments. May cause fever, skin reaction,

Inosine pranobex

headache, dizziness and hypertension. May lower tolerance to infections.

Inosine pranobex. Antiviral active against herpes simplex in skin and mucous membranes. Used for genital warts. Does not act directly against the virus, but increases the body's cellular immune response. Metabolized to uric acid and thus may cause elevated uric acid levels. Caution if used in gout or renal failure.

Inositol. Ingredient of nutritional preparations. It has been considered a vitamin but no nutritional deficiency has been demonstrated.

Inositol nicotinate. Metabolized to NICOTINIC ACID which dilates peripheral blood vessels. Used for chilblains and other conditions where peripheral blood circulation is thought to be poor. Large doses may cause fall in blood pressure and slowing of heart.

Insulin. Hormone. Available as pig or beef insulin derived from animal pancreas and as human insulin now available by synthesis from animal insulin or by genetic engineering from bacterial sources. Causes a fall in blood sugar levels and increased storage of glycogen in the liver. Used to treat diabetes. All products are used by parenteral injection except for inhaled human insulin which was introduced in 2006. Different formulations are produced to provide varied duration of action. Adverse effects include hypoglycaemia and subcutaneous fat atrophy. Products for inhalation are contraindicated in smokers and patients with chronic lung diseases.

Interferon alpha-2a. Antiviral agent produced from bacteria by recombinant techniques (genetic engineering). Used to treat chronic myelogenous leukaemia, 'hairy cell' leukaemia, malignant melanoma and chronic active hepatitis. May cause flu-like syndrome, anorexia, weight loss and effects on the CNS and cardiovascular system. Less likely to cause further suppression of immune system than conven-tional cytotoxics, but full monitoring is needed.

Interferon alpha-2b. Antiviral agent similar to INTERFERON ALPHA-2A but, at present, used for treatment of 'hairy cell' leukaemia and non-Hodgkin's lymphoma, chronic myelogenous leukaemia, malignant melanoma and chronic active hepatitis. Further trials may extend its use to other cancers. Adverse effects similar to those from INTERFERON ALPHA-2A, but may include bleeding.

Interferon alpha-NI. Antiviral agent with actions and adverse effects similar to INTERFERON ALPHA-2B, at present used only for treatment of 'hairy cell' leukaemia, but under investigation for use in other cancers. May also cause liver and kidney damage.

Interferon beta-1a and Interferon beta-1b. Genetically engineered proteins with actions which reduce immune mechanisms. Used to reduce or prevent relapses in multiple sclerosis although the exact mechanism of action is not known. May cause flu-like symptoms, pain at the injection site and CNS effects including convulsions.

Interferon gamma. Used as adjunctive therapy to antibiotics in patients with the rare condition chronic granulomatous disease, in which there is reduced resistance to infection. Produced by biotechnology, it is identical to a human substance involved in resisting infection. Unwanted effects include fever, muscle and joint pains.

Iodine. Halogen, converted to iodide in the body and used in production of thyroid hormone. Low dietary intake leads to reduced thyroid function (myxoedema). Large doses may be given by mouth to suppress thyroid function prior to surgical removal of thyroid tissue when the gland is overactive. May cause hypersensitivity with headache, laryngitis, bronchitis and rashes. May also be used on the skin as a disinfectant.

60

Ipecacuanha. Plant extract used in small doses as an expectorant in cough mixtures. Syrup of ipecacuanha was used in the past as an emetic for emergency treatment of ingested poisons but there is no evidence it reduces absorption and may increase risk of aspiration.

Ipratropium. Anticholinergic used by inhalation for its bronchodilator action in chronic bronchitis and asthma. Used also as intranasal spray for relief of chronic watery nasal discharge. Adverse effects similar to ATROPINE, but much reduced when given by inhalation and are seen only at high doses.

Iprindol. Antidepressant, with actions, uses and adverse effects similar to IMIPRAMINE.

Irbesartan. Antihypertensive. Angiotensin II receptor antagonist with actions, uses and adverse effects similar to LOSARTAN.

Irinotecan. Cytotoxic used in treatment of metastatic colorectal cancer in patients resistant to 5-FLUOROURACIL. It is a pro-drug that is converted to two active metabolites which inhibit DNA replication. May cause nausea, vomiting, bone marrow suppression and 'delayed diarrhoea' 24 hours or more after treatment. This condition could be life threatening and requires hospital treatment.

Iron dextran injection (r). Parenteral formulation for iron-deficiency anaemia. Adverse effects include pain on injection, skin staining, vomiting, headache and dizziness. Anaphylactic reactions may accompany intravenous infusion particularly.

Iron sorbitol injection. Intramuscular formulation for iron-deficiency anaemia. Adverse effects as for IRON DEXTRAN INJECTION.

Isoaminile citrate. Cough suppressant used on its own or in cough linctus. No analgesic or sedative effects. Does not depress respiration. May cause dizziness, nausea and constipation or diarrhoea.

Isocarboxazid. Monoamine oxidase inhibitor/antidepressant. Actions, uses and adverse effects as for PHENELZINE.

Isoconazole. Used to treat fungal and protozoal vaginal infections. Actions and adverse effects similar to METRONIDAZOLE.

Isoflurane. Potent inhalational anaesthetic used for major surgery. Has also analgesic properties. More potent than HALOTHANE in depressing respiration and enhancing effects of muscle relaxants (e.g. TUBOCURARINE) but less likely to sensitize the heart to catecholamines.

Isometheptene. Sympathomimetic agent, with actions and adverse effects similar to ADRENALINE. Used in symptomatic treatment of migraine where it is said to constrict the dilated blood vessels that cause the throbbing headache.

Isoniazid. Synthetic antituberculous agent. About 60 per cent of Caucasians are slow inactivators by acetylation, genetically determined. Adverse effects include peripheral neuropathy, pellagra, mental disturbances and convulsions, which may be reduced by administration of PYRIDOXINE.

Isoprenaline. Beta-adrenoceptor agonist used in bronchial asthma by inhalation or orally. Adverse effects include tachycardia, arrhythmias and tremor. May also be used as intravenous infusion in treatment of shock. More likely to cause cardiac arrhythmias than DOPAMINE or DOBUTAMINE.

Isosorbide dinitrate (Sorbide nitrate). Dilates blood vessels. Similar actions and adverse effects to GLYCERYL TRINITRATE but longer action. Used for symptomatic and prophylactic treatment of angina and in resistant heart failure.

Isosorbide mononitrate. Vasodilator used for prophylaxis of angina. An active metabolite of ISOSORBIDE DINITRATE, it is not metabolized further and may thus have a more predictable effect. Adverse effects are similar to GLYCERYL TRINITRATE.

Isotretinoin

Isotretinoin. VITAMIN A derivative, used to treat severe acne not responsive to antibiotic therapy. Thought to act directly on sebaceous glands in the skin to reduce sebum production. Adverse effects include dryness of skin, mucous membranes and conjunctivae. Teratogenesis, nausea, headache, malaise, joint pains, hair loss and biochemical evidence of liver damage may also occur. Contraindicated in the presence of liver or kidney disease, in pregnancy or in patients with a history or family history of cutaneous epithelioma. Local irritation may occur after topical application. Has been associated with depression.

Ispaghula. Purgative. Dried, ripe seeds of *Plantago ovata*. Increases faecal bulk. Mechanism of action similar to that of METHYLCELLULOSE.

Ispaghula husk. As for ISPAGHULA, but contains only outer layers of dried seeds and is more potent than whole seeds. Also used as an adjunct to diet, for its ability to lower blood cholesterol concentrations by removing cholesterol and fatty acids from the gut. May cause flatulence and bloating.

Isradipine. Antihypertensive which lowers blood pressure by dilating blood vessels. Adverse reactions include headache, flushing, dizziness, tachycardia, palpitations, localized peripheral oedema, weight gain, fatigue and abdominal discomfort. Similar in action to NIFEDIPINE.

Itraconazole. Antifungal agent for oral treatment of vulvovaginal candidiasis, pityriasis versicolour and dermatophytoses. May cause nausea, dyspepsia, abdominal pain and headache. May cause congestive heart failure in patients with a history of congestive heart failure.

Ivabradine (r). Antianginal which acts specifically at the cardiac pacemaker (sinus node) to reduce the electric (If) current and thus reduces both the heart rate and myocardial oxygen consumption. Used to treat stable angina in patients for whom beta-adrenoceptor blocking drugs are contraindicated or are not tolerated. May cause blurred vision and luminous phenomena (phosphenes). Other adverse effects include excessive slowing of the heart and heart block, headaches and dizziness.

K

Kanamycin. Bactericidal aminoglycoside antibiotic with actions and spectrum similar to NEOMYCIN, but less ototoxic. Used in Gram-negative septicaemia, with monitoring of blood levels, particularly in renal failure. Potentiates neuromuscular blockade.

Kaolin. Adsorbent. Used externally as a dusting powder and by mouth as treatment for diarrhoea where it increases faecal bulk and slows passage through the gut. Once thought to have specific adsorbent effect for poisonous substances but it is now known that the adsorbent effect is a general one.

Ketamine (m). Parenteral anaesthetic with analgesic properties in subanaesthetic doses. Rapid onset of action, but may cause psychotic symptoms, including hallucinations, the frequency of which can be reduced by giving DIAZEPAM or DROPERIDOL. Contraindicated in patients with high blood pressure or known psychosis.

Ketoconazole. Used to treat internal and external fungal infections. Adverse effects include nausea, rashes and jaundice.

Ketoprofen. Anti-inflammatory/analgesic, with actions, uses and adverse effects similar to IBUPROFEN.

Ketorolac. Non-steroidal anti-inflammatory analgesic with actions similar to IBUPROFEN. Used intramuscularly or orally to relieve postoperative pain. May cause pain at injection site, drowsiness, sweating and gastro-intestinal symptoms. Dose and duration of use restricted because of severity of gastro-intestinal effects, asthma and anaphylaxis. May also be used topically as eye drops following eye surgery.

Ketotifen. Preventive treatment for asthma. Has the actions of an antihistamine, similar to PROMETHAZINE, and also blocks allergic mechanisms by a mechanism similar to SODIUM CROMOGLICATE. Adverse effects include dry mouth, dizziness and sedation.

L

Labetalol. Antihypertensive. Has both alpha- and beta-adrenoceptor blocking actions. Uses similar to PROPRANOLOL. May be used with care in patients with chronic heart failure. Adverse effects include dizziness, headache, fatigue and, rarely, postural hypotension and liver dysfunction.

Lachesine. Parasympatholytic, similar to TROPICAMIDE. Used in the eye as a mydriatic and cycloplegic.

Lacidipine. Calcium channel antagonist used to treat hypertension. Mode of action and adverse reactions similar to NIFEDIPINE but used only once daily.

Lactic acid. Used intravenously as dilute solution in treatment of acidosis. Acts less rapidly than SODIUM BICARBONATE. Also used topically as strong solutions in treatment of warts.

Lactitol. A semi-synthetic disaccharide consisting of galatose and sorbitol, with actions and uses similar to LACTULOSE.

Lactulose. Laxative. A synthetic disaccharide (galactose plus fructose) that is not absorbed but broken down by gut bacteria to nonabsorbable products that increase the faecal mass by osmotic effects. Effective but expensive. Has been recommended for use in liver failure to reduce absorption of ammonia from the gut.

Laevodopa. *See* LEVODOPA.

Laevulose. Carbohydrate. Used intravenously as a source of calories when oral feeding is not possible. In renal failure it is better tolerated than dextrose. Accelerates metabolism of ethyl alcohol and may be used to treat alcohol poisoning. May cause facial flushing, abdominal pain and localized thrombophlebitis.

Lamivudine. Antiviral agent active against HIV and also used in chronic hepatitis B. Used in combination with other antivirals in progressive disease (AIDS). May cause gastro-intestinal disturbance, muscle and joint pains and bone marrow suppression. Acts synergistically with ZIDOVUDINE and these drugs may be used in combination.

Lamotrigine. Anticonvulsant. Acts by inhibiting excitatory neurotransmitter release and by stabilizing neuronal membranes. Can be used alone or as a second-line, additional treatment in patients not satisfactorily controlled on other anticonvulsants. May cause drowsiness, headache, blurred vision, gastro-intestinal disturbances and skin rashes. Rarely, may cause serious skin reactions, especially in children, and bone marrow depression.

Lanolin. Purified, fat-like substance from the wool of sheep. Used in creams for topical use, it is not absorbed but aids the absorption of drugs carried in the cream. Otherwise used for its emulsifying effect in bland creams and cosmetics. May cause skin sensitization.

Lanreotide. Long-acting analogue of the growth hormone releasing hormone (somatostatin). Used by fortnightly injections to treat acromegaly. May cause pain at injection site, gastro-intestinal upset and gallstones.

Lansoprazole. Suppresses production of gastric acid. Actions, uses and adverse effects similar to OMEPRAZOLE.

L-Asparaginase (Colaspase). Cytotoxic enzyme derived from bacterial culture; used in neoplastic disease. Adverse effects include nausea, vomiting, pyrexia, neurotoxicity, hypersensitivity reactions and bone marrow depression.

Latanoprost. Prostaglandin analogue which increases fluid outflow from the anterior chamber of the eye, thus reducing intraocular pressure. Used as eye drops in the treatment of glaucoma. May cause eye discomfort, reddening and blurred vision.

LAX (levo-acetyl-3,4 methylenedioxyphenyliosprenaline hydrochloride) (m). An illicit drug derivative abused for its euphoriant and hallucinogenic effects. Said to be derived from MDMA.

L-Dopa. *See* LEVODOPA.

Lecithins. Phospholipids found in both animal and vegetable foods. Used as emulsifying and stabilizing agents in skin preparations.

Leflunomide (r). Disease-modifying anti-rheumatoid drug (DMARD). Acts at an early stage in the inflammatory process and thus can take effect earlier than some DMARDs. Used orally to treat rheumatoid and psoriatic arthritis. Needs to be monitored for possible drug interactions due to competition for hepatic metabolism. May cause gastro-intestinal disturbance, headaches and dizziness. Rarely, may cause severe skin reactions including Stevens–Johnson syndrome and impaired liver function.

Lenograstim. Closely related to FILGRAS-TIM, and sharing the same indications. Adverse effects include bone pain and local reactions at the injection site.

Lepirudin. Genetically engineered anticoagulant with actions similar to hirudin, the anticoagulant found in leeches. Acts to prevent clot formation at several stages without the need for co-factors. Used to treat HEPARIN-associated thrombocytopaenia which is characterised by formation of life-threatening blood clots. May cause bleeding, fever and renal failure.

Lercanidipine. Long-acting calcium antagonist with actions similar to NIFEDEPINE. Used as a once-daily treatment for hypertension. May cause flushing, peripheral oedema and headache.

Letrozole (r). Anti-oestrogen. Acts by inhibiting enzymes controlling OESTROGEN production. Used in treatment of advanced breast cancer in patients in whom TAMOXIFEN has failed. Adverse effects include headache, nausea, tiredness, cough and hot flushes.

Leucovorin. FOLINIC ACID derivative used to treat drug-induced folate deficiency, e.g. due to the cytotoxic METHOTREXATE, and thus reduce/prevent anaemia. Not useful in other forms of folate or vitamin B_{12} deficiency.

Leuprorelin. An analogue of gonadotrophin releasing hormone which initially increases but then suppresses sex hormone production. Used to reduce growth of cancer of the prostate, in treatment of endometriosis, and before surgery of the uterus. In women, may cause effects similar to the menopause, in men may cause initial transient increase in bone pain and urinary obstruction and, later, loss of libido, hot flushes and sweating, hypersensitivity reactions, visual disturbances and dizziness.

Levallorphan. Narcotic antagonist similar to NALORPHINE. Less likely to cause severe withdrawal symptoms in 'addicts'.

Levamisole. Antiworm treatment. Used mainly in veterinary practice but also in man against *Ascaris* sp. (roundworm). Adverse effects include nausea, vomiting, abdominal pain and fall in blood pressure.

Levetiracetam (r). Anticonvulsant used as add-on therapy in patients with poorly controlled partial seizures. Mode of action

Levobunolol

uncertain but rapid onset of effectiveness and rapid elimination make the dosage easier to adjust than with many anticonvulsant drugs. May cause gastro-intestinal or CNS adverse effects.

Levobunolol. A nonselective beta-adrenoceptor blocker formulated as eye drops to treat glaucoma by lowering intraocular pressure. Actions and adverse effects similar to TIMOLOL and PROPRANOLOL.

Levocabastine. Antihistamine, potent blocker of H_1. Used topically as nasal spray and eye drops to reduce the symptoms of hay fever (allergic rhinitis/conjunctivitis). May cause local irritation, blurred vision, headache and tiredness.

Levocetirizine (r). Antihistamine: the active isomer of CETIRIZINE with which it shares the same actions, uses and adverse effects.

Levodopa. Amino acid. Converted in body to DOPAMINE, a neurotransmitter substance that is deficient in Parkinson's disease. Controls rigidity and improves movements but less effect on tremor than anticholinergic drugs (e.g. TRIHEXYPHENIDYL). May cause gastro-intestinal symptoms, hypotension, involuntary movements and psychiatric disturbances. Side effects may be reduced by combination with peripheral inhibitors of DOPAMINE synthesis (BENSERAZIDE or CARBIDOPA). Contraindicated/caution in cardiovascular disease and psychiatric disturbance. Effects diminished by phenothiazines (e.g. CHLORPROMAZINE), METHYLDOPA, RESERPINE, PYRIDOXINE.

Levofloxacin (r). Antibiotic with actions, uses and adverse effects similar to CIPROFLOXACIN. The formulation used topically for eye infection is subject to intensive monitoring by the CHM.

Levomepromazine. Antipsychotic, with actions, uses and adverse effects similar to CHLORPROMAZINE.

Levonorgestrel. Sex hormone with actions, uses and adverse effects similar to PROGESTERONE. Also used topically through an intrauterine contraceptive device, when adverse reactions include altered menstrual patterns, lower abdominal and back pain.

Levorphanol (c). Narcotic analgesic similar to MORPHINE, but more reliable when given by mouth. Useful in the management of severe chronic pain in terminal disease.

Levothyroxine. Thyroid hormone. Has a stimulating action in general metabolism which is delayed in onset and prolonged (*see* LIOTHYRONINE). Used in treatment of thyroid deficiency. Doses in excess of requirements may cause thyrotoxic symptoms (e.g. rapid pulse, cardiac arrhythmias, diarrhoea, anxiety features, sweating, weight loss and muscular weakness). Caution if there is pre-existing heart disease.

Lidocaine. Local anaesthetic/antiarrhythmic. Stabilizes nerve cell membranes to prevent impulse conduction. Used topically or by injection for local anaesthesia in minor operations. Intravenous injection or infusion used to treat abnormal heart rhythms. Excessive doses also block motor impulses and normal cardiac conduction. May cause hypotension, CNS depression and convulsions. Metabolized by liver and therefore used with caution in liver disease. Short action prevents use as oral antiarrhythmic.

Lignocaine. *See* LIDOCAINE.

Lindane. Organochlorine insecticide. Used topically on skin/hair for lice and scabies. Safe, providing not ingested, but emergence of resistant strains of the parasites limits its effectiveness.

Liothyronine. Thyroid hormone, probably the active hormone to which THYROXINE is converted. Given by mouth or injection it has effects similar to THYROXINE but more rapid and short-lived. Used when rapid effect is needed (e.g. in myxoedema coma). Used with care if there is evidence of cardiovascular disease as it may precipitate cardiac failure.

Liquid paraffin. Laxative. Lubricates faecal material in colon and rectum. Used when straining is undesirable or defaecation painful (e.g. after operations for haemorrhoids). Reduces absorption of fat-soluble VITAMIN A and VITAMIN D, and in chronic use can cause paraffinomas in mesenteric lymph glands. May leak from anal sphincter. Also used in some topical skin and eye preparations as a lubricant and an aid to removal of crusts.

Liquorice. Dried plant root with expectorant and mild anti-inflammatory properties. Used as a flavouring/expectorant in cough mixtures. DEGLYCYRRHIZINIZED LIQUORICE is used in treatment of peptic ulceration. Large doses may cause salt and water retention leading to hypertension and/or cardiac failure.

Lisinopril. Antihypertensive, with actions, uses and adverse effects similar to CAPTOPRIL.

Lisuride. Dopamine agonist with actions and adverse effects similar to BROMOCRIPTINE. Used in Parkinson's disease where it may add to the effects of LEVODOPA, especially in later stages of the disease when treatment is failing.

Lithium salts. Usually given as carbonate or citrate, provides lithium ions which substitute for sodium in excitable tissues and reduce brain catecholamine levels. Used in prophylactic treatment of mania and depression. Caution in cardiac or renal disease. Needs careful control of plasma levels. Adverse effects include tremor, vomiting, diarrhoea, ataxia, blurred vision, thirst, polyuria leading to confusion and fits, and coma in gross overdosage. Lithium excretion may be enhanced by forced alkaline diuresis, peritoneal dialysis or haemodialysis. Intoxication may be precipitated by diuretic therapy or salt restriction. Lithium succinate has anti-inflammatory and antifungal activity and is used as topical treatment for seborrhoeic dermatitis. It may cause skin irritation but does not have systemic effects.

Liver extracts. Extracts of liver prepared for oral use were used for treatment of pernicious anaemia. Unpalatable and irregularly absorbed. Now replaced by the pure vitamin B$_{12}$ (HYDROXOCOBALAMIN).

Lodoxamide. Anti-allergic, used in treatment of allergic conjunctivitis by topical ocular application. It has actions similar to SODIUM CROMOGLICATE.

Lofepramine. Antidepressant, metabolized to DESIPRAMINE, after absorption. Actions, uses and adverse effects similar to AMITRIPTYLINE.

Lofexidine. Central-acting alpha receptor agonist with actions similar to CLONIDINE. Used in the supportive treatment of withdrawal from opiate addiction where it suppresses the noradrenergic symptoms of withdrawal (e.g. sweating, diarrhoea, muscle cramps). Unlike CLONIDINE is less likely to cause sedation at the doses needed. May cause dry mouth and drowsiness, and could exacerbate existing cardiovascular disease.

Lomefloxacin (r)**.** Broad-spectrum antibiotic with actions similar to CIPROFLOXACIN. Used as eye drops for conjunctivitis. May cause transient burning sensation when first applied. May allow overgrowth of nonsensitive bacteria.

Lomustine (CCNU). Cytotoxic drug used in neoplastic disease. Adverse effects include loss of appetite, nausea, vomiting, liver toxicity and bone marrow depression.

Loperamide. Antidiarrhoeal, with actions, uses and adverse effects similar to DIPHENOXYLATE.

Lopinavir. Antiviral protease inhibitor. Inhibits HIV maturation and proliferation. Used in combination with other antivirals to slow or halt HIV infection. May cause gastro-intestinal disturbances, liver dysfunction, bone marrow suppression, fatigue and muscle disorders, metabolic disorders and skin rashes.

Loprazolam (m). Benzodiazepine, used for short-term treatment of insomnia. Actions and adverse effects similar to DIAZEPAM.

Loratadine. Nonsedating, second generation antihistamine used in the treatment of seasonal affective rhinitis (hay fever). Has proved largely free of sedating effects that affect work and driving performance. Like other drugs of this class has been associated with rare cases of serious cardiac arrhythmias.

Lorazepam (m). Benzodiazepine anxiolytic similar to DIAZEPAM.

Lornoxicam. Non-steroidal anti-inflammatory analgesic with actions and adverse effects similar to PIROXICAM. Used by injection for treatment of postoperative pain and orally for treatment of pain associated with arthritis.

Losartan. Angiotensin II antagonist with effects similar to angiotensin-converting enzyme (ACE) inhibitors, e.g. CAPTOPRIL, but more selective. Used as an antihypertensive where it does not cause dry cough or the allergic reactions associated with ACE inhibitors. May cause dizziness and rashes. Compared to ACE inhibitors this class of drugs appear safer to use in patients with impaired renal function.

Loxapine. Antipsychotic with similar effects to phenothiazines such as CHLORPROMAZINE but chemically different, and less likely to produce extrapyramidal side effects. Adverse effects include dizziness, faintness, muscle twitching, weakness and confusion, peristent tardive dyskinesia, tachycardia, hypo- or hypertension, ECG changes, skin reactions, anticholinergic effects, nausea, vomiting, dyspnoea and headache.

LSD (Lysergic acid diethylamide) (c). Hallucinogen. Not used therapeutically but abused for its psychedelic effects – notably altered visual perception. Consciousness and awareness not altered, but may cause thought disorders, personality changes and apparent psychotic disease. Other 'unwanted' effects include gastro-intestinal disturbance, sweating and incoordination. Delayed 'flashback' adverse effects may occur even months after use and especially in the presence of stress or other CNS-active drugs. Causes tolerance but not physical dependence.

Lumefantrine (r). Antimalarial used in combination with ARTEMETHER to treat acute, uncomplicated infections.

Lumiracoxib (r). Non-steroidal anti-inflammatory analgesic with selective inhibition of the cyclo-oxygenase enzyme-2 (COX-2), similar to CELECOXIB. Used for osteoarthritis and the short-term relief (3–5 days) of acute pain due to orthopaedic surgery, dental surgery or dysmenorrhoea. Better penetration into inflamed tissues and short half-life may make this drug safer than earlier COX-2 inhibitors, but gastro-intestinal effects still occur. Adverse reactions include flu-like symptoms, respiratory and urinary tract infections, fluid retention, dizziness and headache. Should be used with caution if there is pre-existing liver or kidney disease, and must be monitored for possible cardiovascular events.

Lymecycline. Bacteriostatic antibiotic, with actions, adverse effects and interactions similar to TETRACYCLINE.

Lynestrenol. Sex hormone (progestogen) with actions, uses and adverse effects similar to NORETHISTERONE.

Lypressin. Hormone extract from posterior pituitary gland of pigs. Actions, uses and adverse effects similar to VASOPRESSIN.

Lysergic acid diethylamide. *See* LSD.

Lysergide. *See* LSD.

Lysine. Essential AMINO ACID also used as a buffer to reduce acidity/gastric irritation from ACETYL SALICYLIC ACID.

Lysuride. *See* LISURIDE.

M

Magaldrate. Antacid. Complex hydrated form of MAGNESIUM SULPHATE and aluminium sulphate.

Magnesium alginate. Magnesium salt of ALGINIC ACID, used as emulsifying/thickening agent in antacid preparations for treatment of acid reflux.

Magnesium antacids. Range of magnesium salts used alone or complexed with other compounds. Neutralize gastric acid in treatment of peptic ulceration. Large doses have laxative effect which may be reduced by combination with ALUMINIUM ANTACIDS. Very little absorbed but danger of toxic magnesium blood levels in renal failure. May reduce absorption of other drugs (e.g. TETRACYCLINES).

Magnesium carbonate. Nonsystemic antacid with similar actions, uses and adverse effects to MAGNESIUM HYDROXIDE. Releases carbon dioxide in stomach and may cause belching.

Magnesium citrate. Osmotic purgative. Solution used to aid removal or prevent formation of crystals in long-term urinary catheterization.

Magnesium hydroxide. Nonsystemic antacid (only 10 per cent absorbed). Used in treatment of peptic ulceration. Neutralizes gastric acid and acts longer than SODIUM BICARBONATE. May have laxative effect, which can be prevented by simultaneous use of ALUMINIUM ANTACIDS.

Magnesium oxide. Nonsystemic antacid. Converted to MAGNESIUM HYDROXIDE in the stomach and has similar actions and adverse effects.

Magnesium sulphate (Epsom salts). Osmotic purgative. Absorbed only slowly from gut. Magnesium and sulphate ions attract or retain water by osmosis and thus increase bulk of intestinal contents. Effective in 3–6 hours. Produces semi-fluid or watery stools, therefore useful as single treatment but not for repeated dosage. Danger of systemic toxicity from magnesium in patients with reduced renal function.

Magnesium trisilicate. Nonsystemic antacid used in treatment of peptic ulceration. Neutralization of acid is slow in onset but relatively prolonged due to adsorbent properties of silicic acid formed in the stomach. Has a laxative effect in larger doses. Danger of magnesium toxicity in patients with renal failure.

Malathion. Organophosphorus insecticide. Acts by inhibition of cholinesterase and may therefore produce toxic effects due to accumulation of excess ACETYLCHOLINE. One of the least toxic of this group of insecticides, low concentrations of malathion may be used on human skin for infestation (e.g. lice) without systemic effects. Toxic effects may be treated by antidotes ATROPINE SULPHATE and PRALIDOXIME.

Malic acid. Found in apples and pears. Formerly used in tooth-cleaning tablets. Used as part of an astringent skin treatment.

Manganese. Trace element sometimes added to nutritional preparations for supposed increase in the haematinic effects of iron.

Manganese sulphate. Occasionally used as a haematinic. Said to increase the effect of FERROUS SULPHATE in treatment of iron-deficiency anaemia.

Mannitol. Osmotic diuretic. Opposes reabsorption of water which normally accompanies sodium reabsorption from kidney

Maprotiline

tubule. Used when there is danger of renal failure (e.g. shock, cardiovascular surgery) and in fluid overload refractory to other diuretics. May cause cardiac failure owing to increased circulating blood volume.

Maprotiline. Antidepressant, with actions, uses and adverse effects similar to IMIPRAMINE.

Mazindol (c). Anorectic indole derivative with central stimulant properties. Produces tachycardia and rise in blood pressure.

MDA (Methoxydesmethylamfetamine) (c). AMFETAMINE derivative similar to MDMA.

MDEA (Methoxydesethylamfetamine) (c). AMFETAMINE derivative similar to MDMA.

MDMA (Methylenedioxymethamfetamine) (c). AMFETAMINE derivative abused for its euphoriant and hallucinogenic effects. Although thought by users to be safe, when used at dance parties (raves), the combination of excessive exercise and dehydration has been associated with hyperpyrexia, heat stroke and death.

Measles vaccine. Live attenuated measles virus for measles immunization. Adverse effects include mild fever, rash and rare neurological disorders. Use with care if there is a history of convulsions or epilepsy.

Mebendazole. Used in treatment of roundworm. Actions and adverse effects as for TIABENDAZOLE.

Mebeverine. Antispasmodic, with direct action on colonic smooth muscle but no systemic anticholinergic effects. Used for relief of abdominal pain and cramps (e.g. due to irritable colon or nonspecific diarrhoea).

Mecysteine. Mucolytic, with actions, uses and adverse effects similar to ACETYLCYSTEINE. Used orally as well as by aerosol inhalation.

Medazepam (m). Benzodiazepine anxiolytic similar to DIAZEPAM but with less anticonvulsant activity. Used in the treatment of anxiety.

Medium-chain triglycerides. A mixture of triglycerides from straight-chain fatty acids for use in fat malabsorption syndromes.

Medroxyprogesterone. Sex hormone used as treatment for endometriosis, menstrual disorders and for contraception. Used in high doses to treat hormone-dependent malignancies (e.g. of breast, endometrium and prostate). Has been used to prevent threatened abortion but this is no longer recommended. Actions and adverse effects similar to PROGESTERONE. May reduce bone density so not recommended for long-term use in women at risk of osteoporosis.

Mefenamic acid. Anti-inflammatory/analgesic. Mode of action uncertain. Used in treatment of arthritis. May cause severe diarrhoea. Other adverse effects include gastro-intestinal bleeding, exacerbation of asthma, haemolytic anaemia and bone marrow depression. May enhance action of oral anticoagulants (e.g. WARFARIN).

Mefloquine. Antimalarial effective in treatment and prevention of infections resistant to CHLOROQUINE and other antimalarials. Like CHLOROQUINE it is a derivative of QUININE but has longer actions requiring only weekly dosage for prophylaxis. May cause dizziness, gastro-intestinal disturbances, rashes and severe neuropsychiatric reactions. May increase the risk of convulsions in epileptic patients. Also a risk of fatal arrhythmias if given together with HALOFANTRINE.

Mefruside. Diuretic essentially similar to BENDROFLUMETHIAZIDE.

Megestrol. Sex hormone, with actions and effects similar to PROGESTERONE. Used to suppress OESTROGEN-dependent tumours of the breast and uterus by interfering with uptake of OESTROGEN into the tumour. Adverse effects include weight gain, nausea, skin rashes, hair loss and deep venous thromboses in the legs.

Meloxicam. Non-steroidal anti-inflammatory analgesic used in treatment of arthritis and ankylosing spondylitis. Specifically inhibits cyclo-oxygenase 2 (COX-2) rather than COX-1 and thus should be less likely to cause adverse effects on gastric mucosa (bleeding) and kidneys. May cause gastro-intestinal disturbance, skin reactions, CNS or cardiovascular effects and blood dyscrasias.

Melphalan. Cytotoxic drug used in myelomatosis. Actions and adverse effects similar to CHLORAMBUCIL.

Memantine. A receptor-blocking drug that acts centrally to reduce elevated brain levels of glutamate. Persistent elevated glutamate levels impair cognitive function. Used to treat mild to moderate symptoms in Alzheimer's dementia. Long-term benefits are uncertain. Diagnosis and treatment must be undertaken from a specialist clinic. Adverse effects include hallucinations, confusion, dizziness, headache and tiredness. Memantine interacts with a number of other drugs.

Menadiol. Orally active form of VITAMIN K.

Menaphthone. *See* VITAMIN K.

Menotrophin. Preparation of follicle-stimulating hormone, derived from human postmenopausal urine, which also possesses some luteinizing hormone activity. Used to stimulate ovulation.

Menthol. Used as inhalation, orally as pastilles for relief of respiratory symptoms, or topically on skin where it causes dilatation of blood vessels producing a sense of coldness and analgesia.

Mepenzolate. Anticholinergic, with actions and adverse effects similar to ATROPINE. Marked effect upon spasm of colon. Used to relieve pain, distension and diarrhoea associated with gastro-intestinal disorders.

Mepivacaine. Local anaesthetic with actions, adverse effects and uses similar to LIDOCAINE but not used to treat abnormal heart rhythms.

Meprobamate (c). Minor tranquillizer (anxiolytic) with selective action on hypothalamus and spinal cord. Used in treatment of neuroses, alcoholism and functional disorders, such as tension headache. May cause gastro-intestinal disorders, headache, dizziness with hypotension, lowered tolerance to alcohol and withdrawal symptoms. Induces hepatic drug metabolism with danger of drug interactions. Coma with respiratory depression in overdosage. No antidote. Forced alkaline diuresis and haemodialysis may be effective.

Meptazinol. Analgesic with narcotic antagonist activity. Actions, uses and adverse effects similar to PENTAZOCINE, but central adverse effects and dependence appear to be less.

Mequitazine. Antihistamine with actions and adverse effects similar to PROMETHAZINE. Used in treatment of allergic conditions.

Mercaptamine. Formerly used intravenously as an antidote for PARACETAMOL, where it acts as a facilitator of glutathione synthesis and thus replenishes the stores necessary to detoxify PARACETAMOL metabolites. Currently used orally in the treatment of the rare inherited metabolic disorder cystinosis where it binds with the amino acid cystine and reduces its accumulation. May cause troublesome nausea and vomiting.

Mercaptopurine. Cytotoxic drug, inhibiting nucleoprotein synthesis, used in neoplastic disease, particularly leukaemia. Adverse effects include bone marrow depression.

Meropenem. Intravenous broad-spectrum antibiotic with actions, uses and adverse effects similar to IMIPENEM. Unlike IMIPENEM it does not need the addition of CILASTATIN to prolong its action.

Mersalyl

Mersalyl. Organic mercurial diuretic, now seldom used. Depresses active reabsorption of sodium and chloride by kidney tubules. Long-acting; must be administered by intramuscular injection. Danger of excessive loss of sodium and chloride. May cause gastro-intestinal disturbance, skin rashes and, after prolonged use, kidney damage.

Mesalazine (5-Aminosalicylic acid). Active constituent of SULFASALAZINE. Used in ulcerative colitis. Free of sulphonamide adverse effects. Both by mouth and as an enema.

Mescaline (c). A hallucinogenic alkaloid obtained from the Mexican cactus *Lophophora williamsii* (Aztec name, peyote), usually taken by mouth. Actions and adverse effects said to be similar to LSD but milder. Mescaline is abused in USA but less commonly in Europe. Peyote has a long tradition of use by Indians of northern Mexico and southwestern United States as a hallucinogen and medicine. Tolerance may occur but not physical dependence. Overdose does not cause serious physiological effects. No accepted medical usage.

Mesna. Used to protect the bladder mucosa from the irritant effect upon it of CYCLOPHOSPHAMIDE and IFOSFAMIDE. Acts by combining with their toxic metabolite acrolein. Does not prevent their other toxic effects.

Mesterolone (m). Sex hormone, with actions, uses and adverse effects similar to TESTOSTERONE.

Mestranol. Sex hormone, with actions, uses and adverse effects similar to ESTRADIOL.

Metaraminol. Sympathomimetic agent with alpha- and beta-effects similar to ADRENALINE. Alpha-effects predominate and thus it has been used to raise blood pressure in hypotension after myocardial infarction. May cause headache, dizziness, nausea, vomiting and tremor.

Metformin. Oral antidiabetic. Increases use of glucose by peripheral tissues. Used alone or in combination with sulphonylureas (e.g. GLIBENCLAMIDE) or INSULIN. Most useful in overweight subjects, where it suppresses appetite. May cause nausea, vomiting and diarrhoea.

Methacholine. Parasympathomimetic drug, with muscarinic actions of ACETYLCHOLINE.

Methacycline. Antibacterial, with actions, uses and adverse effects similar to TETRACYCLINE.

Methadone (c) (r). Synthetic narcotic analgesic. Actions similar to MORPHINE, but less sedation, euphoria and respiratory depression. Used in control of withdrawal symptoms from narcotic addiction and for relief of chronic pain in terminal disease. NALOXONE is a pure antagonist.

Methallenestril. Sex hormone, with actions, uses and adverse effects similar to ESTRADIOL.

Methamfetamine. CNS stimulant amfetamine similar to DEXAMFETAMINE.

Methaqualone (c). Hypnotic/sedative. General depressant action on CNS. Used in treatment of insomnia. Frequently has 'hangover' effect. May also cause localized loss of sensation with numbness and tingling, as well as skin rashes and gastro-intestinal disturbance. Liable to abuse for so-called 'aphrodisiac' qualities and euphoriant effects. In overdose causes respiratory depression with increased muscle tone and increased reflexes. No antidote. Treatment is supportive.

Methenamine. Antiseptic used topically and for urinary infections. For the latter use, the urine must be rendered acid by also giving AMMONIUM CHLORIDE which liberates formaldehyde from the methenamine. May cause painful micturition, frequency and haematuria.

Methionine. Amino acid, essential constituent of diet. May be used as an antidote in severe poisoning due to PARACETAMOL, where it is thought to prevent liver damage by reducing the concentration of a toxic metabolite. Given orally it causes few side effects, principally nausea. Must not be given more than 10 hours after the overdose as it may then exacerbate liver damage.

Methocarbamol. Muscle relaxant used in treatment of painful muscle spasms. Mode of action uncertain. May cause nausea, dizziness, drowsiness, headache, blurred vision and allergic reactions. Contraindicated in patients with epilepsy or myasthenia gravis.

Methohexital. Ultra-short-acting barbiturate hypnotic. Used for induction of anaesthesia. Actions and adverse effects similar to THIOPENTONE SODIUM.

Methohexitone. See METHOHEXITAL.

Methoserpidine. Antihypertensive. Actions, uses and adverse effects similar to RESERPINE.

Methotrexate. Cytotoxic drug, antagonizing folic acid, used in neoplastic disease, particularly leukaemia. Adverse effects include alopecia, stomatitis, liver toxicity, folate-deficient anaemia and bone marrow depression.

Methotrimeprazine. See LEVOMEPROMAZINE.

Methoxamine. Sympathomimetic. Stimulates alpha-adrenoceptors to cause constriction of blood vessels and rise in blood pressure. Used to reverse hypotension during anaesthesia. May cause pronounced slowing of heart rate and excessive rise in blood pressure.

Methoxydesethylamfetamine. See MDEA.

Methoxydesmethylamfetamine. See MDA.

5-Methoxypsoralen. Sun screen. Used topically to filter out harmful sun rays. May cause photosensitivity and has been suspected of increasing the incidence of skin cancer.

Methylcellulose. Indigestible plant residue used as a lubricating agent in pharmaceutical preparations and as a purgative. Adsorbs water, increases faecal bulk and thus promotes bowel movements. Slow action (0.5–3 days). No important systemic effects.

Methylcysteine. See MECYSTEINE.

Methyldopa. Antihypertensive. Reduces sympathetic tone by central and peripheral mechanisms. Adverse effects include sedation, depression, nasal stuffiness, fluid retention, impotence and haemolytic anaemia.

Methylenedioxymethamfetamine. See MDMA.

Methylephedrine. Sympathomimetic agent, with actions, uses and adverse effects similar to EPHEDRINE.

Methyl nicotinate. Vasodilator/rubefacient used in ointments and creams for topical application at sites of muscle pains in rheumatic conditions (e.g fibrositis, muscular rheumatism).

Methylphenidate (c). Stimulant used to treat narcolepsy and attention deficit disorder. Thought to stimulate brain arousal mechanisms. Sympathomimetic similar in action to DEXAMFETAMINE and AMFETAMINE but considered more effective and easier to control. May cause restlessness, hallucinations, slurred speech, rash and rhabdomyolysis. Physical dependence and withdrawal effects may occur.

Methylphenobarbital (c). Anticonvulsant/ sedative essentially similar to PHENOBARBITAL.

Methylphenobarbitone. See METHYLPHENOBARBITAL.

Methylprednisolone. CORTICOSTEROID with actions, uses and adverse effects similar to PREDNISONE.

Methyl salicylate. Rubefacient used for relief of musculoskeletal pain. Has similar actions and adverse effects to ACETYLSALICYLIC ACID but not used systemically.

Methyltestosterone (m). Sex hormone, with actions, uses and adverse effects similar to TESTOSTERONE.

Methysergide. SEROTONIN antagonist used in preventive treatment for severe migraine. May cause nausea, abdominal cramp, dizziness and psychiatric disturbance. Prolonged use may cause retroperitoneal fibrosis resulting in impairment of renal function.

Meticillin. Antibiotic. Similar properties to CLOXACILLIN, but only active parenterally.

Metildigoxin. Actions, uses and adverse effects similar to DIGOXIN.

Metipranolol. Beta-adrenoceptor blocking drug with actions and adverse effects similar to PROPRANOLOL, but used only as eye drops for glaucoma. *See also* TIMOLOL.

Metirosine. Antihypertensive. Enzyme inhibitor which blocks the synthesis of catecholamines by the adrenal gland. Used to control hypertension caused by the adrenal tumour phaeochromocytoma where the raised blood pressure is caused by excess production of catecholamines. Adverse effects include sedation, diarrhoea and hypersensitivity.

Metoclopramide. Antiemetic with dopamine antagonist actions in brain and peripheral effects on gastro-intestinal tract where it stimulates motility to improve gastric emptying and intestinal transit. May cause drowsiness and involuntary movements. Used to treat nausea and vomiting from most causes and as an adjunct to X-ray examination of the gut.

Metolazone. Diuretic essentially similar to BENDROFLUMETHIAZIDE.

Metoprolol. Beta-adrenoceptor blocking drug, with limited cardioselectivity. Uses, side effects, etc. as for PROPRANOLOL.

Metrifonate. Organophosphorus cholinesterase inhibitor, used as an anti-infective in treatment of schistosomiasis. Active only against S. *haematobium.* May cause unwanted cholinergic symptoms as from ACETYLCHOLINE.

Metronidazole. Antimicrobial. Effective against trichomonas, Vincent's organisms, anaerobic bacteria, giardiasis and amoebiasis. Adverse effects include nausea, metallic taste in mouth, hypersensitivity reactions and DISULFIRAM-like reaction with alcohol.

Metyrapone. Inhibits enzyme responsible for synthesis of adrenocorticosteroids. Used in tests of pituitary gland function. May cause gastro-intestinal disturbance and dizziness.

Mexenone. Absorbs ultraviolet light and protects skin from sunburn.

Mexiletine. Cardiac antiarrhythmic agent similar to LIDOCAINE, but also effective when given by mouth. May cause nausea, vomiting, drowsiness, tremors, convulsions, hypotension and bradycardia.

Mianserin. Antidepressant, with uses similar to IMIPRAMINE, but without its peripheral autonomic adverse effects. Produces sedation and a fall in white blood cell count in some patients.

Mibefradil. Calcium antagonist acting upon the T-type (transient) calcium channels rather than the L (long-lasting) calcium channels. Causes reduced cardiac contraction and conductivity plus vasodilatation. Used in treatment of high blood pressure and prevention of angina. May cause excessive slowing of the heart with consequent arrhythmias and cardiac failure.

Miconazole. Antifungal agent used topically for skin infections.

Midazolam (m). Intravenous benzodiazepine anxiolytic/sedative, with short duration of action. Used for induction of anaesthesia before minor surgery. Actions and adverse effects similar to DIAZEPAM.

Mifepristone. Progesterone antagonist used orally for termination of pregnancy up to 9 weeks gestation. May cause skin rashes, general malaise and gastro-intestinal disturbance. Used only in centres licensed under the Abortion Act. If abortion is not complete after 36–48 hours, treatment with GEMEPROST should be given. Surgical abortion may be used if drug treatment fails.

Milrinone. Phosphodiesterase enzyme inhibitor which reduces breakdown of cyclic AMP and thus prolongs its effects in contraction of cardiac and relaxation of vascular smooth muscle. Used to improve cardiac output in severe congestive cardiac failure. May cause hypotension, angina, cardiac arrhythmias and headache.

Mineral oil. See LIQUID PARAFFIN.

Minocycline. Antibacterial, with actions, uses and adverse effects similar to TETRACYCLINE. May cause dizziness and vertigo.

Minoxidil. Vasodilator/antihypertensive. Reduces muscle tone in peripheral blood vessels. Fluid retention and tachycardia accompany this effect but can be controlled by using concomitant therapy with a diuretic (e.g. BENDROFLUMETHIAZIDE) and a beta-adrenoceptor blocker (e.g. PROPRANOLOL). Other adverse effects include increased hair growth and breast tenderness. Used mainly in severe hypertension when other drugs fail. It is also used topically to treat male pattern baldness, but the effects appear limited and reverse when treatment is stopped.

Mirtazapine. Antidepressant which increases both noradrenergic and serotonergic nerve transmission in the brain. Does not show the unwanted anticholinergic activity of the tricyclic antidepressants,

e.g. AMITRIPTYLINE. May cause drowsiness, weight gain and peripheral oedema. Toxic effects in the liver and bone marrow have been described. In some patients may increase the risk of suicidal thoughts and self-harm.

Misoprostol. Synthetic analogue of endogenously produced prostaglandin PGE_1 that promotes the healing of duodenal and gastric ulcers and ulcers induced by nonsteroid anti-inflammatory drugs. It also protects the gastric mucosa against initial damage. It inhibits production of gastric acid, stimulating bicarbonate and mucus secretion and maintaining mucosal blood flow. May cause diarrhoea, abnormal vaginal bleeding and abortion.

Mithramycin. Cytotoxic antibiotic. No longer used to treat cancer itself, but may be used as emergency therapy to reduce hypercalcaemia due to malignant disease. More effective than chelating agents such as TRISODIUM EDETATE, but causes suppression of bone marrow and cannot be used for more than a few days.

Mitomycin. Cytotoxic antibiotic. Used to treat upper gastro-intestinal and breast cancers. Causes delayed effects on the bone marrow, lung fibrosis and renal damage. Used at 6-week intervals to reduce these effects.

Mitotane. Antineoplastic which selectively inhibits adrenal cortex functions. Used to treat advanced adrenocortical carcinoma. May cause gastro-intestinal disturbance and neurotoxicity.

Mitoxantrone. Cytotoxic drug, with actions against resting-phase tumour, as well as those undergoing DNA synthesis. May thus be effective in both slow and rapid growing tumours. Used in advanced breast cancer. May cause bone marrow suppression, hair loss, gastro-intestinal disturbances, heart failure and impaired liver function.

Mitozantrone. See MITOXANTRONE.

Mivacurium. Skeletal muscle relaxant with actions similar to TUBOCURARINE, but a shorter duration of action.

Mizolastine. Nonsedating antihistamine with actions and uses similar to TERFENADINE. Although minor ECG changes are seen, there have been no reports of cardiac arrhythmias.

Moclobemide. Antidepressant. Acts by selective inhibition of monoamine oxidase enzyme type A (MAO-A) in the brain. Increases brain monoamines by reducing their enzymic breakdown. Acts more rapidly than earlier MAOIs such as PHENELZINE and causes fewer adverse effects. May cause sleep disturbance, agitation, nausea and headache. May interact with tricyclic and tetracyclic antidepressants and with TRAZODONE.

Modafinil (r). Non-AMFETAMINE CNS stimulant used in the treatment of the chronic sleep disorder narcolepsy, excessive sleepiness associated with other chronic pathological conditions, and moderate to severe chronic shiftwork sleep disorder. Acts by blocking the release of the inhibitory neurotransmitter GABA. Does not affect DOPAMINE release and thus hyperkinesia is not a problem. The incidence of euphoria is low and consequently abuse is unlikely. May cause headache and unwanted CNS excitation, e.g. aggression or insomnia.

Moexipril. Prodrug for moexiprilat, a potent ACE inhibitor, with actions similar to CAPTOPRIL. May cause paroxysmal bronchospasm and oral candidiasis but systemic absorption from inhaled corticosteroids is low and systemic adverse effects are infrequent, except when the highest doses are used for a prolonged time.

Molgramostim. Human growth factor made by recombinant DNA technology with actions and uses similar to FILGRASTIM.

Mometasone (r). Potent corticosteroid with actions similar to BECLOMETASONE. Used by inhalation to control persistent asthma. May cause paroxysmal bronchospasm and oral candidiasis but systemic absorption from inhaled corticosteroids is low and systemic adverse effecs are infrequent, except when the highest doses are used for a prolonged time.

Montelukast. Oral leukotriene receptor antagonist. Blocks part of the inflammatory process associated with an asthma attack and thus helps to reduce swelling/constriction of the airways. Used as an add-on therapy in the long-term management of asthma when treatment with inhaled corticosteroids and beta-adrenoceptor stimulants is inadequate. May cause headache and abdominal pain.

Moracizine. Antiarrhythmic with similarities to DISOPYRAMIDE, used to suppress abnormal ventricular rhythms. Has a relatively long duration of action due to active metabolites. May cause dizziness, arrhythmias, gastro-intestinal disturbance, muscle pain and blurred vision.

Morphine (c). Poppy derivative. Centrally acting narcotic analgesic used for relief of severe pain. Other potentially useful effects include euphoria and cough suppression. Adverse effects include respiratory depression, nausea, vomiting, constipation, hypotension, physical dependence and abuse ('addiction'). Coma with danger of death in overdosage. NALOXONE is a specific antagonist.

Moxifloxacin (r). Broad-spectrum antibiotic with actions and adverse effects similar to CIPROFLOXACIN. Used in treatment of community-acquired respiratory infections.

Moxisylyte. Alpha$_{1a}$ adrenoceptor antagonist capable of blocking sympathetic nervous activity in the vascular smooth muscle cells of the penis, used by intrapenile (intracavernous) injection prior to intercourse, as a treatment for failure of erection. Slow onset of action mimics normal intercourse. May cause bruising and pain at site of injection. Occasionally causes systemic effects including headache, dizziness, flushes and dry mouth. Rarely, may cause prolonged erection and priapism. Also used in peripheral vascular disease.

Moxonidine. Antihypertensive acts on imidazoline sub-type 1 receptors to the brain medulla. Used alone or in combination therapy to reduce mild to moderate blood pressure. May cause dry mouth, headache, nausea and insomnia.

Mupirocin. Antibiotic, previously known as pseudomonic acid. Used as an ointment to treat bacterial skin infections. Inactive orally.

Mycophenolate. Immunosupressant, prodrug, metabolized to mycophenolic acid which inhibits lymphocyte production. Used to prevent rejection of liver, kidney or heart transplants. May cause gastro-intestinal upsets, bone marrow suppression, CNS disturbance and increased susceptibility to infection.

N

Nabilone. Derivative of CANNABIS, with antiemetic and anxiolytic properties. Acts on opiate receptors in the brain to block transmission of vomiting impulses. Used to suppress nausea and vomiting from cytotoxic drugs. Adverse effects include drowsiness, postural hypotension, headaches, tremors, psychosis and abdominal cramps.

Nabumetone. Non-steroid anti-inflammatory/analgesic, used in osteoarthritis and rheumatoid arthritis. The drug itself is a relatively weak inhibitor of prostaglandin synthesis, but it is metabolized in the liver to a more active compound. May thus cause less gastro-intestinal irritation than some other drugs in this class such as INDOMETACIN, but is still contraindicated if there is a history of peptic ulceration. May cause diarrhoea, other gastro-intestinal symptoms, headache, dizziness, rashes and sedation.

Nadolol. Beta-adrenoceptor blocking drug. Uses and adverse effects as for PROPRANOLOL.

Nafarelin. Synthetic analogue of gonadotrophin-releasing hormone. Used by nasal spray in the treatment of endometriosis. May cause hot flushes, changes in libido, headaches and muscle pains.

Naftidrofuryl. Peripheral vasodilator said to improve cellular metabolism and to relax muscle cells in blood vessel walls. Recommended for treatment of reduced peripheral blood circulation and dementia caused by reduced blood flow. May cause headache, insomnia and gastro-intestinal disturbance.

Nalbuphine. Narcotic analgesic, with agonist and antagonist properties. Uses and adverse effects similar to PENTAZOCINE.

Nalidixic acid. Urinary antiseptic to which resistance readily occurs. May cause gastro-intestinal symptoms and allergic reactions. May exacerbate epilepsy and respiratory depression.

Nalorphine. Narcotic antagonist. Reverses effects of MORPHINE and other narcotic analgesics but less specific than NALOXONE and has some narcotic activity of its own. Used for reversal of narcotic effects but not when due to PENTAZOCINE. May cause hallucinations and thought disturbances. In 'addicts', causes severe withdrawal symptoms.

Naloxone. Narcotic antagonist. A true antidote to MORPHINE and other narcotic analgesics. Has no narcotic activity in its own right. Used for reversal of narcotic effects from any narcotic drug especially respiratory depression. Danger of severe withdrawal symptoms if given to those physically dependent ('addicted') on narcotics.

Naltrexone. Narcotic antagonist which acts as an antidote to MORPHINE and other narcotic analgesics, with virtually no narcotic activity of its own. Unlike NALOXONE can be given orally and has a long duration of action. Used to promote opioid abstinence in patients who were formerly drug-dependent. May cause drowsiness, anxiety, loss of appetite, nausea, vomiting, diarrhoea or constipation, muscle and joint pains.

Nandrolone (m). Sex hormone, with actions and adverse effects similar to TESTOSTERONE, but anabolic effects greater than androgenic effects. Used in treatment of debilitating illness and carcinoma of the breast. Injection only; not active by mouth.

Naphazoline. Sympathomimetic agent with marked alpha-adrenergic activity. Used topically on nasal mucosa where its vasoconstrictor effect leads to reduced secretion and mucosal swelling (e.g. in allergic rhinitis). Prolonged use may lead to rebound nasal congestion and secretion. Not used systemically but oral overdosage would cause depression of nervous system and coma.

Naproxen. Anti-inflammatory/analgesic, with actions, uses and adverse effects similar to IBUPROFEN.

Naratriptan. Oral 5-HYDROXYTRYPTAMINE agonist with actions and adverse effects similar to SUMATRIPTAN. Used in treatment of acute migraine attacks.

Nateglinide. Short-acting oral antidiabetic with actions similar to the sulphonylureas e.g. GLIBENCLAMIDE. Used as add-on therapy when METFORMIN alone does not give adequate control. Taken before each main meal. May cause hypoglycaemia and skin rashes.

Nebivolol. Cardioselective beta-adrenergic blocker that is metabolized in the liver to an active metabolite. Used once daily as a treatment for high blood pressure. Claimed also to have some vasodilator activity due to actions on the L-arginine/nitric oxide pathway. Precautions and possible adverse effects are similar to those for other beta-blockers such as ATENOLOL. In particular it is noted to cause headaches, dizziness, tiredness, dyspnoea and peripheral oedema.

Nedocromil (r). Preventive treatment for asthma and bronchitis with reversible obstruction of the airways. Acts like SODIUM CROMOGLICATE by blocking allergic mechanisms. Administered by aerosol. May cause headache and nausea. Also used topically as eye drops for allergic conjunctivitis.

Nefazodone. Antidepressant with actions, uses and adverse effects similar to FLUOXE-TINE. May be particularly beneficial in cases with anxiety or insomnia. Rare, but potentially life-threatening liver damage can occur.

Nefopam. Centrally acting analgesic; mode of action unknown, but not related to the narcotics. Used for acute and chronic pain. Adverse effects include gastro-intestinal upsets, palpitations, CNS stimulation, with nervousness, insomnia, headache, blurred vision and sweating. Drowsiness is sometimes seen, but respiratory depression and habituation do not occur. Contraindicated in patients with epilepsy, glaucoma or urinary retention.

Nelfinavir. Antiviral protease inhibitor. Inhibits HIV maturation and proliferation. Used in combination with other antivirals to slow or halt HIV infection. May cause gastro-intestinal disturbances, liver dysfunction, bone marrow suppression, fatigue and muscle disorders, metabolic disorders and skin rashes.

Neomycin. Bactericidal aminoglycoside antibiotic with spectrum similar to STREPTO-MYCIN, but more active against *Staphylococcus* and *Proteus*. Not used systemically because of risk of ototoxicity and nephrotoxicity. Used topically and orally for bowel sterilization and in liver failure. May cause malabsorption if given for long period. Potentiates neuromuscular blockade.

Neostigmine (Prostigmine). Anticholinesterase with actions similar to PHYSO-STIGMINE.

Netilmicin. Aminoglycoside antibiotic, with actions, uses and adverse effects similar to GENTAMICIN.

Nevirapine. Antiviral. Non-nucleoside reverse transcriptase inhibitor used in combination with other antiviral drugs in HIV-1-positive patients with evidence of immunodeficiency. The antiviral activity is very specific and HIV-2 is not sensitive to this drug. May cause skin rashes, impaired concentration, dizziness and psychosis, gastro-intestinal upset and headache. May cause interactions with other drugs that are metabolized in the liver.

Niacin. Vitamin B$_7$. *See* NICOTINIC ACID.

Niacinamide. The active form of vitamin B$_7$. *See* NICOTINAMIDE.

Nialamide. Antidepressant/monoamine oxidase inhibitor with actions, uses and adverse effects similar to PHENELZINE.

Nicardipine. Antianginal, antihypertensive with actions, uses and adverse effects similar to NIFEDIPINE.

Niclosamide. Used in treatment of tapeworms. Adverse effects are uncommon as it is not absorbed from the intestinal tract.

Nicofuranose. *See* TETRANICOTINOYLFRUCTOSE.

Nicorandil. Potassium channel blocker. Acts on muscle cells in coronary arteries and veins to cause dilation and improved blood flow. Used to prevent and treat angina. May cause headaches, flushing and fall in blood pressure.

Nicotinamide. The active form of NICOTINIC ACID (Vitamin B$_7$). Used in multivitamin preparations that are most commonly prescribed in the UK for the treatment of nutritional deficiencies due to alcoholic liver disease or other severe gastro-intestinal dysfunction. Also used topically to reduce the inflammations associated with acne. Causes less troublesome flushing and hypotension than NICOTINIC ACID. Topical use may cause dryness of the skin with burning and irritation.

Nicotine. Plant derivative from the tobacco plant *(Nicotiana* spp). Nicotine is the addictive component in tobacco smoke. Addiction is physiological and psychological and many smokers find it difficult to stop, even when they have illnesses which are made worse by smoking. Nicotine may be administered during the withdrawal period in the form of transdermal patches or chewing gum.

Nicotinic acid (Vitamin B$_7$). Deficiency causes pellagra, with dermatitis, diarrhoea and dementia. Pellagra is only seen in countries where severe nutritional deficiencies have not been eliminated. Nicotinic acid is used in multiple vitamin therapy for alcoholic liver disease and severe gastro-intestinal dysfunction. As a vitamin, nicotinic acid is essential for the production of NAD co-enzyme, which is, in turn, essential for cellular energy-producing processes. In larger doses nicotinic acid has (i) direct relaxant effects on muscle in small blood vessels, (ii) anti-inflammatory properties, and (iii) a number of demonstrable effects in lowering blood cholesterol and other lipids. It has been used to treat reduced peripheral circulation, the inflammatory process in acne and blood lipid disorders. The most common adverse effects from larger doses are vasodilatation with hypotension, flushing and impairment of liver function. NICOTINAMIDE causes less flushing and is the form used in vitamin supplements and as a topical treatment. Nicotinic acid is the form which lowers blood lipids.

Nicotinyl tartrate. Peripheral vasodilator acting directly on muscle in blood vessels. Used for treatment of impaired peripheral blood circulation including chilblains and Raynaud's syndrome. May cause flushing, tachycardia, shivering, gastro-intestinal symptoms and fall in blood pressure.

Nicoumalone. *See* ACENOCOUMAROL.

Nifedipine. Antianginal/antihypertensive vasodilator. Acts by blocking influx of calcium ions into vascular smooth muscle thus reducing peripheral vascular resistance. Adverse effects include flushing, headache and lethargy. In overdosage, causes bradycardia and hypotension, which may be treated by ATROPINE, DOPAMINE and CALCIUM GLUCONATE.

Nikethamide. Respiratory stimulant acting directly on brain respiratory centres. Seldom useful except in respiratory depression due to severe chronic bronchitis. Not used in treatment of respiratory depression due to drug overdosage. May cause sweating, nausea, vomiting, convulsions and depression of the nervous system.

Nimodipine. Vasodilator used after subarachnoid haemorrhage to reverse spasms of the arteries which would cause ischaemia of the brain tissues. Reduces the contraction of vascular smooth muscle by blocking influx of calcium ions, similar in action to NIFEDIPINE.

Nimorazole. Antiprotozoal used to treat certain gastro-intestinal and vaginal infections (e.g. giardiasis, trichomoniasis). Contraindicated in neurological disease. Causes nausea if alcohol taken during treatment.

Niridazole. Used in treatment of infections due to the guinea worm *(Dracunculus medinensis)*. May cause gastro-intestinal symptoms, headache and drowsiness. Rare effects include confusion, convulsions and allergic reactions.

Nisoldipine. Calcium antagonist with actions and adverse effects similar to AMLODIPINE. Used to treat hypertension and angina.

Nitrazepam (m). Benzodiazepine tranquillizer/hypnotic. Depressant action on CNS. Used in treatment of insomnia. May cause dizziness, unsteadiness and slurred speech. In overdosage, respiratory depression much less severe than with barbiturates. Supportive treatment usually adequate. May cause dependence, even in therapeutic doses.

Nitrofurantoin. Urinary antiseptic, producing yellow fluorescence in urine. Adverse effects include hypersensitivity reactions, nausea, vomiting, neuropathy and haemolytic anaemia in G6PD-deficient subjects.

Nitrophenol. Has antifungal activity. Used topically for fungal infections of the skin.

Nitrous oxide. Inhalational anaesthetic. Weak anaesthetic, but strong analgesic. Usually given with at least 30 per cent oxygen (e.g. in dental and obstetric practice for light anaesthesia or for induction only in major surgery).

Nizatidine. Gastric HISTAMINE receptor blocker, with actions and uses similar to CIMETIDINE. May cause headache, tiredness, muscle pains, pharyngitis, cough and sweating.

Nomifensine. Antidepressant, with actions, uses and adverse effects similar to IMIPRAMINE. Withdrawn due to increasing reports of adverse effects, including haemolytic anaemia.

Nonoxynol. Nonionic surfactant used as spermicidal cream.

Nonylic acid. Rubefacient used topically for musculoskeletal pain.

Noradrenaline. Sympathomimetic amine, predominantly alpha-adrenoceptor agonist. Produces general vasoconstriction with rise of blood pressure. Toxicity includes hypertension, cerebral haemorrhage and pulmonary oedema.

Norelgestromin. Progestogen hormone used in combined contraceptive preparations. Actions and adverse effects similar to PROGESTERONE.

Norepinephrine. rINN for NORADRENALINE.

Norethandrolone (m). Sex hormone with actions similar to TESTOSTERONE, but anabolic effects greater than androgenic effects. Active by mouth or by injection. Used to treat debilitating conditions and carcinoma of the breast. Used with caution if liver function is impaired.

Norethisterone. Sex hormone, with actions and adverse effects of PROGESTERONE. Used for contraception and treatment of uterine bleeding.

Noretynodrel. Sex hormone, with actions and adverse effects similar to PROGESTERONE. Used for contraception and treatment of uterine bleeding.

Norfloxacin. Broad-spectrum antibiotic for urinary tract infections, with actions and adverse effects similar to CIPROFLOXACIN, but not available for intravenous use. Adverse effects include photosensitivity, hypersensitivity, pancreatitis, hepatitis, haemolytic anaemia, paraesthesia and confusion. Also used topically as eye drops.

Norgestimate. Synthetic progestogen used as an oral contraceptive, combined with an oestrogen. Adverse effects similar to other progestogens. Experimental studies suggest that it may have a beneficial effect on plasma lipids. Any benefit in reducing cardiovascular disease will only be revealed by long-term epidemiological studies.

Norgestrel. Sex hormone, with actions and adverse effects similar to PROGESTERONE. Used for oral contraception and subdermal long-term depot contraception.

Nortriptyline. Antidepressant, with actions, uses and adverse effects similar to IMIPRAMINE.

Noscapine. Cough suppressant, with actions and adverse effects similar to PHOLCODINE.

Novobiocin. Antibiotic used for infections by PENICILLIN-resistant *Staphylococci*. Adverse effects include hypersensitivity reactions with urticarial rashes and kernicterus in the neonate.

Noxytiolin. Anti-infective with antibacterial and antifungal activity. Used topically for prevention or treatment of infections in bladder or other body cavities (e.g. after bladder operations).

Nystatin. Antibiotic used in treatment of *Candida* infections of skin and mucous membranes, particularly mouth, alimentary tract and vagina.

O

Octocog alfa (r). Blood clotting factor that is deficient in haemophilia and von Willbrand's disease. Used intravenously to stop episodes of uncontrollable bleeding.

Octoxynol. Nonionic surfactant. Used as spermicidal cream.

Octreotide. A synthetic analogue of somatostatin which reduces blood levels of growth hormone and THYROTROPHIN and inhibits INSULIN and GLUCAGON release. Used to relieve the symptoms of gastro-pancreatic endocrine tumours and to treat acromegaly. May cause pain at injection and gastro-intestinal disturbance.

Oestradiol. *See* ESTRADIOL.

Oestriol. *See* ESTRIOL.

Oestrogen. Sex hormone: *see* ESTRADIOL, ESTRIOL and ESTRONE.

Oestrone. *See* ESTRONE.

Ofloxacin. Synthetic antibacterial related to NALIDIXIC ACID, used to treat infections of lower respiratory tract, urinary tract, genital tract and eye. Adverse effects include dizziness, visual disturbances, gastro-intestinal disturbances, tendon damage and allergic reactions.

Olanzapine. Antipsychotic with actions similar to CLOZAPINE but thought to be free of its adverse effects on the bone marrow. Used to treat schizophrenia. May cause drowsiness, weight gain and dizziness. Not recommended for use in patients with dementia because of the increase in risk of cerebrovascular accident.

Oleandomycin. Antibiotic, with similar actions and adverse effects to ERYTHROMYCIN.

Olmesartan medoxomil (r). Prodrug. Converted in the body to the active metabolite olmesartan, an angiotensin II receptor antagonist, used in the treatment of hypertension. Actions, adverse effects and cautions similar to LOSARTAN.

Olopatadine (r). Antihistamine with topical and systemic actions. Used as eye drops to control the symptoms of seasonal allergic conjunctivitis. May cause transient blurred vision and discomfort of the eyes.

Olsalazine. Used to treat and prevent relapse of ulcerative colitis. Consists of two joined molecules of MESALAZINE, the active compound released when SULFASALAZINE is metabolized. This breakdown of the molecule occurs in the colon where it is required. Thought to act by inhibiting prostaglandin synthesis. May cause diarrhoea, abdominal cramps, headache, nausea, dyspepsia, arthralgia and rashes.

Omalizumab (r). Monoclonal antibody injection which counteracts the inflammatory (IgE-mediated) response in allergic asthma. Used as an add-on therapy in adolescents and adults (not children) with severe, persistent, allergic asthma which is not controlled by high dose, daily corticosteroids and long-acting beta-receptor agonists. May cause injection site reactions and, rarely, anaphylaxis.

Omeprazole. Proton pump inhibitor acts directly on gastric cells to reduce acid secretion. Used to treat gastro-oesophageal reflux disease, peptic ulceration and, in combination with antibacterials, for the eradication of *Helicobacter pylori*, the organism associated with many causes of chronic peptic ulcers. Adverse effects include headache, dry mouth, nausea and skin reactions.

Ondansetron

Ondansetron. Antiemetic with actions on 5-HYDROXYTRYPTAMINE receptors in the brain and gastro-intestinal tract, used to treat vomiting induced by anticancer drugs and radiotherapy and occurring after surgery. Adverse effects include constipation, headache and, rarely, hypersensitivity reactions.

Opium tincture (c). Mixture of poppy alkaloids: *see* MORPHINE.

Orciprenaline. Beta-adrenoceptor agonist used in bronchial asthma. Adverse effects include tachycardia, arrhythmias and tremor.

Orlistat. Long-acting inhibitor of gastro-intestinal lipases, the enzymes responsible for breakdown (and thus absorption) of dietary fats. Used in conjunction with a low-calorie diet to aid weight loss. Acts within the gut without being significantly absorbed. May cause fatty, oily stools and flatus with increased frequency of defaecation. Could influence absorption of other drugs, particularly those that are fat-soluble, e.g. some vitamins. May be associated with increased susceptibility to infections.

Orphenadrine. Parasympatholytic/antihistamine. Used as antispasmodic in treatment of parkinsonism. Actions, adverse effects, etc. as for TRIHEXYPHENIDYL.

Oseltamivir (r). Oral antiviral similar to ZANAMIVIR, with specific effects against the influenza virus. Used for both treatment and prevention of influenza in individuals at greater risk from the illness, e.g. the elderly, patients with serious chronic illness and healthcare staff. When used for prevention it is given in addition to the influenza vaccine not instead of it. Adverse effects include nausea, vomiting, abdominal pain and headaches.

Ouabain. Plant derivative with effects on the heart similar to those of DIGOXIN, but only reliably active when given by injection when the onset of action is more rapid than for DIGOXIN.

Oxaliplatin. Cytotoxic with broad antitumour activity, including activity against cells resistant to CISPLATIN. Used by intravenous infusion in combination with 5-FLUOROURACIL in treatment of metastatic colorectal cancer. May cause peripheral nerve damage, bone marrow suppression, hearing loss and impaired liver function.

Oxamniquine. Anti-infective for treatment of schistosomiasis due to *S. mansoni*. Adverse effects include transient fever and dizziness.

Oxatomide. Antihistamine that blocks histamine H_1 receptors and release of allergic mediators from mast cells. Used in treatment of allergies (e.g. hay fever, urticaria) but not asthma. Adverse effects similar to PROMETHAZINE (i.e. drowsiness, potentiation of alcohol). In high doses, causes reversible weight gain.

Oxazepam (m). Benzodiazepine anxiolytic similar to DIAZEPAM.

Ox bile extract. Recommended for treatment of biliary deficiency. Probably of little use, except that it increases bowel activity and helps to relieve constipation.

Oxetacaine. Surface-active local anaesthetic. Added to some antacid mixtures with intention of adding an analgesic effect. Actions and adverse effects similar to LIDOCAINE.

Oxethazaine. *See* OXETACAINE.

Oxitropium. Anticholinergic with a local effect on the lungs used by inhalation as a bronchodilator in chronic asthma and chronic obstructive lung disease. May cause anticholinergic side effects similar to those of ATROPINE SULPHATE, such as dry mouth, blurred vision and urinary retention. Should not be used in patients with glaucoma or prostatic hypertrophy.

Oxolinic acid. Urinary antiseptic for treatment of urine infections. May cause gastro-intestinal symptoms and CNS stimulation. Contraindicated in epilepsy.

Oxpentifylline. *See* PENTOXIFYLLINE.

Oxprenolol. Beta-adrenoceptor blocking drug with partial agonist activity (intrinsic sympathomimetic activity). Uses, side effects, etc. as for PROPRANOLOL.

Oxybuprocaine. Local anaesthetic for topical use. Similar to TETRACAINE, but less likely to cause irritation.

Oxybutynin. Anticholinergic with antispasmodic activity used to relax bladder in treatment of urinary frequency and incontinence, and nocturnal enuresis in children. Side effects similar to those of ATROPINE SULPHATE.

Oxycodone (c). Opioid analgesic used orally and by injection (r) for moderate to severe pain in patients with cancer and after surgery. Adverse effects similar to MORPHINE.

Oxymetazoline. Sympathomimetic with marked alpha-adrenergic effects. Used topically on nasal mucosa as treatment for nasal congestion. Actions and adverse effects similar to NAPHAZOLINE.

Oxymetholone (m). Sex hormone, with similar actions, uses and adverse effects to TESTOSTERONE.

Oxypertine. Tranquillizer used in treatment of schizophrenia, other psychoses and anxiety neuroses. May cause drowsiness (high doses) or hyperactivity (low doses). Gastro-intestinal disturbances, hypotension, and involuntary movements less frequent than with the phenothiazines. Coma with respiratory depression in overdosage. No antidote; supportive treatment only.

Oxyphenbutazone. Anti-inflammatory/analgesic essentially similar to PHENYLBUTAZONE of which it is a metabolite. Now discontinued orally because of high incidence of adverse reactions. Still used topically in eye.

Oxyphenisatin. Laxative used in preparative enemas before radiology, endoscopy or surgery.

Oxyquinoline. Has antibacterial, antifungal, deodorant and keratolytic properties. Used topically on skin or in vagina for minor infections and acne. Sensitivity rashes may occur.

Oxytetracycline. Bacteriostatic antibiotic, with actions, adverse effects and interactions similar to TETRACYCLINE.

Oxytocin. Hormone from the posterior pituitary gland. Causes contraction of uterus. Used for induction of labour. May cause fluid retention and uterine rupture with danger to foetus. Contraindicated in toxaemia of pregnancy, placental abnormalities or foetal distress.

P

Paclitaxel. Cytotoxic agent used in treatment of patients with advanced ovarian cancer resistant to CISPLATIN-based chemotherapy, in metastatic breast cancer and AIDS-related Kaposi's sarcoma resistant to anthracycline therapy, and lung cancer in combination with CISPLATIN. May cause bone marrow suppression, peripheral neuropathy, arthralgia and myalgia.

Palivizumab (r). Monoclonal humanized antibody targeted against respiratory syncytial virus (RSV). Used to prevent RSV lower respiratory tract infections in preterm infants and those up to six months old who are at risk because of underlying serious disease, e.g. congenital heart disease. May cause fever and injection site reactions.

Palonosetron (r). Antiemetic which acts on the 5-HYDROXYTRYPTAMINE receptors in the brain and the gastro-intestinal tract. Used to treat vomiting induced by anti-cancer drugs. Similar to ONDANSETRON, but has a longer duration of action and may be more useful against delayed vomiting. May cause headaches, constipation, diarrhoea and dizziness.

Pamidronate. A biphosphonate with actions similar to ETIDRONATE. Reduces serum calcium in tumour-induced hypercalcaemia but has a slow onset of action so is not suitable for initial treatment of severe hypercalcaemia. Inhibits bone resorption, so is used by infusion to treat Paget's disease, osteolytic lesions and bone pain associated with multiple myeloma and breast cancer. Adverse effects include transient reduction in lymphocyte count, fever and reduced urine output.

Pancreatic enzymes. Extracts of animal pancreas. Used to aid digestion of starch, fats and protein when there is pancreatic deficiency. May cause sore mouth and sensitivity reactions with sneezing, watery eyes or skin rashes. Has been associated with fibrosis of the colon in children under 15 years.

Pancreatin. *See* PANCREATIC ENZYMES.

Pancuronium. Muscle relaxant with actions and uses similar to TUBOCURARINE.

Panthenol. *See* PANTOTHENIC ACID.

Pantoprazole. For benign peptic ulcers, duodenal ulcers and oesophageal reflux. Used in combination with antibiotics to eradicate *Helicobacter pylori* in patients with duodenal ulcer. Reduces gastric acid secretion by acting directly on its production.

Pantothenic acid. Considered a vitamin, but no proven deficiency disease in man. No accepted therapeutic role, but included in some vitamin mixtures.

Papaveretum (c). Mixture of poppy derivatives; 50 per cent is MORPHINE, to which it is similar in all respects.

Papaverine. Muscle relaxant, with action on involuntary muscle. Used in bronchodilator aerosol mixtures and as relaxant in mixtures for gastro-intestinal spasm. Also used by direct injection into the penis to produce erection in erectile impotence. Low toxicity except intravenously when it may cause cardiac arrhythmias.

***para*-Aminobenzoic acid.** Nutrient. Essential metabolite for certain bacteria. Sometimes included in vitamin mixtures but there is no evidence of a deficiency disease in man. Large doses may cause nausea, skin rashes and hypoglycaemia.

para-**Aminosalicylic acid** (PAS). Synthetic antituberculous agent, usually given as the sodium salt. Adverse effects include hypersensitivity reactions, nausea, vomiting, goitre, hypothyroidism and hepatitis.

Paracetamol (Acetaminophen in USA) (r). Analgesic/antipyretic. Inhibits synthesis of prostaglandins in the brain but, unlike ACETYLSALICYLIC ACID, does not have this action in the periphery and therefore has no anti-inflammatory effect. Relieves mild pain but not inflammation. Usually given by mouth; a solubilized preparation is available for short-term intravenous treatment of pain after surgery or fever. Overdosage may cause potentially fatal liver damage. ACETYLCYSTEINE and METHIONINE are antidotes. Subject to intensive monitoring by the CHM when formulated for intravenous use, and when combined with TRAMADOL in an oral preparation.

Paradichlorobenzene. Insecticide included in some ear drops. May irritate the skin. Inhalation or ingestion may cause drowsiness.

Paraldehyde. Anticonvulsant/hypnotic/ sedative. Used in status epilepticus or disturbed patients. Administered by intramuscular injection. Dissolves plastic syringes: glass must be used. Irritant at injection site. Exhaled in breath producing unpleasant odour.

Parathyroid hormone. Extract from parathyroid glands. Increases plasma calcium by mobilizing calcium from bone, reducing urine calcium excretion and increasing its absorption from the gastrointestinal tract. Active only by injection. Used to treat low plasma calcium (tetany). May cause abnormally high plasma calcium with weakness, lethargy and coma.

Parecoxib (r). Non-steroidal anti-inflammatory analgesic with actions similar to ROFECOXIB. Parecoxib is an inactive prodrug which is metabolized in the liver to form the active agent VALDECOXIB. Used intravenously or intramuscularly for the treatment of postoperative pain. Adverse reactions include raised or lowered blood pressure, fluid retention, indigestion and, rarely, bronchospasm, kidney or heart failure.

Paricalcitol. Synthetic VITAMIN D analogue, similar to CALCITROL, the more potent active metabolite of VITAMIN D. Licensed for the treatment of secondary hyperparathyroidism associated with chronic renal failure. Actions and adverse effects similar to VITAMIN D.

Paroxetine. Antidepressant. Actions similar to FLUVOXAMINE. Adverse effects include nausea, somnolence, sweating, tremor, asthenia, dry mouth, insomnia and sexual dysfunction.

PAS. See *para*-AMINOSALICYLIC ACID.

Pectin. Emulsifying agent, used in preparation of pharmaceutical and cosmetic products.

Pegfilgrastim (r). Human granulocyte colony stimulating factor (G-CSF) that stimulates production of white blood cells and is used when production of white blood cells is depressed by cancer chemotherapy. Made by recombinant DNA technology. Actions and adverse effects similar to FILGRASTIM.

Peginterferon alfa-2b. Injectable recombinant interferon for treatment of chronic hepatitis C. Used alone or in combination with RIBAVIRIN. Adverse effects similar to INTERFERON ALPHA-2B.

Pegvisomant (r). Genetically modified growth hormone antagonist which reduces the concentration of insulin-like growth factor-1 (IGF-1). Used by injection in treatment of acromegaly due to pituitary tumours which have not responded adequately to surgery, radiotherapy or SOMATOSTATIN analogues, LANREOTIDE and OCTREOTIDE. May cause gastro-intestinal

Pemetrexed

disorders, flu-like symptoms, injection site rash, weight gain and high blood pressure.

Pemetrexed (r). Cytotoxic. Inhibits folate metabolism. Infused as chemotherapy in combination with CISPLATIN in treatment of metastatic lung cancer and pleural mesothelioma. Pre-treatment with FOLIC ACID, VITAMIN B_{12} and corticosteroids is required in order to reduce toxic effects. May cause a wide range of toxic effects including bone marrow suppression, gastro-intestinal disturbance, urinary disorders and allergic reactions.

Pemoline (c). CNS stimulant with action intermediate between CAFFEINE and AMFETAMINE. Used as treatment for lethargy. May cause insomnia, anxiety and rapid heart rate.

Penamecillin. Similar to PHENOXYMETHYLPENICILLIN.

Penciclovir. Topical antiviral cream for treatment of cold sores (herpes labialis). Actions similar to ACICLOVIR. May cause localized burning or stinging.

Penicillamine. Chelating agent. Binds certain toxic metals (e.g. copper) and increases their excretion. Used in treatment of metal poisoning and rheumatoid arthritis (where its mechanism of action is uncertain). May cause headache, fever, loss of taste, gastro-intestinal symptoms, kidney damage and bone marrow depression.

Penicillins. Group of bactericidal antibiotics that act by inhibiting bacterial cell wall synthesis. All can cause hypersensitivity reactions.

Penicillin V. *See* PHENOXYMETHYLPENICILLIN.

Pentaerithrityl tetranitrate. Vasodilator with longer, but milder, action than GLYCERYL TRINITRATE whose adverse effects it shares. Used to prevent angina attacks.

Pentaerythritol. *See* PENTAERITHRITYL TETRANITRATE.

Pentagastrin. Synthetic gastro-intestinal hormone. Stimulates secretion of gastric acid, pepsin and pancreatic enzymes. Used by injection as test of gastric and pancreatic function. May cause nausea, flushing, dizziness and fall in blood pressure.

Pentamidine. Antiprotozoal used in treatment of protozoal infections including leishmaniasis and *Pneumocystis carnii.* The latter is common in AIDs and HIV-positive individuals for whom treatment and prophylaxis may be given as an inhaled (nebulized) spray. Adverse effects include hypotension, nausea and vomiting.

Pentazocine (c). Narcotic analgesic more potent than CODEINE, but less potent than MORPHINE. Dependence and addiction less common than with MORPHINE. Some activity as a narcotic antagonist like NALOXONE. May cause bad dreams, hallucinations, withdrawal symptoms, also nausea, vomiting, dizziness and drowsiness. Constipation and, rarely, respiratory depression may occur after injections. NALOXONE but not NALORPHINE or LEVALLORPHAN may be used as antagonists.

Pentostatin. Inhibits intracellular enzymes leading to arrest of cell division in 'hairy cell' leukaemia. Adverse effects include rash, bone marrow suppression, heart failure and general malaise.

Pentoxifylline. Vasodilator used in treatment of peripheral vascular disease (e.g. intermittent claudication, Raynaud's syndrome). May reduce blood pressure, lower blood glucose or cause gastro-intestinal symptoms. May cause nausea, dizziness, flushing and hypotension. Caution needed if given with antihypertensives or insulin as it may increase their effects.

Peppermint oil. Essential oil used to relieve gastric and intestinal flatulence and colic (e.g. irritable bowel syndrome).

Adverse effects include heartburn, bradycardia, muscle tremor, anxiety and allergic reactions to its menthol content.

Pepsin. Enzyme found in normal gastric juice. Controls breakdown of proteins. May be given to improve digestion when there is deficiency of pepsin secretion.

Pergolide. DOPAMINE agonist used in Parkinson's disease on its own or as an adjunct to treatment with LEVODOPA when the latter treatment is seen to be losing its effectiveness. Adverse effects include nausea, indigestion, low blood pressure, confusion, hallucinations, dyskinesia and impaired consciousness.

Pericyazine. Tranquillizer, with actions, uses and adverse effects similar to CHLORPROMAZINE.

Perindopril. Antihypertensive with actions, uses and adverse effects similar to CAPTOPRIL. A prodrug, it is converted to perindoprilat before exerting its effect.

Permethrin. Synthetic pyrethroid insecticide used to treat head lice. Has very low toxicity in man but the shampoo may cause irritation if it contacts the eyes.

Perphenazine. Phenothiazine tranquillizer similar to CHLORPROMAZINE, used in treatment of psychotic disorders, agitation and confusion. Not recommended for children.

Pethidine (c). Synthetic narcotic analgesic essentially similar to MORPHINE. Used for relief of severe pain. May produce nausea, vomiting, dry mouth, euphoria, sedation and respiratory depression. Coma with danger of death on overdosage. NALOXONE is a specific antagonist. Long-term use associated with tolerance, physical dependence and abuse ('addiction').

PGI₂. See EPOPROSTENOL.

Phenacetin. Analgesic/antipyretic, but not anti-inflammatory. Converted by the liver to PARACETAMOL which is the main active form. Available only in combined analgesic preparations. Does not cause gastric irritation but may cause haemolytic anaemia and methaemoglobinaemia. Has been associated with kidney damage (analgesic nephropathy) and is now withdrawn in the UK.

Phenazocine (c). Narcotic analgesic similar to MORPHINE, but causes less sedation, vomiting and hypotension. More likely to depress respiration than MORPHINE.

Phenazone. Analgesic/antipyretic. Local anaesthetic action when applied topically. Not much used but found in some analgesic mixtures and in ear drops. May cause skin rashes and bone marrow suppression. Overdose may result in nausea, coma and convulsions. The rate of metabolism (half-life) of single doses is sometimes used as a measure of drug metabolism by the liver.

Phencyclidine (c). Drug of abuse commonly known as 'angel dust'. Originally used as an aid to anaesthesia, but found to cause pronounced psychotic effects which are usually unpleasant.

Phenelzine. Antidepressant; inhibits monoamine oxidase thus increasing tissue concentrations of NORADRENALINE, DOPAMINE and 5-HYDROXYTRYPTAMINE. Adverse effects include hepatitis, interactions with tyramine-containing foods and indirect sympathomimetic amines producing hypertensive crises, and with narcotics to produce profound CNS depression. Hypertensive crisis should be treated with alpha-adrenoceptor blocker (e.g. PHENTOLAMINE).

Phenindamine. Antihistamine, with actions and uses similar to PROMETHAZINE. Unlike most antihistamines, it causes stimulant side effects and may be used when sedation is a problem. May cause insomnia, convulsions, dry mouth and gastro-intestinal disturbances.

Phenindione

Phenindione. Anticoagulant, with actions and interactions similar to WARFARIN. Adverse effects include allergic reactions, jaundice and steatorrhoea.

Pheniramine. Antihistamine, with actions, uses and adverse effects similar to PROMET-HAZINE.

Phenmetrazine (c). Anorectic/sympatho-mimetic amine, widely abused, with actions and adverse effects of AMFETAMINE.

Phenobarbital (c). Long-acting barbiturate anticonvulsant. Depresses epileptic discharges in the brain. Used orally as preventive treatment in epileptics and occasionally by injection to control a severe fit. Danger of sedation and impairment of learning capacity. Induces its own metabolism by the liver. Given only with caution in liver disease. Danger of drug interaction. Coma with respiratory depression in overdose. No antidote. Treatment is supportive, sometimes plus forced alkaline diuresis or haemodialysis to promote excretion of the drug.

Phenobarbitone. *See* PHENOBARBITAL.

Phenol. Disinfectant in dilute solution; in strong solutions it denatures cell proteins and damages sensory nerves. Uses include injection for the sclerosis of haemorrhoids and alleviation of intractable pain by localized effects in the nerves involved.

Phenolphthalein. Purgative that acts by direct stimulation of colonic muscle. Action prolonged by absorption of drug from the gut and recirculation in bile. Produces pink urine and faeces (red if alkaline). May cause skin rashes in sensitive individuals.

Phenoperidine (c). Narcotic analgesic, with actions and adverse effects similar to MOR-PHINE. Used with DROPERIDOL to produce neuroleptanalgesia – a state of consciousness but calmness and indifference – allowing the patient to cooperate with the surgeon.

Phenothrin. Synthetic pyrethroid insecticide used for topical application against head lice. Active against lice and eggs. Shampoo is irritant to eyes but systemic toxicity is unlikely.

Phenoxybenzamine. Alkylating agent with alpha-adrenoceptor blocking and antihistamine effects. Used in phaeochromocytoma. Side effects include sedation, nausea and vomiting.

Phenoxybenzylpenicillin (Phenbenicillin). As for PHENOXYMETHYLPENICILLIN.

Phenoxyethylpenicillin (Phenethicillin). As for PHENOXYMETHYLPENICILLIN.

Phenoxymethylpenicillin (Penicillin V). Acid-resistant PENICILLIN used orally. Shares actions and adverse effects of BENZYLPENICILLIN.

Phenoxypropanol. Preservative/anti-infective for skin preparations.

Phenoxypropylpenicillin (Propicillin). As for PHENOXYMETHYLPENICILLIN.

Phensuximide. Anticonvulsant essentially similar to ETHOSUXIMIDE.

Phentermine (c). Anorectic/sympathomimetic amine. Actions and adverse effects similar to DIETHYLPROPION. No longer recommended because of lack of efficacy and unfavourable risk/use ratio.

Phentolamine. Alpha-adrenoceptor blocking drug with partial agonist and smooth muscle relaxant activity. Used in phaeochromocytoma to manage high blood pressure and as a diagnostic test. May be used with PAPAVERINE in erectile impotence. Side effects include tachycardia, gastro-intestinal disturbance and nasal stuffiness.

Phenylbutazone. Anti-inflammatory/analgesic used in treatment of inflammatory joint disorders. Adverse effects include nausea, vomiting, skin rashes, peptic ulceration, sodium retention and hypotension. Occasionally causes bone marrow depression with thrombocytopaenia, agranulocytosis and aplastic anaemia. May enhance action of oral anticoagulants (e.g. WARFARIN). Owing to high incidence of adverse effects, its use has been restricted to one condition only, ankylosing spondylitis.

Phenylephrine. Sympathomimetic amine, with actions, uses and toxicity of NORADRENALINE. Also used as mydriatic and nasal decongestant.

Phenylpropanolamine (m). Sympathomimetic, with actions, uses and adverse effects similar to EPHEDRINE.

Phenytoin. Anticonvulsant. Suppresses epileptic discharge in the brain. Used orally to prevent convulsions and by injection to control convulsions or to suppress irregular heart rhythms. Long-term use may cause gum hypertrophy, acne, hirsutism, folate deficiency, anaemia, osteomalacia and liver enzyme induction with danger of drug interactions. In mild overdosage, causes ataxia, dysarthria and nystagmus. Coma and respiratory depression occur in severe cases. No antidote; supportive therapy only.

Pholcodine (m). Narcotic derivative related to CODEINE but with little analgesic activity. Used only for cough suppression. May cause constipation. Similar to CODEINE in overdosage.

Phosphoric acid. In dilute form acts as a stimulant to gastric secretion.

Phosphorylcolamine. Synthetic amino acid with high phosphorus content. Said to promote improved metabolism. Used as a 'tonic' in debilitated patients.

Physostigmine (Eserine). Anticholinesterase, allowing accumulation of ACETYLCHOLINE. Actions those of ACETYLCHOLINE. Effects of overdose antagonized by ATROPINE.

Phytomenadione. *See* VITAMIN K.

Pilocarpine. Parasympathomimetic drug, with actions of ACETYLCHOLINE. Used as eye drops in the treatment of glaucoma where it reduces ocular pressure by constricting the pupils to improve drainage. Also used to stimulate tear and saliva production associated with radiotherapy or chronic inflammatory autoimmune disease Sjorgren's syndrome.

Pimecrolimus (r). Blocks the synthesis of inflammatory substances (cytokines) in the active cells (T cells) in atopic dermatitis (eczema). Used as a topical cream for short-term treatment or intermittent long-term treatment. Safety in continuous use is not established. May cause skin reactions (burning and redness) or infections at the site of application.

Pimozide. Tranquillizer, with uses, adverse effects, etc. similar to CHLORPROMAZINE.

Pindolol. Beta-adrenoceptor blocking drug with partial agonist activity (intrinsic sympathomimetic activity). Uses, side effects, etc. as for PROPRANOLOL.

Pioglitazone. Antidiabetic acts by a complex mechanism to reduce INSULIN resistance and thus to improve control of blood glucose by endogenous INSULIN. Used in combination with METFORMIN or a sulphonylurea. May cause weight gain, dizziness, flatulence, liver toxicity, headache, joint pains and impotence.

Pipenzolate. Anticholinergic, with actions and adverse effects similar to ATROPINE. Used to reduce gastric acid secretion and intestinal spasm.

Piperacillin. Broad-spectrum, injectable PENICILLIN similar to CARBENICILLIN, particularly effective against Gram-negative organisms including *Pseudomonas, Proteus,* anaerobes. Used in combination with TAZOBACTAM, a penicillinase inhibitor, in severe, life-threatening infections. Adverse effects include pseudomembranous colitis, leucopenia and interstitial nephritis. Dosage reduction needed in renal failure.

Piperazine

Piperazine. Used in treatment of threadworms and roundworms. Adverse effects include dizziness and ataxia.

Pipothiazine. *See* PIPOTIAZINE.

Pipotiazine. Phenothiazine tranquillizer, with indications, actions and adverse effects similar to FLUPHENAZINE.

Piracetam. Anticonvulsant used as an adjunct to other drug treatment in cortical myoclonus (spontaneous disabling jerking movements associated with an epileptic focus in the brain). May cause abnormal movements, insomnia, nervousness, drowsiness, depression and weight gain.

Pirbuterol. Bronchoselective beta-adrenoceptor agonist, with actions, uses and adverse effects similar to SALBUTAMOL.

Pirenzepine. Anticholinergic with selective effects on gastric mucosa. Reduces gastric acid secretion while causing less of the adverse effects normally associated with such compounds (*see* ATROPINE). May cause dry mouth and blurred vision.

Piretanide. Diuretic, with actions, uses and adverse effects similar to FUROSEMIDE.

Piroxicam. Non-steroid anti-inflammatory/analgesic with long duration of action needing only once-daily dosage. Actions and uses similar to IBUPROFEN. Adverse effects include gastro-intestinal intolerance and oedema.

Pituitary gland extract. Extract of animal pituitary tissue used for its antidiuretic activity. *See* VASOPRESSIN.

Pivampicillin. Prodrug antibiotic. Readily absorbed from gastro-intestinal tract and rapidly metabolized to the active drug AMPICILLIN, whose actions, uses and adverse effects it shares.

Pivmecillinam. Prodrug antibiotic. Readily absorbed from gastro-intestinal tract and rapidly metabolized to the active drug MECILLINAM, whose actions, uses and adverse effects it shares.

Pizotifen. For prevention of migraine. Has antiserotonin and antihistamine properties. May cause drowsiness, weight gain, dizziness and nausea.

Podophyllin. Plant extract resin, with antimitotic and purgative actions. Used topically to treat warts and by mouth as an irritant purgative (mainly succeeded by less irritant compounds).

Podophyllotoxin. Purified extract of PODOPHYLLUM used to treat genital warts. Local adverse effects are fewer and milder compared with PODOPHYLLIN. May cause local irritation.

Podophyllum. Purgative. Pronounced irritant effect on the bowel or skin. Because of its violent effects has been replaced by milder drugs. Still used as a paint for warts where it prevents growth.

Poldine. Parasympatholytic, with actions, etc. similar to ATROPINE. Used to reduce gastric acid secretion in treatment of peptic ulceration.

Poloxalene. Purgative. Lowers surface tension of intestinal fluids and softens faeces.

Poloxamer '188'. *See* POLOXALENE.

Polyacrylic acid. Gel used as a tear fluid substitute for management of dry eye conditions.

Polyestradiol. Sex hormone. Used in treatment of carcinoma of the prostate. Adverse effects similar to ETHINYLESTRADIOL.

Polyethylene glycol. Used as a solvent and/or moisturizing agent in topical preparations.

Polymyxin B. Antibiotic active against Gram-negative bacteria. Not absorbed when taken by mouth but effective topically (e.g. within gut or on skin or eyes). May also be given by intramuscular injection. Rarely causes skin sensitivity but injections may be painful and associated with neurological symptoms.

Polynoxylin. Antiseptic, with wide antibacterial and antifungal actions. Used topically for skin, throat and external ear infections.

Polysaccharide–iron complex. Haematinic, with actions, uses and adverse effects similar to FERROUS SULPHATE.

Polysorbate 60. Emulsifying agent. Aids water-in-oil mixtures and solubilizing of fat-soluble substances.

Polythiazide. Thiazide diuretic similar to BENDROFLUMETHIAZIDE.

Polyvinyl alcohol. A synthetic resin with strong hydrophilic properties used in eye drops to lubricate dry eyes and in jelly skin preparations which dry rapidly to form a soluble plastic film.

Poractant. Extract from porcine lung used to treat lung damage (respiratory distress syndrome) in preterm infants. Similar to COLFOSCERIL.

Porfimer (r). Cytotoxic. Used by intravenous injection as palliative treatment for obstruction lesions in lung and oesophageal cancers. May cause photosensitivity reactions, constipation and respiratory symptoms.

Posaconazole (r). Broad-spectrum antifungal used to treat invasive fungal infections in patients who are either resistant to, or intolerant of, treatment with AMPHOTE-RACIN B or ITRACONAZOLE. Acts by inhibiting a step in fungal cell wall synthesis. Used in immunocompromised patients, e.g. those who have advanced HIV disease, are receiving chemotherapy, or have had organ transplants. May cause bone marrow suppression, gastro-intestinal disturbance, headaches and fever.

Posterior pituitary extract. Mixed hormonal extract, with actions of OXYTOCIN and VASOPRESSIN whose toxic effects it also shares. Used by injection or nasal absorption to treat diabetes insipidus.

Potassium aluminium sulphate. *See* ALUM.

Potassium benzoate. Used topically for mild fungal infections of the skin: *see* BENZOIC ACID. Also used in mixtures of potassium salts for oral treatment of potassium deficiency.

Potassium bicarbonate. Antacid. Has been used as gastric antacid as SODIUM BICARBONATE, but unsuitable for intravenous use.

Potassium canrenoate. Potassium-sparing diuretic, related, and with similar actions, uses and adverse effects, to SPIRONOLAC-TONE.

Potassium chloride. Potassium supplement. Used when there is a danger of hypokalaemia (e.g. treatment with potassium-losing diuretics) and fluid overload in liver failure. Oral potassium chloride itself causes nausea and gastric irritation. Usually administered as slow-release preparation or in an effervescent solution of bicarbonate and trimethylglycine. May be given by slow intravenous infusion. Danger of hyperkalaemia in renal failure. Treated by haemodialysis and ion exchange resins.

Potassium citrate. Renders urine less acid. Used to reduce bladder inflammation. May produce adverse effects similar to POTASSIUM CHLORIDE.

Potassium glycerophosphate. A source of additional dietary potassium and phosphate used in 'tonics'.

Potassium *para*-aminobenzoate. Nutrient. *See para*-AMINOBENZOIC ACID. Has been used to treat skin disorders where there is excessive fibrosis (e.g. scleroderma).

Potassium perchlorate. Treatment for overactive thyroid gland. Reduces formation of thyroid hormone by interfering with uptake of iodine into the gland. May cause nausea, vomiting, rashes, kidney damage and bone marrow suppression.

Povidone. Mixture of synthetic polymers mainly used in tablet formulations for its binding, suspending and dispersing effects. May also be used in artificial tears and contact lens solutions.

Povidone-iodine. Antiseptic. Liberates inorganic iodine slowly on to the skin or mucous membranes. Used pre-operatively and in treatment of wounds.

Practolol. Cardioselective beta-adrenoceptor blocking drug. Withdrawn because of adverse effects on eye, ear and peritoneum.

Pralidoxime (P2S). Cholinesterase reactivator used in treatment of organophosphorus cholinesterase poisoning.

Pramipexole. DOPAMINE agonist with selectivity for the receptors in the brain responsible for many of the symptoms of parkinsonism. Used in Parkinson's disease when LEVODOPA no longer achieves satisfactory benefits. May cause dyskinesias and similar adverse effects to other DOPAMINE agonists used for this indication, i.e. nausea, constipation, drowsiness, uncontrolled movements, low blood pressure and hallucinations.

Pramocaine. Surface-active local anaesthetic, with actions and adverse effects similar to LIDOCAINE. Used topically on skin or mucous membranes.

Pramoxine. *See* PRAMOCAINE.

Pravastatin. Statin. Enzyme inhibitor with actions, uses, precautions and adverse effects similar to SIMVASTATIN.

Praziquantel. Anti-infective for treatment of schistosomiasis. Active against *S. haematobium* and *S. japonicum*. Effective both in urinary tract and hepatic infections. Adverse effects, usually transient, include nausea, epigastric pain, dizziness and drowsiness.

Prazosin. Vasodilator/antihypertensive. Adverse effects include tachycardia and headache. Excessive fall in blood pressure may occur early in treatment.

Prednisolone. Synthetic CORTICOSTEROID, with actions, etc. as for PREDNISONE.

Prednisone. Synthetic CORTICOSTEROID, with similar actions, etc. to CORTISONE, but has greater anti-inflammatory activity with less salt and water retention.

Pregabalin (r). Binds to voltage-gated calcium channels in the central nervous system and thus reduces the release of the excitatory neurotransmitter substances involved in pain (glutamate, NORADRENALINE, and substance P) and epilepsy (glutamate, and NORADRENALINE). Used to treat neuropathic pain and as an addition to standard therapy in refractory epilepsy. May cause drowsiness, memory disturbance, impaired coordination and gastrointestinal disturbance, including increased appetite and weight gain.

Prenalterol. Synthetic beta-adrenoceptor agonist which increases the force of cardiac contraction with only minor increases in heart rate and little, if any, peripheral vascular actions. Used in intractable heart failure. May be useful as antidote in overdosage of beta-adrenoceptor antagonists.

Prenylamine. Vasodilator used to prevent angina attacks. May cause gastro-intestinal symptoms, flushing, skin rashes and hypotension. Contraindicated in cardiac or liver failure.

Prilocaine. Local anaesthetic similar to LIDOCAINE, but less toxic. Used in dentistry.

Primaquine. Antimalarial agent. Adverse effects include nausea, methaemoglobinaemia and haemolytic anaemia.

Primidone. Anticonvulsant. Similar to barbiturates; partly metabolized by liver to PHENOBARBITAL. Suppresses epileptic discharges in the brain. Used orally to prevent convulsions. Additive effect with PHENO-BARBITAL, to which it is otherwise essentially similar.

Probenecid. For prevention of gout. Increases urine excretion of uric acid and thus reduces its levels in the body. May cause nausea, vomiting and skin rashes. Reduces excretion of PENICILLIN.

Probucol. Reduces elevated concentrations of serum CHOLESTEROL with lesser effect on triglycerides. Used in hypercholesterolaemia.

Procainamide. Antidysrhythmic/local anaesthetic similar to PROCAINE but longer acting and with less CNS stimulation. Used to treat cardiac dysrhythmias, but contraindicated in heart block. May cause dose-related hypotension, mental depression and hallucinations. Hypersensitivity may cause arthritis and rash (systemic lupus erythematosus-like syndrome).

Procaine. Local anaesthetic. Stabilizes nerve cell membranes to prevent impulse transmission. Used by injection for anaesthesia in minor operations. Poor activity if applied topically. Short action (due to rapid removal in the blood) may be prolonged by combination with a vasoconstrictor (e.g. ADRENALINE). May cause CNS stimulation with euphoria and convulsions. Metabolite of procaine interferes with antimicrobial activity of sulphonamides (e.g. SULFADIMIDINE). Preparations containing ADRENALINE are contraindicated in heart disease, hyperthyroidism or treatment with tricyclic antidepressants (e.g. AMITRIPTYLINE) where it may cause cardiac dysrhythmias.

Procaine benzylpenicillin. Long-acting form of BENZYLPENICILLIN, with similar actions and adverse effects.

Procaine penicillin. *See* PROCAINE BENZYLPENICILLIN.

Procarbazine. Cytotoxic drug used in neoplastic disease. Adverse effects include nausea, vomiting, diarrhoea, stomatitis, alopecia, neurotoxicity and bone marrow depression.

Prochlorperazine. Phenothiazine similar to CHLORPROMAZINE, but less sedative and more potent antiemetic actions. Used mainly as an antiemetic. More likely than CHLORPROMAZINE to cause extrapyramidal side effects. May be given orally, by buccal absorption, by injection or as a suppository.

Procyclidine. Parasympatholytic used in treatment of parkinsonism. Actions, etc. similar to TRIHEXYPHENIDYL.

Progesterone. Sex hormone acts on the uterus (in sequence with OESTROGEN) to prepare the endometrium to receive the fertilized ovum. Has been used in treatment of uterine bleeding, for contraception, for breast and uterine tumours, and for threatened abortion. In low doses used as a hormone supplement to treat menstrual disorders, premenstrual syndrome and infertility. Has to be injected and therefore largely replaced by newer progestational agents which are active by mouth. May cause acne, weight gain, enlargement of the breasts, headache, gastro-intestinal symptoms, ovarian cysts and jaundice.

Proguanil. Antimalarial agent. Adverse effects include vomiting and renal irritation.

Prolintane. CNS stimulant claimed to have effect intermediate between CAFFEINE and AMFETAMINE. Used to treat lethargy. May cause nausea, rapid heart rate and insomnia.

Promazine. Phenothiazine/antihistamine similar to CHLORPROMAZINE.

Promethazine. Phenothiazine/antihistamine with actions similar to CHLORPRO-

MAZINE. Used as an antiemetic and in treatment of allergic reactions, but has little antipsychotic effects. Marked sedative effects make it useful as a hypnotic in children and in pre-operative medication. Adverse effects and overdosage effects similar to CHLORPROMAZINE.

Propafenone. Antiarrhythmic used to prevent and treat life-threatening irregular cardiac rhythms.

Propamidine. Antiseptic, with antibacterial and antifungal actions. Used topically for infections of skin and conjunctiva. Treatment should not be prolonged more than one week or tissue damage may occur.

Propantheline. Parasympatholytic, with peripheral and toxic effects similar to ATROPINE. Used to reduce gastric acid secretion in peptic ulceration and as an antispasmodic for gastro-intestinal and urinary complaints. Contraindications and overdosage effects as for ATROPINE.

Propicillin. Essentially similar to PHEN-OXYMETHYLPENICILLIN.

Propiverine. Smooth muscle relaxant with actions combining the effects of anticholinergics (e.g. ATROPINE) and calcium channel blockers (e.g. NIFEDIPINE). Used orally to relax the bladder muscle (detrusor) in incontinence from spinal cord lesions or unstable bladder conditions. May cause dry mouth, blurred vision and drowsiness.

Propranolol. Beta-adrenoceptor antagonist used in angina, hypertension, arrhythmias, hyperthyroidism, migraine, anxiety and to prevent recurrence of myocardial infarction. May cause bronchoconstriction, cardiac failure, cold extremities and sleep disturbances.

Propylene glycol. Solvent used in extract of some crude drugs and as a vehicle for some injections and topical applications. May cause local irritation but less toxic than other glycols owing to rapid breakdown and excretion.

Propylhexedrine. Sympathomimetic used as inhalation for treatment of nasal congestion. Actions and adverse effects similar to NAPHAZOLINE.

Propylthiouracil. Depresses formation of thyroid hormone. Used in treatment of hyperthyroidism. Adverse effects include allergic rashes, headache, nausea, diarrhoea and blood dyscrasias, including tendency to bleeding.

Prostacyclin. See EPOPROSTENOL.

Protamine sulphate. Specific antidote to anticoagulant effect of HEPARIN. Derived from fish protein. Adverse effects include hypotension and dyspnoea.

Prothionamide. See PROTIONAMIDE.

Protionamide. Antituberculous agent, with actions and uses similar to ETHIONAMIDE. May be better tolerated.

Protirelin. Also known as thyrotrophin-releasing hormone (TRH). Used intravenously as a diagnostic agent in difficult cases of hypothyroidism where it causes a rapid rise of plasma THYROTROPHIN (TSH) in normal cases.

Protriptyline. Antidepressant, with similar action and adverse effects to IMIPRAMINE but has central stimulating effects. Used to treat depression associated with withdrawal and lack of energy. May aggravate anxiety and insomnia.

Proxymetacaine. Surface-active, local anaesthetic, with actions and adverse effects similar to LIDOCAINE. Used in ophthalmology.

Pseudoephedrine (m). Sympathomimetic, with actions, uses and adverse effects similar to EPHEDRINE. Used mainly as decongestant. Said to have less effect on increasing blood pressure.

Psilocybine (m). The hallucinogenic alkaloid obtained from *Psilocybe semi-*

lanceate, the liberty cap mushroom or 'magic mushroom', and from related species. Metabolized to the active compound psilocin. Actions and adverse effects similar to LSD but of shorter duration.

Psyllium. Purgative. Increases faecal bulk by same mechanism as METHYLCELLULOSE.

Pumactant. Synthetic, protein-free, pulmonary surfactant administered into the airways to treat the surfactant deficiency which is the cause of respiratory distress syndrome in premature babies. Surfactant (natural or synthetic) coats the airways and reduces surface tension at the air/alveoli interface, thus making easier the mechanical effort involved in breathing. Used as an adjunct to artificial ventilation. Suspended due to association with higher mortality than other lung surfactants.

Pyrantel. Antiworm treatment. Acts by paralysing mature and immature forms, thus allowing their excretion. Little absorbed from the gut so that its activity is concentrated where needed at the site of the infection. Used as a single dose for threadworm, hookworm, roundworm, whipworm and trichostrongyliasis. May cause gastro-intestinal disturbances, headache, dizziness, drowsiness, insomnia and rashes.

Pyrazinamide. Antituberculous drug. High incidence of adverse effects, particularly liver toxicity.

Pyridostigmine. Anticholinesterase, with actions similar to PHYSOSTIGMINE.

Pyridoxine (Vitamin B$_6$). Vitamin used in treatment of specific deficiency and other anaemias and in ISONIAZID-induced neuropathy. Recommended also for depression due to the oral contraceptive but true pyridoxine deficiency is not universal in such cases.

Pyrimethamine. Antimalarial agent. Adverse effects include skin rashes and folate-deficient anaemia.

Q

Quetiapine. Antipsychotic/tranquillizer with actions and uses similar to CLOZAPINE. Does not appear to cause bone marrow depression but may cause drowsiness, dry mouth, dizziness and constipation.

Quinagolide. DOPAMINE antagonist. Suppresses hyperprolactinaemia and thus can be used to stop galactorrhoea and to assist return to a normal menstrual cycle and normal fertility. Adverse effects include nausea, vomiting, other gastro-intestinal effects, headache and hypotension.

Quinalbarbitone. *See* SECOBARBITAL.

Quinapril. Antihypertensive with actions, uses and adverse effects similar to CAPTOPRIL.

Quinidine. Antidysrhythmic agent, with local anaesthetic activity. Depresses myocardial contractility and impulse conduction. Reduces cardiac output. Used to prevent recurrent dysrhythmias or to convert established dysrhythmias back to normal sinus rhythm. Dose-dependent effects include vertigo, tinnitus, deafness, blurred vision, confusion, gastro-intestinal symptoms, cardiac arrhythmias and cardiac arrest. Rashes and bruising are dose-independent. Contraindicated when dysrhythmia is due to DIGOXIN or when there is heart block.

Quinine. Antimalarial agent. Used to reduce skeletal muscle spasms. Adverse effects include vomiting, psychosis, visual and auditory disturbances, haemolytic anaemia and thrombocytopenia. Toxic doses may cause abortion.

Quinupristin. Antibiotic derived from *Streptomyces pristinaespiralis.* Used in combination with DALFOPRISTIN, another antibiotic from the same source. This combination acts synergistically against Gram-positive organisms. Used by injection only when specifically indicated in order to reduce the potential for development of bacterial resistance. Adverse reactions include injection site pain, headache, itching and joint pain.

R

Rabeprazole. Proton-pump inhibitor used to suppress acid production in peptic ulceration and gastro-oesophageal reflux. Actions, uses and adverse effects similar to OMEPRAZOLE.

Raloxifene. Selective oestrogen receptor modulator with oestrogenic and anti-oestrogenic activities. Prevents postmenopausal bone loss without stimulating reproductive tissues. Used in women who are at greater risk of postmenopausal osteoporosis. May cause hot flushes, leg cramps and peripheral oedema.

Raltitrexed. Cytotoxic used in palliative treatment of large bowel (colorectal) cancer. May cause gastro-intestinal disorders, bone marrow suppression, CNS symptoms, muscle pains, weakness and hair loss.

Ramipril. Antihypertensive with actions, uses and adverse effects similar to CAPTOPRIL. Also used to reduce the risk of stroke. A prodrug which is converted to ramiprilat before exerting its effect.

Ranitidine. Selectively blocks histamine receptors mediating gastric acid secretions. Uses and adverse effects similar to CIMETIDINE, but may cause less CNS effects or breast enlargement in males. Has fewer interactions with other drugs.

Ranitidine bismuth citrate. A complex of ranitidine and bismuth for treatment of peptic ulcers. May be used in combination with antibiotics in patients with *Helicobacter pylori* infection. Ranitidine reduces gastric acid secretions by selectively blocking histamine receptors and bismuth inhibits growth of *H. pylori* and has antacid properties. May cause blackening of tongue and stools, gastro-intestinal disturbance and headache. Prolonged use may allow sufficient absorption of bismuth to cause kidney damage, liver damage and CNS effects.

Rasagiline (r). Selective monoamine oxidase inhibitor, which prevents the breakdown of DOPAMINE in the brain. Used as monotherapy to treat early Parkinson's disease or as an adjunct to LEVODOPA to prevent end-of-dose symptom fluctuations in more advanced disease. May cause headache, flu-like symptoms, allergic reactions and a wide range of symptoms in the gastro-intestinal, musculoskeletal and nervous systems.

Rauwolfia. Indian shrub. *See* RESERPINE for main derivative.

Razoxane. Antimitotic used in treatment of certain bone and soft-tissue tumours together with radiotherapy. May cause gastro-intestinal disturbance, bone marrow suppression and hair loss.

Reboxetine. Selective NORADRENALINE reuptake blocker used in the treatment of depression. Less likely to cause troublesome anticholinergic effects than the tricyclic antidepressants but may cause dry mouth, constipation, insomnia, sweating, palpitations, urinary retention and impotence.

Remifentanil (c). Short-acting opioid analgesic similar to FENTANYL and ALFENTANIL. Used in induction and maintenance of anaesthesia. The short action allows for more rapid recovery after surgery. May cause respiratory depression, bradycardia, nausea and vomiting.

Remoxipride

Remoxipride. Antipsychotic, with actions and uses similar to CHLORPROMAZINE. Adverse effects include sedation, involuntary movements, agitation and anticholinergic effects. Withdrawn due to risk of bone marrow suppression (aplastic anaemia).

Repaglinide. Rapid-onset/short-acting oral hypoglycaemic that releases INSULIN from the pancreas. Similar to the sulphonylureas e.g. GLIBENCLAMIDE. Used in treatment of non-insulin-dependent diabetes alone or in combination with other drugs. It is taken shortly before meals and dosage is thus related to the eating pattern. May reduce the long-term cardiovascular, cerebrovascular and renal effects of diabetes. May interact with a wide range of drugs that are metabolized in the liver leading to increased or decreased effectiveness. Adverse effects may include hypoglycaemia, skin rash, gastro-intestinal upset and visual disturbances.

Reproterol. Beta-adrenoceptor agonist, with actions, uses and adverse effects as for SALBUTAMOL.

Reserpine. Rauwolfia derivative. Reduces sympathetic tone by NORADRENALINE depletion. Depletes brain NORADRENALINE, DOPAMINE and 5-HYDROXYTRYPTAMINE. Used in hypertension and as antipsychotic. Adverse effects include depression, Parkinsonism, nasal stuffiness, fluid retention and impotence.

Resorcinol. Dermatological treatment. Reduces itching and helps remove scaly skin. Used topically in treatment of acne and dandruff. Also as ear drops where used for antiseptic effects. If absorbed over long term, may cause suppression of thyroid gland. If ingested, is corrosive and may cause kidney damage, coma and convulsions.

Retinol. See VITAMIN A.

Ribavirin. Antiviral agent. Administered by inhalation to treat infants and children with severe chest infection caused by the respiratory syncytial virus (RSV). Given orally (r), in combination with INTERFERON ALFA or PEGINTERFERON ALFA preparations, to treat chronic hepatitis C.

Riboflavin (Vitamin B$_2$). Deficiency leads to mucosal ulceration and angular stomatitis.

Riboflavine. See RIBOFLAVIN.

Ricinoleic acid. Acid that forms stable soaps with alkalis. Used in contraceptive creams and jellies.

Rifabutin. Antibiotic used prophylactically to prevent infection with tuberculosis and related organisms in patients with impaired immunity. Adverse effects include anaemia, gastro-intestinal disturbances and discolouration of skin, urine and body secretions.

Rifampicin. Bactericidal antibiotic, used in tuberculosis. Adverse effects include liver toxicity and influenza-like symptoms. Induces liver enzymes, so reducing effectiveness of some other drugs including oral contraceptives and corticosteroids.

Riluzole. Reduces glutamate levels in the CNS and thus protects vulnerable neurones in motor neurone disease where it is used prophylactically. May cause gastro-intestinal disturbance, headache and dizziness.

Rimexolone. Corticosteroid used as eye drops to treat postoperative inflammation. Less likely to cause raised intraocular pressure than earlier drugs. May cause blurred vision and pain in the eye.

Rimiterol. Beta-adrenoceptor agonist. Actions, uses and adverse effects as for SALBUTAMOL.

Risedronate. Biphosphonate with actions, uses and adverse effects similar to ETIDRONATE. Thought to be less likely to cause gastro-intestinal upsets.

Risperidone (r). Antipsychotic used in schizophrenia. Effective against both positive and negative symptoms, e.g. delusions and poverty of speech respectively. Acts as antagonist against dopaminergic, adrenergic and 5HT receptors. Said to be well tolerated but may cause postural hypotension, extrapyramidal disturbances and other adverse effects associated with antipsychotic drugs, e.g. CHLORPROMAZINE. Not recommended for use in patients with dementia because of the increase in risk of cerebrovascular accident. The formulation for depot injection is subject to intensive monitoring by the CHM.

Ritodrine. Beta-adrenoceptor agonist. Actions, uses and adverse effects as for ISOXSUPRINE.

Ritonavir. Antiviral protease inhibitor. Inhibits HIV maturation and proliferation. Used in combination with other antivirals to slow or halt HIV infection. May cause gastro-intestinal disturbances, liver dysfunction, bone marrow suppression, fatigue and muscle disorders, metabolic disorders and skin rashes.

Rituximab. Monoclonal antibody which causes breakdown of lymphocytes. Used by infusion to treat follicular lymphoma that has not responded to established treatments. May cause infusion-related reactions, including fever, nausea, vomiting, allergic reactions and pain at the site of the tumour. These reactions can be reduced by prior treatment with antihistamines, analgesics and corticosteroids.

Rivastigmine. Central acetylcholinesterase inhibitor used to improve cognitive function in mild to moderate Alzheimer's dementia. Brain ACETYLCHOLINE, which is involved in memory storage and retrieval, is deficient in this condition. Inhibition of acetylcholinesterase reduces breakdown of ACETYLCHOLINE and thus increases levels. Low peripheral anticholinesterase activity improves tolerance but may still cause gastro-intestinal disturbance, anorexia,

weight loss, tremor, confusion and depression. Rarely, cardiac arrhythmias have been reported. Diagnosis and treatment must be undertaken in a specialist clinic. Long-term benefits remain uncertain and care is needed in case there are interactions with other drugs.

Rizatriptan. Selective 5-HYDROXYTRYPTA-MINE agonist with actions similar to SUMA-TRIPTAN. Given orally for the treatment of acute migraine. May cause flushing, drowsiness, dizziness, palpitations and abdominal or chest pain. Contraindicated if there is a history of heart disease.

Rocuronium. Nondepolarizing skeletal muscle relaxant used as an adjunct to anaesthesia. Actions, uses and adverse effects similar to TUBOCURARINE.

Rofecoxib. Non-steroidal anti-inflammatory analgesic with selective inhibition of the cyclo-oxygenase enzyme-2 (COX-2). Thus it reduces prostaglandin production at the sites of inflammation without affecting the protective effects of COX-1 prostaglandins on the gastro-intestinal tract. It has been found to be associated with increased problems from cardiac, renal and hepatic disease and has been withdrawn because of an adverse risk-benefit ratio.

Ropinirole. DOPAMINE agonist used to treat the DOPAMINE deficiency in Parkinson's disease, where its effects are similar to BROMOCRIPTINE. May cause nausea, vomiting, drowsiness, hypotension and bradycardia.

Ropivacaine. Local anaesthetic similar to LIDOCAINE and BUPIVACAINE but with more prolonged effects.

Rose bengal. Staining agent. Used for detection of damage to the cornea.

Rosiglitazone (r). Antidiabetic acts by a complex mechanism to reduce INSULIN resistance and thus to improve control of blood glucose by endogenous INSULIN.

Rosoxacin

Used in combination with METFORMIN or a sulphonylurea. May cause weight gain, dizziness, flatulence, headache, joint pains and impotence.

Rosoxacin. Antibiotic used only in treatment of gonorrhoea where the patient is allergic to PENICILLIN or organism is resistant to penicillins and other antibiotics. Needs only single dose. May cause dizziness, drowsiness, headache and gastro-intestinal disturbances.

Rosuvastatin (r). Statin. Enzyme inhibitor with actions, uses, precautions and adverse effects similar to SIMVASTATIN.

Rotigotine (r). Dopamine agonist used as monotherapy to treat DOPAMINE deficiency in early Parkinson's disease. Effects similar to ROPINIROLE and BROMOCRIPTINE, but formulated as transdermal patches to provide steady sustained concentrations over 24 hours. May cause anorexia, drowsiness, dizziness, headaches, postural hypotension, hypertension, abnormal movements, gastro-intestinal disturbance and patch-site reactions.

Rubella vaccine. Live attenuated rubella virus for immunization against rubella (German measles). Used routinely in girls before puberty. May be used in non-pregnant women of childbearing age. Adverse effects include rash, fever, enlarged lymph glands and joint pains. Must not be given to pregnant women or those receiving drugs to suppress the immune response.

Rubidomycin. *See* DAUNORUBICIN.

S

Salbutamol. Bronchoselective beta-adrenoceptor agonist used in bronchial asthma by inhalation, intravenous infusion or orally. Used also by intravenous infusion or orally to inhibit premature labour. Adverse effects include tachycardia, arrhythmias, tremors and muscle cramps.

Salcatonin. *See* CALCITONIN (SALMON).

Salicylamide. Analgesic/antipyretic, with actions and adverse effects similar to ACETYLSALICYLIC ACID but less effective and used only infrequently. In overdosage, does not cause acidosis but depression of respiration and loss of consciousness.

Salicylic acid. Anti-inflammatory/analgesic; an active metabolite of ACETYLSALICYLIC ACID whose adverse effects it shares. Not used systemically as it causes marked gastric irritation. Topically on skin it acts as a keratolytic and has bacteriostatic and antifungal properties. Used to treat warts, skin ulcers, psoriasis and other skin conditions.

Salmeterol. A bronchoselective beta-adrenoceptor agonist used in bronchial asthma and chronic obstructive pulmonary disease, similar to SALBUTAMOL but with a longer duration of action. May also inhibit the underlying inflammatory disease. Should only be used in addition to inhaled or oral steroids and should not replace them. Adverse effects similar to SALBUTAMOL.

Salsalate. Anti-inflammatory/analgesic. After absorption is broken down to SALICYLIC ACID. Uses and adverse effects similar to ACETYLSALICYLIC ACID.

Saquinavir. Antiviral protease inhibitor. Inhibits HIV maturation and proliferation. Used in combination with other antivirals to slow or halt HIV infection. May cause gastro-intestinal disturbances, liver dysfunction, bone marrow suppression, fatigue and muscle disorders, metabolic disorders and skin rashes.

Secobarbital (c). Barbiturate hypnotic usually prescribed in combined preparation with AMOBARBITAL. No major differences from AMOBARBITAL.

Selegiline. Selective monoamine oxidase inhibitor, which prevents breakdown of DOPAMINE in the brain and so increases and prolongs the action of LEVODOPA. Used in conjunction with LEVODOPA in the treatment of Parkinson's disease. Adverse effects include hypotension, nausea, vomiting, confusion, agitation and involuntary movements.

Selenium sulphide. Reduces formation of dandruff and other forms of eczema of the scalp. Used as a shampoo. Highly toxic if ingested, causing anorexia, garlic breath, vomiting, anaemia and liver damage.

Senna (m). Plant extract purgative, with actions, adverse effects, etc. as for CASCARA.

Sennosides A and B. Active principles of SENNA.

Sermorelin. Synthetic growth hormone releasing factor. Used intravenously as a diagnostic agent in investigation of function of the anterior pituitary gland.

Serotonin. *See* 5-HYDROXYTRYPTAMINE.

Sertindole. Antipsychotic with actions similar to CLOZAPINE but thought to be free of its adverse effects on the bone marrow. Used to treat schizophrenia. May cause nasal congestion, dizziness, weight gain, fluid retention and shortness of breath. Suspended following reports of serious cardiac arrhythmias and sudden death.

Sertraline. Antidepressant similar to FLU-VOXAMINE which acts by blocking re-uptake of SEROTONIN into nerve cells. Unlike tricyclic antidepressants it does not cause anticholinergic or cardiac side effects. The most common side effects are dry mouth, gastro-intestinal disturbances, tremor and male sexual dysfunction.

Sibutramine. Anti-obesity agent. Non-AMFETAMINE appetite suppressant. Acts by blocking uptake of catecholamines, specifically NORADRENALINE, into brain cells. Used as an adjunct to dietary management of nutritional obesity. May cause constipation, insomnia, hot flushes, rapid pulse, hypertension and anxiety.

Sildenafil (m). Enzyme inhibitor that acts specifically in the penis to block break-down of cyclic guanosine monophosphate (cGMP), the substance that promotes local vasodilation and thus erection. Used to treat erectile dysfunction. Should be avoided or used only with special care in patients with pre-existing heart or kidney disease. May cause headache, flushing, dizziness, indigestion and altered colour vision. Contraindicated with a wide range of other drugs because of the danger of interactions. Now also demonstrated to have vasodilator effects on the blood vessels in the lung. Licensed to treat pulmonary arterial hypertension, both primary and secondary to connective tissue disease. Improves exercise capacity, but carries the same risk of adverse effects as when used for erectile dysfunction.

Silver nitrate. Disinfectant/cleansing agent, used in wet dressings or baths for suppurating lesions. Must only be used short term. The lotion should not be used if a precipitate is present.

Silver protein. Has mild antibacterial properties. Used in eye drops or nasal sprays for treatment of minor infections.

Silver sulfadiazine. Sulphonamide deriv-ative, with actions similar to SULFADIMI-DINE. Used topically in treatment of burns to prevent infection.

Simeticone (activated DIMETICONE). Liquid silicone polymer (DIMETICONE) plus finely divided silicon dioxide used as an anti-foaming agent to relieve gas bubbles from gastro-intestinal tract (e.g. in flatulence or dyspepsia).

Simvastatin. Statin. Enzyme inhibitor which reduces the synthesis of CHOLES-TEROL without reducing uptake into cells. Used to reduce blood cholesterol concen-trations in both primary and secondary pre-vention of cardiovascular disease, when diet and other lifestyle changes are not sufficient. Adverse effects include head-aches, gastro-intestinal disturbance, altered liver function, tiredness and allergy. Myalgia, myositis and myopathy occur rarely, notably in patients with a history of liver disease and where multiple lipid-low-ering drugs have been used. In extreme cases this has led to rhabdomyolysis and renal failure. Has recently been licensed for non-prescription use.

Sirolimus (r). Immunosuppressant. Cyto-toxic antibiotic with immunosuppressive, antitumour and antifungal activities. Used to prevent rejection of renal transplants. May cause bone marrow suppression, diar-rhoea and joint pains.

Soap spirit. Soft soap in alcohol used in some dermatological preparations for its cleaning and descaling actions.

Sodium acid citrate. Anticoagulant. Now preferred to SODIUM CITRATE.

Sodium edetate

Sodium acid phosphate. Saline purgative, with actions and uses similar to SODIUM PHOSPHATE.

Sodium alkyl sulphoacetate. Wetting agent/laxative. Used mainly as an enema for treatment of persistent constipation and pre-operative bowel evacuation.

Sodium antimonylgluconate (Triostam). Used in schistosomiasis. Adverse effects include anorexia, nausea, vomiting, diarrhoea, muscle and joint pains and cardiotoxicity.

Sodium aurothiomalate (gold salt). Used in rheumatic diseases, notably severe rheumatoid arthritis where it is capable of halting the disease process. Given intramuscularly in weekly doses, it takes up to 4–6 months to achieve maximum effect. Adverse effects include mouth ulcers, skin rashes, oedema, proteinuria, blood dyscrasias, colitis, peripheral neuritis and pulmonary fibrosis. The high incidence of adverse effects can be reduced if use of this drug is controlled from specialist rheumatology centres.

Sodium bicarbonate. Absorbable (systemic) antacid. Rapidly dissolves and neutralizes acid in stomach. Produces quick relief of dyspepsia due to peptic ulceration but is not retained in stomach and therefore has short duration of action. Absorbed from small intestine, may cause systemic alkalosis. If used in large doses, with large doses of milk may cause renal damage (i.e. 'milk-alkali syndrome'). Danger of fluid retention in patients with cardiac failure or renal disease.

Sodium calcium edetate. Chelating agent. Exchanges its calcium for other metal ions in the blood. Most effective exchange is for lead and it may be used by injection or by mouth for treatment of lead poisoning. May cause nausea, diarrhoea, abdominal cramps, and pain and thrombophlebitis at site of injection. Renal damage and dermatitis have occurred with prolonged treat-

ment. Used with caution if there is pre-existing renal disease.

Sodium cellulose phosphate. Nonabsorbable powder taken by mouth in treatment of hypercalcaemia. Adsorbs calcium ions in the intestine and prevents their absorption, thus reducing the dietary intake of calcium.

Sodium chloride. Essential component of body fluids and tissues. Used intravenously to replace lost fluids when rapid treatment is needed or orally when replacement is less urgent (e.g. for sweat loss in tropics). Hyperosmolar solutions have been recommended as an emetic for first aid treatment of poisoning, but saline is a poor emetic and may cause death due to hypernatraemia. This use is no longer recommended.

Sodium citrate. Mild purgative used in some enemas. Was used as an anticoagulant in blood for transfusion but now superseded by SODIUM ACID CITRATE. Used as alkalizing agent in treatment of cystitis.

Sodium clodronate. Biphosphonate similar to ETIDRONATE. Acts on bone mineral metabolism to suppress bone reabsorption without affecting absorption. Used in malignant disease to treat hypercalcaemia caused by bone dissolution. Adverse effects include gastro-intestinal upsets and occasionally hypocalcaemia.

Sodium cromoglicate. Preventive treatment for asthma, rhinitis (hay fever) and conjunctivitis due to allergy. Also used for ulcerative colitis. Acts by blocking allergic mechanisms. Administered orally, by inhalation of powder or topically in eye. May cause bronchial irritation and spasm, and contact dermatitis.

Sodium cromoglycate. See SODIUM CROMOGLICATE.

Sodium edetate. Chelating agent used intravenously to reduce high blood calcium

105

levels. Actions and adverse effects similar to SODIUM CALCIUM EDETATE. May cause excessive lowering of calcium levels.

Sodium feredetate. Haematinic with actions, uses and adverse effects similar to FERROUS SULPHATE.

Sodium fluoride. Used for the prevention of dental caries in areas where the intake of fluoride from drinking water is low. May be given in water or fruit juice or applied to the teeth in solution or toothpaste. Adverse effects occur only in overdosage or from high environmental fluoride levels. Large overdoses may cause gastro-intestinal symptoms, paralysis and convulsions, with death from cardiac and respiratory failure. Chronic poisoning may cause increased bone density and eye damage.

Sodium glycerophosphate. A source of additional dietary sodium and phosphate used in 'tonics'.

Sodium hyaluronate. Transparent, high viscosity sodium salt of high molecular weight carbohydrate. Used in ophthalmic surgery to replace aqueous and vitreous humour.

Sodium hypochlorite. Source of chlorine, which has antimicrobial action for cleansing and desloughing of skin ulcers.

Sodium iodide. Expectorant. Causes increased and more watery bronchial secretion. Included in some cough mixtures. Acts also as a source of iodine (essential for production of thyroid hormone). Added to table salt to prevent endemic goitre and may be used pre-operatively to prepare hyperactive goitre for removal. Should not be given in pulmonary tuberculosis, where it may reactivate the disease.

Sodium iron edetate. *See* SODIUM FEREDETATE.

Sodium lactate. Salt administered intravenously to increase the alkali reserve. Metabolized to bicarbonate. Contraindi-

cated in liver failure, where conversion to bicarbonate is impaired.

Sodium lauryl sulphate. Detergent/wetting agent. Used for cleaning properties in skin preparations and in enemas to aid softening of faeces.

Sodium lauryl sulphoacetate. Similar to SODIUM LAURYL SULPHATE.

Sodium morrhuate. Sclerosing agent used for injection treatment of varicose veins; causes obliteration of the dilated vessels. May cause allergic reactions. A test dose is recommended.

Sodium nitrite. Used in treatment of cyanide poisoning in conjunction with SODIUM THIOSULPHATE. The nitrite produces methaemoglobin which reacts with cyanide ions to produce cyanmethaemoglobin. Cyanmethaemoglobin does not damage cell respiration but slowly breaks down, releasing cyanide in smaller amounts which are converted to the less toxic thiocyanate by the thiosulphate.

Sodium nitroprusside. Potent, rapid-acting antihypertensive used by intravenous infusion for severe hypertensive crisis or for controlled hypotension during surgical procedures. Acts by direct dilatation of blood vessels. Duration brief as metabolized to cyanide and then thiocyanate. Adverse effects include sweating, nausea, vomiting, weakness and muscle twitching. Excessive dosage may lead to 'cyanide poisoning' (i.e. tachycardia, hyperventilation, cardiac arrhythmias plus the above symptoms). DICOBALT EDETATE or SODIUM NITRITE plus SODIUM THIOSULPHATE are antidotes.

Sodium perborate. Mild disinfectant/deodorant used for mouth infections. Prolonged use may cause blistering and swelling in mouth.

Sodium phosphate. Saline purgative. Poorly absorbed from the gastro-intestinal tract. Retains water in the intestine and thus increases faecal mass.

Sodium picosulfate. Saline purgative with actions and uses similar to MAGNESIUM SULPHATE.

Sodium picosulphate. *See* SODIUM PICOSULFATE.

Sodium polystyrene sulphonate. Ion exchange resin used in treatment of high plasma potassium levels where it exchanges sodium ions for potassium. May be used orally or rectally. Adverse effects include nausea, vomiting, constipation, and sodium overload which may cause cardiac failure.

Sodium pyrrolidone-carboxylate. Hygroscopic salt. Used as a moisturizing agent for dry skin.

Sodium ricinoleate. Surface-active agent used in some toothpastes for its cleaning properties.

Sodium salicylate. Analgesic/anti-inflammatory/antipyretic, with actions, uses and adverse effects similar to ACETYLSALICYLIC ACID. Usually taken in solution. Danger of sodium overload in patients with cardiac failure or renal failure.

Sodium sulphate (Glauber's salts). Saline purgative. Actions and uses similar to MAGNESIUM SULPHATE. Unpleasant taste. Danger of sodium retention with congestive heart failure in susceptible subjects.

Sodium tetradecyl sulphate. Injection used for treatment of varicose veins.

Sodium thiosulphate. Used in treatment of cyanide poisoning together with SODIUM NITRITE.

Sodium valproate. Anticonvulsant used in all forms of epilepsy and to treat various psychiatric conditions including mania and panic disorders. May cause gastro-intestinal symptoms, weight gain, liver necrosis, allergic reactions, ranging from rash to hypersensitivity, and prolonged bleeding times. Before surgery, check for bleeding tendencies. May potentiate effects of antidepressant drugs whose dose should be reduced in combined treatment. Rarely, hirsutism, acne and reversible extrapyramidal symptoms have been reported. Should not be used by women of childbearing age without specialist neurological or psychiatric advice because of the risk to the developing foetus.

Soft paraffin. Topical emollient and protective used on skin in 'barrier creams' and wound dressings where it aids removal of the dressing.

Solifenacin (r). Anticholinergic with actions, uses and adverse effects similar to TOLTERODINE.

Somatotrophin (growth hormone). Human growth hormone. Extracted from pituitary glands. Was used to treat short stature when the epiphyses remain open. Now withdrawn because of association with transmission of viral infections and replaced by SOMATROPIN.

Somatropin (m). Synthetic human growth hormone produced by bacteria using recombinant DNA technology. Identical in structure to endogenous human growth hormone.

Sorbic acid. Preservative with antibacterial and antifungal properties.

Sorbide nitrate. *See* ISOSORBIDE DINITRATE.

Sorbitol. Carbohydrate poorly absorbed by mouth, but used as intravenous infusion it is a useful source of calories. May also be used as sweetening agent in diabetic foods, in dialysis fluids and as a laxative.

Sotalol. Beta-adrenoceptor blocking drug. Uses, side effects, etc. as for PROPRANOLOL.

Soya oil. Vegetable oil used intravenously for nutrition in debilitating conditions and topically as an emollient for dry skin. Adverse effects from intravenous use include rash, fever, chills, bone marrow depression and jaundice.

Spectinomycin. Antimicrobial active against a wide range of bacteria. Offers no advantages over other antimicrobials, except in treatment of gonorrhoea where a single injection may be adequate.

Spiramycin. Antibiotic with similar actions and adverse effects to ERYTHROMYCIN.

Spironolactone. Potassium-sparing diuretic. Acts by antagonism of the sodium-retaining hormone ALDOSTERONE and thus prevents exchange of sodium for potassium in the kidney tubule. Diuretic action is weak. Used when ALDOSTERONE is an important cause of fluid overload (e.g. liver cirrhosis and nephrotic syndrome). Toxic effects include headache, nausea, vomiting and swelling of the breasts (especially in men). Danger of excessive potassium retention which, if severe, is treated with haemodialysis and ion exchange resins. Indications now limited to treatment of oedema in liver cirrhosis, nephrotic syndrome and heart failure, and primary hyperaldosteronism.

Squalane. Ingredient of skin ointments that increases skin permeability to drugs.

Squill. Expectorant. Has irritant action on gastric mucosa and produces reflex expectorant action. Used in cough mixtures for chronic bronchitis when sputum is scanty, but too irritant for use in acute bronchitis. May cause nausea, vomiting, diarrhoea and slowing of heart rate.

Stanozolol (m). Sex hormone, with actions, uses and adverse effects similar to TESTO-STERONE. Used in Behcet's disease and for prevention of hereditary angio-oedema. Long-term use may cause jaundice; used with caution in liver disease.

Starch. Polysaccharide prepared from maize, wheat or potato. Used as an absorbent in dusting powders for skin lesions. Also used as a disintegrating agent in tablets, a mucilage in infant feeds and an antidote in iodine poisoning.

Stavudine. Antiviral agent with actions against HIV. Similar to ZIDOVUDINE. Used in patients with AIDS for whom ZIDOVUDINE is inappropriate. May cause headache, malaise, skin irritation, damage to peripheral nerves and neoplasia. Potentially fatal lactic acidosis has been reported.

Stearyl alcohol. Used in ointments and creams where its solubility aids the incorporation of water or aqueous solution.

Sterculia. Plant extract. Takes up moisture and increases faecal mass which promotes peristalsis. Used as a purgative and a bulking agent in treatment of obesity.

Stibogluconate sodium. Antimony derivative. Used in treatment of leishmaniasis. Adverse effects include nausea, vomiting, diarrhoea, muscle and joint pains, and cardiotoxicity.

Stibophen. Used in schistosomiasis. Actions and adverse effects as for SODIUM ANTIMONYLGLUCONATE.

Stilboestrol. See DIETHYLSTILBESTROL.

Storax. Balsam obtained from trunk of *Liquidambar orientalis*. Has mild antiseptic action. Used topically to assist healing of skin (e.g. for bed sores and nappy rash).

Streptodornase. Enzyme derived from streptococcal bacteria. Breaks down proteins in exudates. Used together with STREPTOKINASE to help remove clotted blood or fibrinous/purulent accumulations. Administered topically, intramuscularly or by instillation into body cavities (e.g. for haemothorax). May cause pain, fever, nausea, skin rashes and more severe allergic reactions. If haemorrhage occurs, the treatment is as for STREPTOKINASE.

Streptokinase. Plasminogen activator/ fibrinolytic agent derived from *Strepto-*

coccus. Given intravenously in thrombotic or embolic disease. May produce allergic reactions or haemorrhage which can be reversed by an antifibrinolysin such as TRANEXAMIC ACID.

Streptomycin. Bactericidal aminoglycoside antibiotic, active against tubercle bacillus, many Gram-negative and some Gram-positive organisms. Poorly absorbed orally. Administered intramuscularly. Excreted mainly by kidneys, so accumulates if renal function impaired. Adverse effects include hypersensitivity reactions (particularly contact dermatitis), ototoxicity and potentiation of neuromuscular blockade.

Strontium ranelate (r). Mineral salt which, in experimental models, affects bone metabolism to both increase new bone formation and decrease resorption of existing bone. Used in postmenopausal osteoporosis to reduce the incidence of vertebral and hip fractures. Kidney function must be carefully monitored if there is evidence of chronic renal disease. May cause nausea, diarrhoea, headache and eczema.

Styramate. Centrally acting muscle relaxant. May cause drowsiness, dizziness and rashes.

Succinic acid. Said to promote absorption of iron from the intestine.

Succinylsulfathiazole. Sulphonamide antibacterial, with actions, etc. of SULFADIMIDINE. Poorly absorbed. Used mainly for gut infections and sterilization of bowel prior to surgery.

Sucralfate. Aluminium–sucrose complex used for treatment of peptic ulcers. Protects gastro-duodenal mucosa by forming complex with pepsin which adheres to active ulcers. May cause constipation after prolonged use, possibly due to release of aluminium.

Sulconazole. Antifungal, with broad spectrum of activity. Used topically for fungal infections of skin (e.g. tinea, pityriasis and candidiasis). May cause hypersensitivity reactions with itching, burning, redness and swelling.

Sulfabenzamide. Sulphonamide antibacterial with actions, uses and adverse effects similar to SULFADIMIDINE.

Sulfacetamide. Sulphonamide antibacterial, with actions similar to SULFADIMIDINE, but used only as eye drops for eye infections.

Sulfadiazine. Sulphonamide antibacterial, with actions, etc. similar to SULFADIMIDINE.

Sulfadimidine. Sulphonamide antibacterial, which inhibits conversion of *para*-AMINOBENZOIC ACID to FOLIC ACID. Broad spectrum of activity. Mainly used in urinary tract infections. Adverse effects include crystalluria, skin rashes, polyarteritis and Stevens–Johnson syndrome. May produce kernicterus in newborn. Potentiates WARFARIN by competitive displacement from plasma proteins.

Sulfadoxine. Long-acting sulphonamide antibacterial with actions, uses and adverse effects similar to SULFADIMIDINE. Has been used in treatment of leprosy and in prevention of malaria. Mainly replaced by safer, more effective products.

Sulfaguanidine. Sulphonamide antibacterial, with actions, etc. of SULFADIMIDINE. Poorly absorbed. Used mainly for gut infections and sterilization of bowel prior to surgery.

Sulfamethizole. Sulphonamide antibacterial, with actions, etc. similar to SULFADIMIDINE.

Sulfamethoxazole. Sulphonamide antibacterial, with actions, etc. of SULFADIMIDINE, but somewhat longer action.

Sulfametopyrazine. Sulphonamide antibacterial with actions, etc. similar to SULFADIMIDINE. Long-acting. Side effects may be more serious than SULFADIMIDINE.

Sulfametoxydiazine

Sulfametoxydiazine. Sulphonamide antibacterial, with actions, etc. of SULFADIMIDINE, but only once-daily administration required.

Sulfapyridine. Sulphonamide antibactieral with actions and adverse effects similar to SULFADIMIDINE. Toxic effects are common and its use is generally limited to treatment of dermatitis herpetiformis and other skin conditions.

Sulfasalazine. Compound of SULFAPYRIDINE and SALICYLIC ACID. Used in ulcerative colitis. Broken down in the intestine to SULFAPYRIDINE and MESALAZINE, the latter being active in reducing local prostaglandin synthesis. Adverse effects as for SULFADIMIDINE.

Sulfasomizole. Sulphonamide antibacterial, with actions, etc. of SULFADIMIDINE, but somewhat longer action.

Sulfathiazole. Sulphonamide antibacterial, with actions, etc. of SULFADIMIDINE.

Sulfinpyrazone. Prophylactic treatment for gout. Promotes renal excretion of urates by reducing reabsorption in renal tubules. Reduces blood uric acid levels and gradually depletes urate deposits in tissues. Should never be started during an acute attack. The initiation of treatment may precipitate an acute attack. Reduces platelet stickiness and is used to prevent thrombosis in the coronary and cerebral circulations. May cause nausea, vomiting and abdominal pain. May aggravate peptic ulcer and so should be used with caution in patients with peptic ulcer. Long-term use may suppress bone marrow activity. Caution in renal disease. May interact to enhance actions of oral anticoagulants and oral hypoglycaemics.

Sulindac. Non-steroid anti-inflammatory agent with actions, uses and adverse effects similar to IBUPROFEN.

Sulphacetamide. *See* SULFACETAMIDE.

Sulphadiazine. *See* SULFADIAZINE.

Sulphadimidine. *See* SULFADIMIDINE.

Sulphaguanidine. *See* SULFAGUANIDINE.

Sulphamethoxazole. *See* SULFAMETHOXAZOLE.

Sulphanilamide. Sulphonamide antibacterial, with actions and adverse effects similar to SULFADIMIDINE but more toxic. Now used only for topical infections (e.g. in eye or ear drops).

Sulphasalazine. *See* SULFASALAZINE.

Sulphathiazole. *See* SULFATHIAZOLE.

Sulphinpyrazone. *See* SULFINPYRAZONE.

Sulphormethoxine. Sulphonamide antibacterial, with actions, etc. of SULFADIMIDINE, but only once-weekly administration required.

Sulphur. Used topically in skin lotions or ointments as an antiseptic.

Sulpiride. Antipsychotic, with actions (including antiemetic) and uses similar to CHLORPROMAZINE. Adverse effects include sedation, extrapyramidal symptoms, sleep disturbance, agitation and hypertension.

Sultiame. Anticonvulsant. Carbonic anhydrase inhibitor similar to ACETAZOLAMIDE. Used in prevention of epilepsy, usually in addition to other drugs. May cause paraesthesia of face and extremities, hyperventilation and gastric upsets. Inhibits PHENYTOIN metabolism and may cause PHENYTOIN toxicity. In overdosage causes vomiting, headache, hyperventilation and vertigo but not coma. May cause crystalluria with renal damage which is treated by alkaline diuresis.

Sumatriptan. 5-HYDROXYTRYPTAMINE agonist administered orally or by subcutaneous auto-injection to relieve migraine attacks. Acts at receptors in the cranial blood vessels to reduce vasodilation associated with throbbing headache. May cause pain at the injection site, flushing, feelings of chest tightness and tiredness, transient hypertension and rebound headaches. Contraindicated if there is a history of heart disease or other vascular disease.

Suramin. Antiworm treatment. Used in filiariasis. May cause impairment of kidney function. Use reserved for cases resistant to less toxic drugs.

Suxamethonium. Muscle relaxant. Acts by depolarization of muscle end plate, rendering the tissue incapable of responding to the neurotransmitter. Action limited by destruction by pseudocholinesterase. Used as an adjunct to anaesthesia for surgery. Short-acting, but effects are prolonged in patients with reduced pseudocholinesterase levels. May cause bradycardia, cardiac arrhythmias, fever and bronchospasm. Prolonged respiratory paralysis is treated by assisted ventilation and *not* by anticholinesterases.

T

Tacalcitol. Synthetic analogue of CALCITROL (the active form of Vitamin D$_3$). Inhibits skin cell proliferation without the unwanted effects of CALCITROL on calcium balance. Used topically in the treatment of psoriasis. May cause local itching and burning sensation. Calcium balance needs to be monitored if there is pre-existing kidney disease.

Tacrolimus (r). Topical immunomodulator that acts to suppress lymphocyte cell activity. Used in atopic dermatitis when conventional treatments, including corticosteroid creams, have failed. May cause a burning/itching of the skin but, unlike corticosteroids, will not cause thinning of the skin with long-term use. May exacerbate acne or herpes simplex infections.

Tadalafil (r). Enzyme inhibitor used to treat erectile dysfunction. Actions and adverse effects similar to SILDENAFIL. Contraindicated with a wide range of other drugs because of the danger of interactions.

Talc. Has lubricant and anti-irritant properties. Used topically on skin and as an aid to the manufacture of some tablets.

Tamoxifen. Anti-oestrogen. Competes with OESTROGEN for tissue receptor sites. Used as palliative treatment for breast cancer and in treatment of infertility due to failure of ovulation. May cause gastrointestinal disturbance, fluid retention, hot flushes and vaginal bleeding.

Tamsulosin. Selective alpha-adrenoceptor antagonist with actions on the smooth muscle of the prostate and the lower urinary tract. Used to facilitate micturition/passing urine when there is an obstruction due to benign prostatic hypertrophy. May cause dizziness, headache, hypotension and abnormal ejaculation.

Tannic acid. Astringent. Precipitates proteins and forms complexes with some heavy metals and alkaloids. May be used topically on skin for minor burns, abrasions or chilblains. Formerly used orally to reduce absorption of some poisons. May cause liver damage, nausea and vomiting.

Tartrazine. Orange-coloured dye. Used to colour some foods and medicines. May cause hypersensitivity reactions. Shows cross-sensitivity with ACETYLSALICYLIC ACID.

Tazarotene. Retinoid prodrug applied topically to the skin where it is absorbed and converted by skin protease enzymes to form tazarotenic acid. Used in psoriasis where it reduces the excess production of keratin by the skin cells. Unlike other retinoids ETRETINATE or ACITRETIN it does not have systemic effects. May cause local itching, stinging, redness and dry skin.

Tazobactam. Inhibits the enzyme penicillinase which inactivates the PENICILLIN antibiotics. Used in combination with PIPERACILLIN to increase its spectrum of activity.

Tegafur (r). Prodrug for the cytotoxic 5-FLUOROURACIL. Used orally for a range of cancers including colorectal, head and neck, breast and liver. Adverse effects similar to 5-FLUOROURACIL but usually less severe.

Teicoplanin. Antibiotic with actions, uses and adverse effects similar to VANCOMYCIN.

Telithromycin (r). Antibiotic with actions, uses and adverse effects similar to ERYTHROMYCIN.

Telmisartan. Antihypertensive with actions, uses and adverse effects similar to LOSARTAN.

Temazepam (c). Benzodiazepine tranquillizer/hypnotic similar to NITRAZEPAM, but with shorter duration of action and therefore less tendency to impair CNS function on the following day.

Temocillin. Injectable PENICILLIN broad-spectrum antibiotic with activity against penicillin-resistant organisms. Used in severe, life-threatening infections. Adverse effects similar to other PENICILLINS.

Tenecteplase. Antithrombotic. Used intravenously to dissolve blood clots which are suspected of causing myocardial infarction. Adverse effects include haemorrhage and, rarely, hypersensitivity reactions. Should be used once only.

Tenofovir (r). Antiviral used in combination with other antiretroviral agents in the treatment of active HIV infection. Appears relatively well tolerated for this class of drugs. May cause gastro-intestinal upsets.

Tenoxicam. Non-steroid anti-inflammatory/ analgesic with a long duration of action suitable for once-daily dosing, for use in arthritis. Adverse effects include gastro-intestinal symptoms, oedema, headache, dizziness, skin rash, blood dyscrasias and prolonged bleeding time.

Terazosin. Vasodilator/antihypertensive, with actions, uses and adverse effects similar to PRAZOSIN. May also be used to reduce symptoms of urinary obstruction caused by benign prostatic hypertrophy.

Terbinafine. Topical and orally active antifungal for treating ringworm (tinea) infections of skin and nails. May cause gastro-intestinal symptoms including irreversible taste loss and liver dysfunction. May also cause skin rashes associated with myalgia and arthralgia. Rarely, may cause serious skin reactions such as toxic epidermal necrosis.

Terbutaline. Beta-adrenoceptor agonist. Actions, uses and adverse effects as for SALBUTAMOL.

Terebene. Pleasant-smelling oil used to mask unpleasant odours or tastes and as a vapour to relieve nasal decongestion. Large doses are irritant to the gastro-intestinal tract.

Terfenadine. Antihistamine, with actions and adverse effects similar to PROMETHAZINE but is claimed to produce less sedation. Serious cardiac arrhythmias can occur if taken with certain antibiotics, antifungals or grapefruit juice. Contraindicated in patients with cardiac or hepatic disease. Used for hay fever and allergic skin conditions.

Teriparatide (r). Recombinant fragment of human parathyroid hormone that has similar actions on calcium and phosphate metabolism in bone and the kidneys. Used by injection in the treatment of established osteoporosis in postmenopausal women. In contrast to earlier therapies it appears to increase not only calcium concentrations but also bone mass and bone strength. It may thus reduce the incidence of bone fracture. Must be used with care in patients with renal impairment and previous hypercalcaemia. May cause limb pain, headaches, tiredness and anaemia.

Terlipressin. Prodrug which, after injection, is converted in the body into VASOPRESSIN.

Terodiline. Relaxes smooth muscle through several mechanisms, including anticholinergic and calcium antagonist actions. Used to reduce bladder tone in treatment of urinary frequency and incontinence. Adverse effects include dry mouth, blurred vision, constipation, tachycardia and life-threatening ventricular heart arrhythmias.

Testosterone (m) (r). Male sex hormone. Controls development and maintenance of male sex hormones and secondary sex characteristics (androgenic effects). Also produces metabolic effects that lead to increased growth of bone, water retention, increased production of red blood cells and increased blood vessel formation in the skin (anabolic effects). Used in the male to speed sexual development, but of no value in treating sterility or impotence unless related to sexual underdevelopment. In the female used to treat some menstrual disorders, for suppression of lactation and to reduce growth of breast tumours. Has also been used for anabolic effects in debilitated patients, but now superseded by new drugs. Unwanted effects include excess fluid and water retention, stimulation of growth of prostate tumours and virilization in females. May be administered orally, by buccal tablet, injection, implant, topical gel, or transdermal patch. Gel preparations and some products for injection are subject to intensive monitoring by the CHM.

Tetanus vaccine. Vaccine for prevention of tetanus. Prepared from the tetanus toxin which has been deactivated by chemical treatment.

Tetrabenazine. Used to suppress abnormal movements (e.g. Huntington's chorea). Adverse effects include drowsiness, gastrointestinal upsets and depression.

Tetracaine. Local anaesthetic similar to LIDOCAINE. Powerful surface activity but toxic by injection. Used topically in ophthalmology.

Tetrachloroethylene. Used in treatment of hookworms. Adverse effects include nausea, vomiting, diarrhoea and vertigo.

Tetracosactide. Synthetic polypeptide, with actions, uses and adverse effects similar to CORTICOTROPHIN. Used intravenously as a test of adrenal function or by depot injection for treatment of inflammatory or degenerative disorders.

Tetracosactrin. *See* TETRACOSACTIDE.

Tetracycline. Bacteriostatic antibiotic, active against many Gram-positive and Gram-negative organisms, some viruses and chlamydia. Adverse effects include diarrhoea and *Candida* bowel superinfection, yellow discolouration of teeth,

inhibition of bone growth in children and exacerbation of renal failure. Interacts in the bowel with compounds of iron, calcium and aluminium to produce insoluble chelates that are not absorbed.

Thenyldiamine. Antihistamine, with actions, uses and adverse effects similar to PROMETHAZINE but shorter duration of action.

Theobromine. Xanthine derivative. No useful CNS stimulant effects. Has been used as a diuretic or to dilate coronary or peripheral arteries. Now superseded by more effective agents but still found in some mixtures.

Theophylline. May be used as a bronchodilator, but AMINOPHYLLINE and other derivatives are more commonly used as bronchial muscle relaxants.

Theophylline ethylenediamine. *See* AMINOPHYLLINE.

Thiabendazole. *See* TIABENDAZOLE.

Thiamine. *See* ANEURINE.

Thiethylperazine. Phenothiazine with actions similar to CHLORPROMAZINE but with little tranquillizing effect. Used as an antiemetic. Given orally, by injection or as suppository. Adverse effects, etc. as for CHLORPROMAZINE.

Thioacetazone. Antituberculous agent, used as a cheap alternative to *para*-AMINOSALICYLIC ACID. May cause gastrointestinal symptoms, blurred vision, conjunctivitis and allergic reactions.

Thioguanine. *See* TIOGUANINE.

Thiopental. Very short-acting barbiturate used intravenously for anaesthesia of short duration or induction of anaesthesia prior to use of other anaesthetics. Mode of action and adverse effects similar to AMOBARBITAL.

Thiopentone. *See* THIOPENTAL.

Tioconazole

Thioridazine. Phenothiazine tranquillizer similar to CHLORPROMAZINE. Should only be used as second-line therapy for schizophrenia. Contraindicated in patients with cardiac disorders.

Thio-TEPA. Cytotoxic drug used in neoplastic disease. Adverse effects include bone marrow depression.

Thonzylamine. Antihistamine, with actions, uses and adverse effects similar to PROMETHAZINE but shorter duration of action.

Threitol dimethane sulphonate. Cytotoxic drug used for treatment of ovarian cancer. May cause gastro-intestinal disturbance, bone marrow suppression and allergic rashes.

Threonine. Essential amino acid.

Thymol. Disinfectant, similar to but less toxic than PHENOL. Used in mouthwashes.

Thymoxamine. *See* MOXISYLYTE.

Thyrotrophin (TSH). Pituitary hormone that stimulates production of thyroid hormones. Used in tests of thyroid function.

Thyroxine. *See* LEVOTHYROXINE.

Tiabendazole. Used in treatment of roundworms. Adverse effects include nausea, drowsiness and vertigo.

Tiagabine. Anticonvulsant. Acts by selective inhibition of nerve cell uptake of gamma-aminobutyric acid (GABA), the main inhibitory neurotransmitter. The increased synaptic concentrations of GABA thus decrease nerve cell excitability. Used as add-on therapy in patients where epilepsy is not adequately controlled by conventional drugs. May cause dizziness, tiredness, nervousness, tremor, depression and slow speech.

Tiaprofenic acid. Non-steroid anti-inflammatory/analgesic, with actions, uses and adverse effects similar to IBUPROFEN.

Tibolone. A steroid with effects which mimic the action of OESTROGEN, androgen

and PROGESTERONE. Used to treat menopausal hot flushes caused by deficiency of OESTROGEN and PROGESTERONE and to prevent postmenopausal osteoporosis. Adverse effects include changes in body weight, dizziness, headache, dermatitis, gastrointestinal disturbances and increased facial hair growth.

Ticarcillin. Broad-spectrum PENICILLIN injection reserved for the treatment of severe, life-threatening infections. Dosage must be reduced in the presence of severe renal impairment. Adverse effects similar to other PENICILLINS.

Ticlopidine. Antiplatelet drug that appears to act by causing irreversible changes to the platelet membrane, thus reducing their ability to form blood clots with fibrin. Used in combination with other antiplatelet drugs to prevent further thromboembolic events. Increases bleeding time and has been associated with bone marrow suppression and drug interactions. Must therefore be used with care if there is a history of previous bleeding tendency and if other drugs are used.

Tiludronic acid. Biphosphonate with actions and adverse effects similar to ETIDRONATE. Used to treat Paget's disease.

Timolol. Beta-adrenoceptor blocking drug. Uses and adverse effects as for PROPANOLOL, but mainly used by local conjunctival instillation as eye drops for glaucoma and orally to prevent recurrence of myocardial infarction.

Tinidazole. Antimicrobial used for prevention of postoperative anaerobic and acute gum infections. May cause nausea, vomiting and bone marrow suppression.

Tinzaparin. Low molecular weight HEPARIN similar to ENOXAPARIN.

Tioconazole. Topical antifungal used to treat fungal infections of the nails. Similar to KETOCONAZOLE. May cause local irritation.

Tioguanine. Cytotoxic drug, with actions, uses and adverse effects similar to MERCAPTOPURINE.

Tiothixene. Tranquillizer essentially similar to CHLORPROMAZINE.

Tiotropium (r). Long-acting anticholinergic similar to IPRATROPIUM. Used by inhalation as maintenance therapy for obstructive airways disease. Adverse effects include constipation, candidiasis, sinusitis, pharyngitis, dry mouth and, rarely, urine retention and abnormal heart rhythms.

Tipranavir (r). Oral antiviral used in combination with other antivirals to treat HIV infection.

Tirofiban. Prevents platelet aggregation. Used intravenously in conjunction with ASPIRIN and unfractionated HEPARIN to prevent myocardial infarction in patients with unstable angina or other evidence of threatened infarction. May cause bleeding at any vulnerable site, therefore contra-indicated if there is a recent history of haemorrhagic stroke or other bleeding. Should be used with care if there is a history of peptic ulceration or recent surgery.

Titanium dioxide. Dermatological treatment. Reduces itching and absorbs ultra-violet rays. Used topically to prevent sunburn and to treat some forms of eczema.

Tizanidine. Centrally acting alpha$_2$ receptor agonist which reduces muscle spasticity without affecting muscle power. Used in patients with spinal injury or disease and in multiple sclerosis. May cause drowsiness, dry mouth, insomnia and hallucinations.

Tobramycin. Antimicrobial. Actions and adverse effects similar to GENTAMICIN.

Tocainide. Cardiac antiarrhythmic drug with actions similar to LIDOCAINE, but active after oral administration. May cause blood dyscrasias in long-term use. Reserved for acute life-threatening arrhythmias.

Tolazamide. Antidiabetic, with actions, uses and adverse effects similar to CHLORPROPAMIDE.

Tolazoline. Alpha-adrenoceptor blocking drug with partial agonist activity and smooth muscle relaxant properties. Used in peripheral vascular disease. Side effects include flushing, tachycardia, nausea and vomiting.

Tolbutamide. Oral antidiabetic drug, with actions, uses and adverse effects similar to CHLORPROPAMIDE, but excreted more rapidly and thus shorter acting. Recommended when there is greater danger of hypoglycaemia (e.g. in the elderly).

Tolcapone (r). Enzyme inhibitor active against catecholamine-o-methyltransferase (COMT). Added to treatment in Parkinson's disease when therapy with LEVODOPA plus CARBIDOPA or BENSERAZIDE no longer provides adequate control, e.g. the on-off phenomenon. Helps to stabilize LEVODOPA concentrations in the periphery without causing an unwanted increase. Can only be used in patients with advanced Parkinson's disease who failed to respond to, or cannot tolerate, other COMT inhibitors. In rare instances has caused potentially fatal acute liver injury, so liver function must be monitored and treatment discontinued if liver damage is suspected. May be associated with movement disorders, insomnia and gastro-intestinal disturbance.

Tolfenamic acid. Non-steroidal anti-inflammatory agent with structural similarities to MEFENAMIC ACID. Used in treatment of migraine. Adverse reactions include gastro-intestinal disturbance, skin reactions and bronchospasm. Liver disturbance has been described.

Tolmetin. Non-steroid anti-inflammatory/analgesic, with actions, uses and adverse effects similar to IBUPROFEN.

Tolnaftate. Antifungal agent used as cream or powder for skin infections.

Tolterodine. Anticholinergic with increased selectivity for bladder muscle receptors used to treat urinary frequency, urge and incontinence, and when other causes of frequent urination have been excluded. Similar to OXYBUTYNIN but less likely to cause troublesome adverse effects. May cause dry mouth, constipation, drowsiness, headache, dry skin and dry eyes.

Tolu. Balsam obtained from trunk of *Myroxylon balsamum.* Used in cough mixtures for expectorant action and flavour.

Topiramate (r). Anticonvulsant. Mode of action not fully understood but enhances the activity of the inhibitory neurotransmitter GABA. Used as an adjunct when existing treatment fails to control convulsions. Also used for prophylaxis of migraine headache. Adverse effects include confusion, unsteadiness and dizziness.

Topotecan. Cytotoxic used in treatment of advanced (metastatic) ovarian cancer. May cause gastro-intestinal disturbance, hair loss and bone marrow suppression.

Torasemide. Diuretic. Actions, uses and adverse effects similar to FUROSEMIDE but has a longer duration of action and relative sparing of potassium loss.

Toremifene. Anti-oestrogen with actions and adverse effects similar to TAMOXIFEN. Used in treatment of advanced (metastatic) breast cancer.

Tragacanth. Laxative. Increases faecal bulk by the same mechanism as METHYL-CELLULOSE. Occasionally causes allergic rashes or asthma.

Tramadol (r). Synthetic opioid used in the treatment of moderate to severe pain. Actions, uses and adverse effects similar to PETHIDINE but with a low abuse potential. Not a controlled drug. The compound preparation of tramadol with PARACETAMOL is subject to intensive monitoring by the CHM.

Tramazoline. Sympathomimetic agent used topically as nasal decongestant. Actions and adverse effects similar to NAPHAZOLINE.

Trandolapril. ACE inhibitor used to treat hypertension. Actions and adverse effects similar to CAPTOPRIL.

Tranexamic acid. Antifibrinolytic agent, used to reverse effects of STREPTOKINASE or other fibrinolytic activity.

Tranylcypromine. Antidepressant. Inhibits monoamine oxidase. Actions and adverse effects similar to PHENELZINE, but more likely to cause hypertensive crisis, and less likely to cause hepatitis. Also has AMFETAMINE-like properties.

Trastuzumab (r). Monoclonal humanized antibody directed against epidermal growth factor that is important in tumour growth in specific cases of breast cancer. Used in monotherapy or combination therapy in cases where response is predicted. May cause widespread aches and pains, flu-like symptoms, skin reactions and bone marrow suppression.

Travoprost. Prostaglandin analogue (a prostamide) thought to regulate ocular pressure by a natural mechanism. Used as eye drops in glaucoma when beta-blocker drugs are contraindicated or inadequate. May cause redness and itching of the eyes, iris discolouration and headache.

Trazodone. Antidepressant. Blocks neuronal uptake of 5-HYDROXYTRYPTAMINE (serotonin). Unlike the tricyclic antidepressants (e.g. AMITRYPTILINE) does not have anticholinergic properties. Thus, tends to be better tolerated in dose and overdose. Adverse effects include gastric discomfort, dry mouth, headache, dizziness, drowsiness, insomnia and slight hypotension.

Treosulfan. Cytotoxic drug, used in treatment of ovarian cancer. Metabolized by liver to active, epoxide form. Acts

Tretinoin

by damaging DNA and thus interfering with cell replication. Adverse effects include gastro-intestinal symptoms, skin reactions, hair loss and bone marrow depression.

Tretinoin. VITAMIN A derivative. Used topically for acne and to reduce photodamage due to excessive exposure to sunlight. Acts by reducing rate of cell turnover and increasing skin thickness. When used topically may cause local skin irritation, peeling and hypo- or hyperpigmentation. Used in conjunction with chemotherapy in treatment of acute leukaemia.

Triamcinolone. Potent synthetic CORTICOSTEROID, with actions, etc. similar to CORTISONE. Used mainly for topical treatment of certain skin rashes (e.g. eczema). Also used for relief of hay fever symptoms.

Triamterene. Potassium-sparing diuretic similar to AMILORIDE.

Triazolam (m). Benzodiazepine tranquillizer/hypnotic, with actions, uses and adverse effects similar to TEMAZEPAM. Licence withdrawn on the grounds that this drug may cause more adverse effects than other benzodiazepines.

Tribavirin. See RIBAVIRIN.

Trichloroethylene. Weak inhalational anaesthetic with good analgesic but poor muscle relaxant properties. Used mostly in short surgical procedures (e.g. in obstetrics). May slow the heart and lead to irregular rhythms. Anaesthesia is sometimes followed by nausea, vomiting and headache. When used as a solution in industry, excessive concentrations may depress liver and kidney function. High concentrations may cause acute poisoning, coma and death.

Trichlorofluoromethane. Aerosol propellant/refrigerant. Produces intense cold by its rapid evaporation and thus makes tissues insensitive to pain. Used for relief of muscle pain and spasm.

Triclocarban. Disinfectant used in skin preparations and shampoo for prevention/treatment of certain bacterial and fungal infections. Large doses may cause methaemoglobinaemia.

Triclofos. Hypnotic/sedative. Hydrolysed in stomach to trichloroethanol and absorbed as such. More palatable and causes less gastric irritation than CHLORAL HYDRATE to which it is otherwise similar.

Triclosan. Antiseptic solution for preoperative hand and skin disinfection.

Triethanolamine. Emulsifying agent used as ear drops to soften wax for removal. May cause localized skin rashes.

Trifluoperazine. Phenothiazine tranquillizer/antiemetic similar to CHLORPROMAZINE.

Trifluperidol. Butyrophenone tranquillizer, with actions, uses and adverse effects similar to HALOPERIDOL.

Trihexyphenidyl. Antispasmodic parasympatholytic used in parkinsonism of all causes. Like ATROPINE, it may produce dry mouth, blurred vision, constipation, hesitancy of micturition, confusion and hallucinations. Contraindicated in glaucoma and prostate hypertrophy. In overdosage, dry mouth, nausea, vomiting, excitement, confusion, hot dry skin, rapid pulse and fixed dilated pupils. Depression of respiration and hypotension with loss of consciousness in late stages.

Tri-iodothyronine. See LIOTHYRONINE.

Tri-isopropylphenoxy-polyethoxyethanol. Dispersant/emulsifying agent. Used to stabilize oil-in-water mixtures and to disperse and repel spermatozoa thus preventing conception.

Trilostane. Used to inhibit synthesis of hormones in the adrenal cortex in conditions such as Cushing's syndrome.

Trimeprazine. See ALIMEMAZINE.

Trimethoprim. Antimicrobial. Inhibits conversion of FOLIC ACID to FOLINIC ACID. Combined with SULFAMETHOXAZOLE in CO-TRIMOXAZOLE. May also be used on its own for prevention of urinary tract infections. Adverse effects include nausea, vomiting, skin rashes and bone marrow depression.

Trimipramine. Antidepressant, with actions and adverse effects similar to AMITRIPTYLINE.

Triostam. *See* SODIUM ANTIMONYLGLU-CONATE.

Tri-potassium di-citrato bismuthate. Bismuth chelate. Used in treatment of peptic ulcer. May cause blackening of the tongue and faeces, constipation, nausea and vomiting.

Triprolidine. Antihistamine, with actions, uses and adverse effects similar to PROMETHAZINE.

Triptorelin. Depot intramuscular injection of growth hormone analogue. Suppresses the release of pituitary growth hormone and reduces circulating concentrations of TESTOSTERONE. Used for this effect in the suppression of advanced cancer of the prostate. Adverse effects include hot flushes, decreased libido, feminization and bone pain.

Tri-sodium edetate. Chelating agent, used intravenously in hypercalcaemia and locally for lime burns in the eye. Exchanges sodium ions for calcium ions. May cause nausea, diarrhoea, cramp and pain in the limb receiving the infusion. Excessive doses may cause renal damage.

Tropicamide. Parasympatholytic, used in the eye as a mydriatic and cycloplegic. Actions, etc. similar to ATROPINE SULPHATE, but has rapid onset and short duration of action.

Tropisetron. Antiemetic, selective 5-HYDROXYTRYPTAMINE antagonist, which blocks peripheral reflexes from relaying messages to the vomiting centre in the brain. Used to prevent nausea and vomiting during cancer chemotherapy. May cause headache, constipation, diarrhoea and dizziness and, rarely, hypersensitivity reactions.

Trospium. Anticholinergic with dominant muscarinic effects. Used orally to relax the muscle in the bladder and urinary tract and thus reduce urinary frequency and urgency and incontinence. May cause dry mouth and constipation.

Troxerutin. Vitamin derivative claimed to improve strength and reduce permeability of blood vessels. Used to treat haemorrhoids and venous disorders in the legs.

Tryptophan. Amino acid, essential component of diet. Converted in the body to 5-HYDROXYTRYPTAMINE (serotonin), a neurotransmitter substance that may be depleted in depression. Used in treatment of depression. May cause nausea, drowsiness and may interact with monoamine oxidase inhibitors (e.g. PHENELZINE). Can only be prescribed by hospital specialists.

Tuberculin. Diagnostic agent for tuberculosis. Intradermal injection produces skin reaction in positive cases. May cause skin necrosis in highly sensitive cases.

Tubocurarine. Nondepolarizing skeletal muscle relaxant. Blocks passage of impulses at the neuromuscular junction. Used as an adjunct to anaesthesia. May cause fall in blood pressure and paralysis of respiration. NEOSTIGMINE and ATROPINE SULPHATE plus assisted respiration may be used in treatment of toxic effects.

Tulobuterol. An orally active beta-adrenoceptor agonist with bronchodilator activity similar to SALBUTAMOL. Used prophylactically in reversible obstructive airways disease. Adverse effects similar to SALBUTAMOL include hypokalaemia, tremor and tachycardia.

Turpentine oil. Extract of pine used externally as a rubefacient. May cause rashes and vomiting. Rarely used internally but acts as an evacuant if given rectally.

Tyloxapol. Mucolytic. Administered by inhalation from a nebulizer. Liquefies mucus and aids expectoration where viscid mucus is troublesome (e.g. chronic bronchitis). May cause inflammation of eyelids. If left open, the solution is prone to bacterial infections.

Typhoid vaccine. Available as inactivated vaccine prepared from the polysaccharide of the capsule of *Salmonella typhi* bacteria or as a live vaccine containing the live attenuated strain of the bacteria. The former is given by parenteral injection and may produce fever, headaches, malaise and local soreness. The latter is taken by mouth as a powder in capsule form and is contra-indicated in patients whose immunity is suppressed by drugs or disease.

Tyrothricin. Antimicrobial. Too toxic for systemic use but used for topical treatment of skin, mouth or ear infections.

U

Undecenoic acid. Antifungal. Applied topically to skin, for example in treatment of tinea pedis (athlete's foot).

Urea. Osmotic diuretic, with actions and uses similar to MANNITOL. May cause gastric irritation with nausea and vomiting. Intravenous use may cause fall in blood pressure and venous thrombosis at site of injection. Largely superseded by MANNITOL and other diuretics. Topically in a cream it is used to reduce excess scaling (ichthyosis) and soften the skin.

Urea hydrogen peroxide. Disinfectant/deodorant used as a source of HYDROGEN PEROXIDE.

Urethane. Cytotoxic drug. Used in treatment of certain neoplastic diseases but largely superseded by newer drugs. May cause gastro-intestinal disturbance and bone marrow depression. Has also mild hypnotic properties and is used as an anaesthetic for small animals.

Urofollitrophin. *See* UROFOLLITROPIN.

Urofollitropin. Follicle-stimulating hormone that stimulates ovulation and spermatogenesis in men, extracted from human postmenopausal urine. Discontinued because of a theoretical risk of contracting Creutzfeldt-Jakob disease from products derived from human urine.

Urokinase. Enzyme produced by the kidney and excreted in urine. Like STREPTOKINASE, it activates plasminogen and is used intravenously to break down blood clots in pulmonary embolism. Adverse effects and their treatment similar to STREPTOKINASE.

Ursodeoxycholic acid. Used to aid dissolution of CHOLESTEROL gallstones and to treat primary biliary cirrhosis. May produce diarrhoea.

V

Valaciclovir. Prodrug of ACICLOVIR with the same actions and adverse effects. Improves the bioavailability and thus improves effectiveness in the treatment of herpes zoster (shingles), herpes simplex and genital herpes. Also used to prevent the spread of genital herpes.

Valdecoxib (r). Non-steroidal anti-inflammatory analgesic with selective inhibition of the cyclo-oxygenase enzyme-2 (COX-2). Thus it reduces prostaglandin production at the sites of inflammation without affecting the protective effects of COX-1 prostaglandins on the gastro-intestinal tract. Used for symptomatic relief of pain in osteoarthritis and rheumatoid arthritis. Gastro-intestinal effects are reduced but not eliminated. May also cause dizziness, fluid retention, hypertension, headache and itching. Should be used with caution in patients with renal, cardiac or hepatic impairment, and renal function should be monitored. Contraindicated in moderate or severe congestive heart failure.

Valganciclovir (r). Antiviral. Prodrug rapidly converted in the body to GANCICLOVIR with the same actions and adverse effects. Used to treat and maintain suppression of cytomegalovirus (CMV) in CMV retinitis in immunocompromised patients, e.g. with AIDS.

Valproic acid. Anticonvulsant. *See* SODIUM VALPROATE.

Valsartan. Angiotensin II receptor antagonist used in the treatment of hypertension. Actions, adverse effects and contraindications similar to LOSARTAN.

Vancomycin. Antibiotic, used in infections with PENICILLIN-resistant *Staphylococci* and other potentially serious bacteria. Must be given intravenously. Adverse effects include ototoxicity, pain at injection site, rash, nausea and vomiting.

Vardenafil. Enzyme inhibitor used to treat erectile dysfunction. Actions and adverse effects similar to SILDENAFIL. Contraindicated with a wide range of other drugs because of the danger of interactions.

Vasopressin (Antidiuretic hormone). Posterior pituitary hormone. Has anti-diuretic action on kidney and constricts peripheral blood vessels. Used by injection in diagnosis and treatment of diabetes insipidus and by infusion to control bleeding from oesophageal varices. May cause excessive fluid retention, pallor, sweating, nausea, headache, angina and abdominal cramps. DESMOPRESSIN is a synthetic analogue.

Vecuronium. Skeletal muscle relaxant with uses and adverse effects similar to TUBOCURARINE.

Venlafaxine. Antidepressant with novel chemical structure, but actions similar to tricyclic antidepressants (e.g. AMITRIPTYLINE), i.e. it blocks neuronal uptake of the neurotransmitters NORADRENALINE and SEROTONIN but has no anticholinergic effects at therapeutic doses. It is less likely, therefore, to cause cardiac effects or convulsions in therapy or overdose. Rare adverse effects include speech and movement disorders.

Verapamil. Used in prevention of angina of effort, hypertension and in treatment of cardiac dysrhythmias. May cause nausea, dizziness and fall in blood pressure. Contraindicated in heart failure.

Veratrum. Natural product. Reduces sympathetic tone. Was used in hypertension, but seldom used now because of adverse effects which include nausea, vomiting, sweats, dizziness, respiratory depression and abnormal heart rhythms.

Vigabatrin. Anticonvulsant used in treatment of epilepsy not satisfactorily controlled by other drugs. Acts as an analogue of gamma-aminobutyric acid (GABA), a neurotransmitter thought to be deficient in epilepsy, and able to stabilize discharges from epileptic foci. May cause drowsiness, dizziness, irritability, headache and memory disturbances. Agitation may occur in children. Severe persistent visual field disturbances have been reported infrequently.

Viloxazine. Antidepressant with some anticonvulsant properties. Unlike the tricyclic antidepressants (e.g. IMIPRAMINE), it is said to have no anticholinergic or sedative properties. Used in treatment of depression, especially when those effects occur from other drugs. May cause nausea and vomiting. If given with PHENYTOIN may induce toxicity due to that drug. No antidote; overdosage treated symptomatically.

Vinblastine. Cytotoxic alkaloid from West Indian periwinkle, used in neoplastic disease. Adverse effects include neuropathy and bone marrow depression.

Vincristine. Cytotoxic, with actions and adverse effects as for VINBLASTINE.

Vindesine. Semi-synthetic cytotoxic derived from VINBLASTINE. Has a broader spectrum of antitumour activity than the parent compound and apparently does not share cross-resistance with VINBLASTINE or VINCRISTINE. Used mainly for leukaemia and malignant melanoma. Adverse effects include haematological, neurological, cutaneous and gastro-intestinal effects.

Vinorelbine. Semi-synthetic vinca alkaloid with actions and adverse effects similar to VINBLASTINE/VINCRISTINE. Used

in the treatment of lung and breast cancers, usually in combination with other drugs.

Viomycin. Antibiotic, with actions and adverse effects similar to STREPTOMYCIN.

Viprynium. Used in treatment of threadworms. Adverse effects include red stools, vomiting and diarrhoea.

Vitamin A. Fat-soluble vitamin present in liver, dairy products and some vegetables, essential for normal visual function and maintenance of epithelial surfaces. Overdosage produces mental changes, hyperkeratosis, hypoprothrombinaemia and foetal abnormalities if taken early in pregnancy.

Vitamin B$_1$. *See* ANEURINE.

Vitamin B$_2$. *See* RIBOFLAVINE.

Vitamin B$_6$. *See* PYRIDOXINE.

Vitamin B$_7$. *See* NICOTINIC ACID.

Vitamin B$_{12}$. *See* HYDROXOCOBALAMIN.

Vitamin C (Ascorbic acid). Vitamin found in fruit and vegetables, necessary for normal collagen formation. Deficiency causes scurvy with mucosal bleeding and anaemia. High-dose administration in prophylaxis against common cold is controversial. Similarly, although vitamin C influences the formation of haemoglobin and red cell maturation, its addition to haematinics is of questionable value for most patients.

Vitamin D (Calciferol). Group of fat-soluble vitamins found in dairy products and formed in skin exposed to sunlight. Includes ERGOCALCIFEROL (calciferol, vitamin D$_2$) and COLECALCIFEROL (vitamin D$_3$). Promotes gut absorption of calcium and its mobilization from bone. Deficiency produces rickets and bone softening. Excess produces hypercalcaemia, ectopic calcification and renal failure.

Vitamin E

Vitamin E (Tocopheryl). Vitamin with no clearly defined requirements or deficiency disease in man. Has been suggested as treatment for habitual abortion, cardiovascular disease and other conditions.

Vitamin K (Menaphthone, Menadiol, Phytomenadione, Acetomenaphthone). Fat-soluble vitamin responsible for formation of prothrombin and other clotting factors. Used to reverse oral anticoagulants and in bleeding diseases including haemorrhagic disease in the newborn. Excessive dosing may produce haemolysis.

Voriconazole. Antifungal with actions similar to FLUCONAZOLE. Used orally and intravenously to treat severe fungal infections in immunocompromised patients. It may cause a wide range of adverse effects including skin rash, flu-like symptoms, hepatic and renal dysfunction, CNS disturbance and arrhythmias including, rarely, torsade de pointes and QT prolongation.

W X Y

Warfarin. Coumarin anticoagulant that interferes with synthesis of clotting factors by the liver. May produce allergic reactions. Overdosage produces haemorrhage controlled by VITAMIN K. Drugs such as ACETYLSALICYLIC ACID and PHENYLBUTAZONE potentiate the anticoagulant action of warfarin by displacing it from plasma protein binding sites. Hepatic enzyme inducers, such as barbiturates, cause warfarin to be metabolized more quickly and so reduce the anticoagulant action. Caution if used in liver disease.

Wheat husk. Concentrated extract of nonabsorbable fibre content of wheat. Used as bulking agent in treatment of constipation. May cause flatulence and abdominal distension.

Wool fat. Fat/grease recovered from wool. Resembles the secretion from human sebaceous glands in the skin. Mixed with vegetable or soft paraffin oils it produces emollient creams which penetrate the skin and aid drug absorption through the skin. May cause skin sensitization.

Xamoterol. Partial agonist at cardiac beta-adrenoceptors. It therefore stimulates the force and rate of cardiac contraction, but reduces potentially harmful effects of circulating NORADRENALINE on the heart. It is used to improve cardiac efficiency in patients with mild heart failure. Adverse effects include palpitations, rashes, dizziness and gastro-intestinal symptoms.

Xipamide. Diuretic with potency similar to FRUSEMIDE but slower onset and longer duration of action. Uses and adverse effects similar to BENDROFLUMETHIAZIDE.

Xylometazoline. Sympathomimetic, used topically as nasal decongestant. Actions and adverse effects similar to NAPHAZOLINE.

Yohimbine. Plant extract with alpha-adrenoceptor blocking actions. Said to have aphrodisiac properties but not proven.

Z

Zafirlukast. Leukotriene antagonist used orally in prevention of asthma. Not useful in acute asthma attacks. May cause sore throat, headache and gastro-intestinal disturbance.

Zalcitabine. Antiviral drug which prevents replication of the human immunodeficiency virus (HIV) involved in AIDS. Adverse effects include peripheral neuropathy, pancreatitis, gastro-intestinal disorders, rash, pruritus, sweats and, rarely, liver failure, oesophageal ulcers and anaphylaxis.

Zaleplon. Hypnotic with early onset of effects and short (5–6 hours) duration of effect. Uses and adverse effects similar to ZOLPIDEM and ZOPICLONE.

Zanamivir. Antiviral that acts by inhibiting an enzyme responsible for the replication and spread of the influenza virus. Active against influenza types A and B but has to be given by inhalation since the drug has no effect when given by mouth. If used in treatment within 24–48 hours of onset of flu symptoms, it can reduce the duration of the attack, allow earlier return to work and possibly reduce spread through the community. Any adverse effects appear to be similar to flu symptoms. No resistant influenza viruses have been demonstrated.

Zidovudine. Antiviral drug which prevents replication of retroviruses, including the human immunodeficiency virus (HIV) involved in AIDS. It does not eliminate the infection, and cannot be regarded as a cure. Adverse effects are common and include nausea, abdominal pain, headache, rash, muscle pains and anaemia. Acts synergistically with LAMIVUDINE and these drugs may be used in combination.

Zinc acetate (r). Zinc salt used for treatment of Wilson's disease (hepatolenticular degeneration), an inherited metabolic defect which results in reduced excretion of dietary copper intake. Copper is subsequently deposited in the liver and the brain, causing damage in both sites. Once the salt is absorbed, the zinc cation is released. This induces the production of an intestinal protein that binds copper and prevents its absorption. The effectiveness of treatment is monitored by measuring blood copper levels. Adverse effects include gastro-intestinal disturbance and, rarely, anaemia. May interfere with the absorption of other metals and thus lead to deficiencies. Since zinc has a slow onset of action, symptomatic patients should also be treated at first with a chelating agent such as PENICILLAMINE.

Zinc chloride. Astringent/deodorant. Used in mouthwash and for application to wounds. Caustic in higher concentrations.

Zinc ichthammol. Mixture of ZINC OXIDE and ICHTHAMMOL used for treatment of eczema.

Zinc naphthenate. Used topically for fungal infections of the skin.

Zinc oleate. Topical treatment for eczema. Actions similar to ZINC OXIDE.

Zinc oxide. Dermatological treatment. Has mild astringent, soothing and protective effects. Used topically in treatment of eczema and excoriated skin.

Zinc powder. See ZINC OXIDE.

Zinc salicylate. Dermatological treatment, with actions and uses similar to ZINC OXIDE.

Zinc sulphate. Astringent used topically for skin wounds/ulcers to assist healing. Also included in some eye drops for minor allergic conjunctivitis. Orally it is an emetic, but is not used for this purpose due to toxic effects. In smaller, sustained-release doses, it is used for nutritional zinc deficiency. For zinc-deficiency states, a soluble formulation causes less gastro-intestinal disturbance.

Zinc undecenoate. Antifungal used topically for fungal infections of the skin.

Zolmitriptan. Orally active selective serotonin (5-HT) antagonist used in the symptomatic treatment of migraine. Actions and adverse effects similar to SUMATRIPTAN.

Zolpidem (m). Hypnotic with similar actions and adverse effects to the benzodiazepine hypnotics (e.g. TEMAZEPAM).

Zonisamide (r). Anticonvulsant which is chemically distinct from other drugs in this class, but contains a sulphonamide group. Appears to have a broad range of actions, including inhibition of neuronal firing and improved neurotransmitter modulation. Used as an additional therapy in adult patients who do not respond adequately to first-line treatments. May cause sulpho-namide-related hypersensitivity, gastro-intestinal disturbance and a wide range of psychiatric disorders, including agitation, confusion and depression.

Zopiclone (m). A non-benzodiazepine hypnotic used for short-term treatment of insomnia. May cause a bitter metallic aftertaste, minor gastro-intestinal disturbances and drowsiness. Has similar adverse psychiatric reactions to DIAZEPAM.

Zotepine. Antipsychotic with actions against both the positive and negative features of schizophrenia. Uses and effectiveness similar to CLOZAPINE. May cause a wide range of gastro-intestinal, CNS, haematological and biochemical adverse effects. Use should be carefully monitored.

Zuclopenthixol. Major tranquillizer with actions similar to CHLORPROMAZINE. Used in treatment of schizophrenia. Sedation and hypotension are predictable adverse effects. Extrapyramidal (parkinsonian) symptoms are less frequent than with CHLORPROMAZINE.

PART II

Trade Names

A

AAA. Mouth and throat spray. Local anaesthetic/antiseptic for sore throat: *see* BENZOCAINE, CETALKONIUM.

Abelcet. Antifungal: *see* AMPHOTERICIN.

Abidec. Vitamin mixture: *see* ANEURINE, NICOTINAMIDE, PYRIDOXINE, RIBOFLAVIN, VITAMIN A, VITAMIN C, VITAMIN D.

Accolate. Leukotriene antagonist used for treatment of asthma: *see* ZAFIRLUKAST.

Accupro. Antihypertensive: *see* QUINAPRIL.

Accuretic. Antihypertensive: *see* HYDROCHLOROTHIAZIDE, QUINAPRIL.

Acepril. Antihypertensive: *see* CAPTOPRIL.

Acezide. Antihypertensive combination: *see* CAPTOPRIL, HYDROCHLOROTHIAZIDE.

Acidex. Liquid, sugar-free antacid: *see* ALGINATES, SODIUM BICARBONATE.

Aci-Jel (d). Jelly for topical treatment of vaginal infection.

Acnecide. Topical gel treatment for acne: *see* BENZOYL PEROXIDE.

Acorvio. Antifungal cream: *see* MICONAZOLE.

Actal. Antacid: *see* ALEXITOL SODIUM.

Actifed. Decongestant: *see* PSEUDOEPHEDRINE, TRIPROLIDINE.

Actifed Compound Linctus. As Actifed plus DEXTROMETHORPHAN for cough suppression.

Actifed Expectorant. As Actifed with GUAIFENESIN.

Actilyse. Fibrinolytic: *see* ALTEPLASE.

Actinac. Topical treatment for acne: *see* ALLANTOIN, BUTOXYETHYL NICOTINATE, CHLORAMPHENICOL, HYDROCORTISONE, SULPHUR.

Actiq (c). Analgesic lozenge for chronic pain: *see* FENTANYL.

Actonel. For treatment and prevention of postmenopausal osteoporosis: *see* RISEDRONATE.

Actonorm gel. Antacid: *see* ALUMINIUM HYDROXIDE, MAGNESIUM HYDROXIDE, SIMETICONE.

Actos. Oral hypoglycaemic: *see* PIOGLITAZONE.

Actrapid. Synthetic human crystalline insulin: *see* INSULIN.

Acular. Non-steroidal anti-inflammatory used to reduce pain and inflammation after eye surgery: *see* KETOROLAC.

Acupan. Analgesic: *see* NEFOPAM.

Adalat. Antianginal: *see* NIFEDIPINE.

Adalat LA. Controlled-release antianginal antihypertensive: *see* NIFEDIPINE.

Adalat retard. Sustained-release vasodilator antihypertensive: *see* NIFEDIPINE.

131

Adcal-D₃. For vitamin deficiency or treatment of osteoporosis or osteomalacia: *see* CALCIUM, VITAMIN D.

Adcortyl. Corticosteroid for topical or systemic use: *see* TRIAMCINOLONE.

Addiphos. Source of phosphate during parenteral feeding.

Adenocor. Antiarrhythmic: *see* ADENOSINE.

Adipine. Antihypertensive, antianginal: *see* NIFEDIPINE.

Adizem-XL/Adizem SR. Controlled-release antianginal/antihypertensive: *see* DILTIAZEM.

Adriamycin. Cytotoxic antibiotic: *see* DOXORUBICIN.

Aerodiol. Nasal spray for hormone deficiency in postmenopausal women: *see* ESTRADIOL.

Agenerase. Antiviral: *see* AMPRENAVIR.

Aggrastat. To prevent coronary thrombosis and myocardial infarction: *see* TIROFIBAN.

Airomir. CFC-free aerosol bronchodilator for asthma: *see* SALBUTAMOL.

Aknemycin Plus. Topical treatment for acne: *see* ERYTHROMYCIN, TRETINOIN.

Alcobon. Antifungal for systemic yeast infections: *see* FLUCYTOSINE.

Aldactide. Diuretic/antihypertensive: *see* HYDROFLUMETHIAZIDE, SPIRONOLACTONE.

Aldactone. Diuretic: *see* SPIRONOLACTONE.

Aldara. Topical treatment for genital warts and basal cell carcinoma: *see* IMIQUIMOD.

Aldomet. Antihypertensive: *see* METHYLDOPA.

Alembicol D (b). Lipid extract of coconut oil; substitute for long-chain fats in fat malabsorption.

Algesal. Rubefacient: *see* DIETHYLAMINE SALICYLATE.

Algipan. Rubefacient: *see* CAPSICUM, NICOTINIC ACID, SALICYLIC ACID.

Alimta (r). Cytotoxic. Used to treat pleural mesothelioma and non-small cell lung cancer: *see* PEMETREXED.

Alkeran. Cytotoxic: *see* MELPHALAN.

Allegron. Antidepressant: *see* NORTRIPTYLINE.

Almogran. For migraine: *see* ALMOTRIPTAN.

Alomide. Anti-allergic for allergic conjunctivitis: *see* LODOXAMIDE.

Aloxi (r). Anti-emetic injection used to prevent/reduce both acute and delayed nausea and vomiting associated with chemotherapy: *see* PALONOSETRON.

Alphaderm. Topical corticosteroid cream: *see* HYDROCORTISONE, UREA.

Alphagan. Eye drops for treatment of glaucoma: *see* BRIMONIDINE.

Alpha Keri Bath. Emollient bath additive for dry skin: *see* LIQUID PARAFFIN, WOOL FAT.

Alphosyl. Topical treatments for psoriasis and other scaly disorders: *see* ALLANTOIN, COAL TAR.

Alphosyl HC. Topical steroid treatment for psoriasis: *see* ALLANTOIN, COAL TAR, HYDROCORTISONE.

Altacite Plus. Antacid: *see* CO-SIMALCITE.

Alu-Cap. Antacid: *see* ALUMINIUM HYDROXIDE.

Aludrox. Antacid: *see* ALUMINIUM HYDROXIDE.

Alupent. Sympathomimetic bronchodilator: *see* ORCIPRENALINE.

Alvedon. Analgesic/antipyretic suppository: *see* PARACETAMOL.

Alvesco (r). Inhaled corticosteroid for prophylaxis of asthma: *see* CICLESONIDE.

Ambisome. Antifungal: *see* AMPHOTERICIN.

Ametop. Anaesthetic gel for use prior to taking a blood sample (venepuncture): *see* TETRACAINE.

Amias. Antihypertensive also used in treatment of heart failure: *see* CANDESARTAN CILEXETIL.

Amikin. Antibiotic: *see* AMIKACIN.

Amil-Co. Diuretic combination: *see* AMILORIDE, HYDROCHLOROTHIAZIDE.

Aminogran (b). Low AMINO ACIDS food substitute for phenylketonuria.

Aminoplasmal. Intravenous AMINO ACIDS and electrolytes for parenteral nutrition.

Aminoplex 5 and 14. Intravenous AMINO ACIDS, SORBITOL, MALIC ACID, vitamins and electrolytes.

Amoxil. Antibiotic: *see* AMOXICILLIN.

Amphocil. Antifungal: *see* AMPHOTERICIN.

Amsidine. Cytotoxic: *see* AMSACRINE.

Amytal (c). Hypnotic/minor tranquillizer: *see* AMOBARBITAL.

Anabact. Topical antibacterial: *see* METRONIDAZOLE.

Anacal. Topical treatment for haemorrhoids: *see* HEPARINOID.

Anaflex lozenges. Antiseptic for mouth and throat: *see* POLYNOXYLIN.

Anaflex topical preps. Skin antiseptic: *see* POLYNOXYLIN.

Anafranil. Antidepressant: *see* CLOMIPRAMINE.

Analog (b). Range of oral dietary supplements for management of inherited metabolic disorders in infants.

Anapen. Single-use automatic injection system for first-line emergency treatment for acute allergic reactions: *see* ADRENALINE.

Ancotil. Antifungal: *see* FLUCYTOSINE.

Androcur. For male sexual disorders: *see* CYPROTERONE.

Andropatch. Transdermal patch for male sex HRT in both primary or secondary deficiency: *see* TESTOSTERONE.

Anectine. Muscle relaxant during anaesthesia: *see* SUXAMETHONIUM.

Anexate. Benzodiazepine antagonist: *see* FLUMAZENIL.

Angeliq (r). For relief of menopausal symptoms and to prevent endometrial hyperplasia: *see* DROSPIRENONE, ESTRADIOL.

Angettes. Enteric-coated aspirin to reduce the risk of thrombosis: *see* ACETYLSALICYLIC ACID.

Angilol. Beta-adrenoceptor blocker: *see* PROPRANOLOL.

Angiopine MR. Sustained-release antianginal, antihypertensive: *see* NIFEDIPINE.

Angiox (r). To prevent blood clotting in patients undergoing percutaneous coronary intervention: *see* BIVALIRUDIN.

Angitil. Antianginal/antihypertensive: *see* DILTIAZEM.

Anhydrol forte. Antiperspirant: *see* ALUMINIUM CHLORIDE.

Anodesyn. Local treatment for haemorrhoids: *see* ALLANTOIN, LIDOCAINE.

Anquil. Tranquillizer: *see* BENPERIDOL.

Antabuse. For treatment of alcoholism: *see* DISULFIRAM.

Antepsin. Mucosal protective for treatment of peptic ulceration: *see* SUCRALFATE.

Anturan. Increases urate excretion in gout: *see* SULFINPYRAZONE.

Anugesic-HC. Topical treatment for haemorrhoids: *see* BENZYL BENZOATE, BISMUTH OXIDE, BISMUTH SUBGALLATE, HYDROCORTISONE, PRAMOCAINE, ZINC OXIDE.

Anusol. Local treatment for haemorrhoids: *see* BISMUTH BENZOATE, BISMUTH OXIDE, BISMUTH SUBGALLATE, ZINC OXIDE.

Anusol HC. As Anusol plus HYDROCORTISONE.

APO-go. Antiparkinsonian: *see* APOMORPHINE.

Apresoline. Antihypertensive: *see* HYDRALAZINE.

Aprinox. Diuretic: *see* BENDROFLUMETHIAZIDE.

Aproten (b). GLUTEN-free products for coeliac disease.

Aprovel. Antihypertensive: *see* IRBESARTAN.

Apsin VK. Antibiotic: *see* PHENOXYMETHYLPENICILLIN.

Apsolol. Beta-adrenoceptor blocker: *see* PROPRANOLOL.

Aptivus (r). Oral antiviral: *see* TIPRANAVIR.

Aquadrate. Keratolytic for thickened, dry skin: *see* UREA.

Aranesp (r). To treat anaemia associated with chronic renal failure and some cancers: *see* DARBEPOETIN.

Arava (r). To treat rheumatoid and psoriatic arthritis: *see* LEFLUNOMIDE.

Arcoxia (r). For pain relief in arthritis, and a range of acute and chronic conditions: *see* ETORICOXIB.

Aredia. For treatment of tumour-induced hypercalcaemia, Paget's disease, osteolytic lesions and bone pain associated with multiple myeloma and breast cancer: *see* PAMIDRONATE.

Aricept. To improve cognitive function in mild to moderate Alzheimer's dementia: *see* DONEPEZIL.

Arilvax (d). Vaccine for immunization against yellow fever.

Arimidex. Anti-oestrogen for treating advanced breast cancer in postmenopausal women: *see* ANASTROZOLE.

Arixtra (r). Antithrombotic for prevention of venous thromboembolism in orthopaedic surgery for deep vein thrombosis and pulmonary embolism: *see* FONDAPARINUX.

Aromasin. Hormone antagonist used for treatment of advanced breast cancer: *see* EXEMESTANE.

Arpicolin. Syrup formulation. Anticholinergic/antiParkinsonian: *see* PROCYCLIDINE.

Arret. Antidiarrhoeal: *see* LOPERAMIDE.

Arthrotec. Anti-inflammatory with prostaglandin analogue for protection against ulceration of the stomach: *see* DICLOFENAC, MISOPROSTOL.

Arythmol. Antiarrhythmic for treatment and prophylaxis of ventricular arrhythmias: *see* PROPAFENONE.

Asacol. For ulcerative colitis: *see* MESALAZINE.

Asasantin retard. For ischaemic heart disease: *see* DIPYRIDAMOLE.

Ascabiol. Topical treatment for scabies and lice: *see* BENZYL BENZOATE.

Asendis (d). Tricyclic antidepressant: *see* AMOXAPINE.

Aserbine. Desloughing cream/solution for removal of clots and slough in wounds or ulcers: *see* BENZOIC ACID, MALIC ACID, PROPYLENE GLYCOL, SALICYLIC ACID.

Asilone. Antacid: *see* ALUMINIUM HYDROXIDE, SIMETICONE, MAGNESIUM OXIDE.

Asmabec. Steroid aerosol for asthma: *see* BECLOMETASONE.

Asmabec Clickhaler. CFC-free aerosol bronchodilator/corticosteroid combination for asthma: *see* BECLOMETASONE, SALBUTAMOL.

Asmanex (r). Corticosteroid powder inhaler for prevention of asthma: *see* MOMETASONE.

Asmasal. Sympathomimetic bronchodilator aerosol: *see* SALBUTAMOL.

Asmaven. Sympathomimetic bronchodilator: *see* SALBUTAMOL.

Aspav. Water-dispersable, analgesic tablets: *see* ACETYLSALICYLIC ACID, PAPAVERETUM.

AT 10. For vitamin D deficiency or resistance: *see* DIHYDROTACHYSTEROL.

Atarax. Sedative/tranquillizer: *see* HYDROXYZINE.

Atimos Modulite. Long-acting, selective beta-adrenoceptor agonist for treatment of asthma: *see* FORMOTEROL.

Ativan. Sedative/tranquillizer: *see* LORAZEPAM.

Atrovent. Bronchodilator for inhalation: *see* IPRATROPIUM.

Audax. Drops for middle and outer ear infection: *see* CHOLINE SALICYLATE.

Augmentin. Antibacterial: *see* AMOXICILLIN, CLAVULANIC ACID.

Aureocort. Topical treatment for allergic/infective skin conditions: *see* CHLORTETRACYCLINE, TRIAMCINOLONE.

Avastin (r). Intravenous antineoplastic used to treat metatastic colorectal cancer: *see* BEVACIZUMAB.

Aveeno. Bath additive for skin allergy.

Avelox (r). Broad-spectrum antibiotic for respiratory tract infections: *see* MOXIFLOXACIN.

Avloclor. Antimalarial: *see* CHLOROQUINE.

Avodart. To relieve symptoms of benign prostatic hyperplasia: *see* DUTASTERIDE.

Avomine. Antihistamine/antiemetic: *see* PROMETHAZINE.

Avonex. To reduce relapses in multiple sclerosis: *see* INTERFERON BETA-1A.

Axid. Gastric histamine receptor blocker; reduces acid secretion: *see* NIZATIDINE.

Axsain. Topical treatment for post-herpetic neuralgia (pain persisting after

Azactam

resolution of shingles) and relief of painful diabetic neuropathy: *see* CAPSAICIN.

Azactam. Antibiotic: *see* AZTREONAM.

Azilect (r). Antiparkinsonion: *see* RASAGILINE.

Azopt. Eye drops for glaucoma: *see* BRINZOLAMIDE.

B

Bactigras. Impregnated wound dressing: *see* CHLORHEXIDINE.

Bactroban. Topical antibiotic: *see* MUPIROCIN.

Balmosa. Rubefacient: *see* CAMPHOR, CAPSICUM, METHYL SALICYLATE, MENTHOL.

Balneum. Topical application for dry skin: *see* COAL TAR, SOYA OIL.

Bambec. Bronchodilator: *see* BAMBUTEROL.

Baratol. Antihypertensive: *see* INDORAMIN.

Baxan. Antibiotic: *see* CEFADROXIL.

Beclazone. Steroid aerosol for asthma: *see* BECLOMETASONE.

Becloforte. Steroid aerosol for asthma: *see* BECLOMETASONE.

Becodisks. Inhalation system for treatment of asthma: *see* BECLOMETASONE.

Beconase. Nasal aerosol for allergic rhinitis: *see* BECLOMETASONE.

Becotide. Steroid aerosol for asthma: *see* BECLOMETASONE.

Bedranol. Beta-adrenoceptor blocker: *see* PROPRANOLOL.

Benefix. Clotting factor concentrate for treatment of haemophilia B or Christmas disease: *see* FACTOR IX.

Benerva. Vitamin B_1 for deficiency: *see* ANEURINE.

Benerva compound. Vitamin B mixture for deficiency: *see* ANEURINE, NICOTINAMIDE, RIBOFLAVIN.

Benylin Chesty Cough. Cough suppressant: *see* DIPHENHYDRAMINE, MENTHOL.

Benylin with codeine. As Benylin Chesty Cough with CODEINE.

Benylin Cough and Congestion. As Benylin Chesty Cough with DEXTROMETHORPHAN, PSEUDOEPHEDRINE.

Benzamycin. Tropical treatment for acne: *see* BENZOYL PEROXIDE, ERYTHROMYCIN.

Berkozide (d). Diuretic: *see* BENDROFLUMETHIAZIDE.

Beta-Adalat. Antihypertensive: *see* ATENOLOL, NIFEDIPINE.

Betacap. Topical treatment for scalp psoriasis: *see* BETAMETHASONE.

Beta-Cardone. Beta-adrenoceptor blocker: *see* SOTALOL.

Betadine. Antiseptic: *see* POVIDONE-IODINE.

Betaferon. For reduction of frequency and severity of relapses in multiple sclerosis: *see* INTERFERON BETA-1B.

Betagan. Beta-adrenoceptor blocker eye drops for treatment of glaucoma: *see* LEVOBUNOLOL.

Betaloc. Beta-adrenoceptor blocker: *see* METOPROLOL.

Beta-Prograne. Sustained-release antihypertensive: *see* PROPRANOLOL.

Betim. Beta-adrenoceptor blocker: *see* TIMOLOL.

Betnelan. Corticosteroid: *see* BETAMETHASONE.

Betnesol. Soluble corticosteroid tablets and injection: *see* BETAMETHASONE.

Betnesol-N. Topical corticosteroid/ antibiotic: *see* BETAMETHASONE, NEOMYCIN.

Betnovate. Topical corticosteroid: *see* BETAMETHASONE.

Betnovate C. Topical corticosteroid/ anti-infective: *see* BETAMETHASONE, CLIOQUINOL.

Betnovate N. Topical corticosteroid/ antibiotic: *see* BETAMETHASONE, NEOMYCIN.

Betoptic. Eye drops for glaucoma: *see* BETAXOLOL.

Bezalip. Lipid-lowering agent: *see* BEZAFIBRATE.

Bi-Aglut (b). GLUTEN-free biscuits for gluten-sensitive bowel disorders.

BICNU. Cytotoxic: *see* CARMUSTINE.

Biltricide. Antischistosomiasis: *see* PRAZIQUANTEL.

BiNovum. Oral contraceptive: *see* ETHINYLESTRADIOL, NORETHISTERONE.

Bioplex. Mouthwash for treatment of oral aphthous ulcers: *see* CARBENOXOLONE.

Biorphen. Anticholinergic/ antiparkinsonian: *see* ORPHENADRINE.

Bonefos. For treatment of hypercalcaemia induced by malignant disease: *see* SODIUM CLODRONATE.

Bonjela. Topical therapy for mouth ulcers: *see* CETALKONIUM, CHOLINE SALICYLATE.

Bondronat (r). Intravenous biphosphonate to treat tumour-induced hypercalcaemia: *see* IBANDRONIC ACID.

Bonviva (r). For postmenopausal osteoporosis: *see* IBANDRONIC ACID.

Botox. To treat spasms of muscles of the face, eye and limbs: *see* BOTULINUM TOXIN.

Bradosol. Antiseptic for mouth and throat infections: *see* DOMIPHEN.

Brasivol. Topical abrasive/cleansing paste for acne: *see* ALUMINIUM OXIDE.

Brevinor. Oral contraceptive: *see* ETHINYLESTRADIOL, NORETHISTERONE.

Brexidol. Non-steroid anti-inflammatory/ analgesic: *see* PIROXICAM.

Bricanyl. Sympathomimetic bronchodilator: *see* TERBUTALINE.

Britlofex. For relief of symptoms during withdrawal from opiate addiction: *see* LOFEXIDINE.

Broflex. Antiparkinsonian/anticholinergic: *see* TRIHEXYPHENIDYL.

Brolene ophthalmic preps. Anti-infective drops/ointment for use in the eye: *see* PROPAMIDINE.

Brufen. Non-steroid anti-inflammatory/ analgesic: *see* IBUPROFEN.

Brulidine. Topical anti-infective for burns, wounds: *see* DIBROMPROPAMIDINE.

Buccastem. Antiemetic tablet for buccal absorption: *see* PROCHLORPERAZINE.

Budenofalk. Oral corticosteroid treatment for Crohn's disease: *see* BUDESONIDE.

Burinex. Diuretic: *see* BUMETANIDE.

Burinex A. Diuretic: *see* AMILORIDE, BUMETANIDE.

Burinex K. As Burinex plus POTASSIUM CHLORIDE supplement.

Buscopan. Anticholinergic/antispasmodic for gastro-intestinal spasm: *see* HYOSCINE BUTYLBROMIDE.

Buspar. Anxiolytic: *see* BUSPIRONE.

BuTrans. Analgesic transdermal patch: *see* BUPRENORPHINE.

C

Cabaser. To control symptoms of Parkinson's disease: *see* CABERGOLINE.

Cacit. Effervescent calcium supplement for treatment of deficiency states and osteoporosis: *see* CALCIUM CARBONATE, CALCIUM CITRATE.

Cacit D3. For vitamin and calcium deficiency, or for osteoporosis: *see* CALCIUM CITRATE, VITAMIN D.

Cafergot. Vasoconstrictor for migraine: *see* CAFFEINE, ERGOTAMINE.

Calaband. Impregnated bandage for dressing skin wounds and ulcers: *see* BORIC ACID, CALAMINE, CASTOR OIL, GLYCERIN, ZINC OXIDE.

Caladryl. Cream or lotion for skin irritation (e.g. sunburn, insect bites): *see* CALAMINE, CAMPHOR, DIPHENHYDRAMINE.

Calceos. For vitamin and calcium deficiency, or for osteoporosis: *see* CALCIUM, VITAMIN D.

Calcichew. Antacid: *see* CALCIUM CARBONATE.

Calcichew D3. Calcium supplement with vitamin D_3 for treatment of deficiency states, osteoporosis and osteomalacia: *see* COLECALCIFEROL.

Calcijex. Vitamin for intravenous administration in patients with chronic renal failure: *see* CALCITRIOL.

Calcimax. Calcium/vitamin supplements for calcium deficiencies: *see* ANEURINE, CALCIUM CHLORIDE, CALCIUM

LAEVULINATE, NICOTINIC ACID, PANTOTHENIC ACID, PYRIDOXINE, RIBOFLAVIN, VITAMIN C.

Calciparine. Anticoagulant: *see* HEPARIN.

Calcium Resonium. Ion exchange resin: *see* CALCIUM POLYSTYRENE SULPHONATE.

Calcium-Sandoz. Calcium supplement for deficiency (e.g. tetany).

Calgel. Anaesthetic/antibacterial gel for teething pain in infants: *see* CETYLPYRIDINIUM, LIDOCAINE.

Calmurid. Keratolytic cream for removal of dry, scaly skin: *see* LACTIC ACID, UREA.

Calmurid HC. Corticosteroid cream for eczema: *see* HYDROCORTISONE, LACTIC ACID, UREA.

Calogen (b). Contains arachis oil, a source of high energy for use in renal failure.

Caloreen (b). Protein-free, high-calorie powder for use when low-protein diet is needed (e.g. kidney failure).

Calpol. Analgesic elixir: *see* PARACETAMOL.

Calpol Fast Melts. Analgesic tablet formulated to dissolve on the tongue: *see* PARACETAMOL.

CAM. Bronchodilator elixir for children: *see* EPHEDRINE.

Camcolit. Antidepressant for manic depressive psychosis: *see* LITHIUM SALTS.

Campral EC. A synthetic GABA analogue for maintaining abstinence after alcohol withdrawal: *see* ACAMPROSATE.

Campto. Cytotoxic: *see* IRINOTECAN.

Canesten. Antifungal: *see* CLOTRIMAZOLE.

Canesten HC. Topical anti-infective/corticosteroid. As Canesten plus HYDROCORTISONE.

Capasal. Shampoo for dry and scaly scalp conditions: *see* COAL TAR, SALICYLIC ACID.

Capastat. Antituberculous antibiotic: *see* CAPREOMYCIN.

Caplenal. For gout: *see* ALLOPURINOL.

Capoten. Antihypertensive: *see* CAPTOPRIL.

Capozide. Antihypertensive combination: *see* CAPTOPRIL, HYDROCHLOROTHIAZIDE.

Caprin. Slow-release analgesic: *see* ACETYLSALICYLIC ACID.

Carace. Antihypertensive: *see* LISINOPRIL.

Carace plus. Antihypertensive: *see* HYDROCHLOROTHIAZIDE, LISINOPRIL.

Carbalax. Phosphate enema: *see* SODIUM ACID PHOSPHATE.

Carbellon. Antacid/sedative: *see* CHARCOAL, MAGNESIUM HYDROXIDE, PEPPERMINT OIL.

Carbo-Dome. Topical treatment for psoriasis: *see* COAL TAR.

Carbomix. Oral adsorbant for treatment of acute poisoning and drug overdose: *see* ACTIVATED CHARCOAL.

Cardene. Antianginal, antihypertensive: *see* NICARDIPINE.

Cardene SR. Sustained-release antianginal, antihypertensive: *see* NICARDIPINE.

Cardilate MR. Antihypertensive, antianginal: *see* NIFEDIPINE.

Cardura. Antihypertensive: *see* DOXAZOSIN.

Carisoma. Muscle relaxant: *see* CARISOPRODOL.

Carobel (b). Carob seed flour for thickening feeds in the treatment of vomiting.

Carylderm. Insecticide lotion shampoo for treatment of lice: *see* CARBARYL.

Casilan (b). High-protein, low-salt food for hypoproteinaemia.

Casodex. Antiandrogen used in treatment of carcinoma of the prostate gland: *see* BICALUTAMIDE.

Catapres. Antihypertensive: *see* CLONIDINE.

Caverject. Prostaglandin injection for intracavernous (penile) injection in treatment of erectile dysfunction: *see* ALPROSTADIL.

Ceanel (b). Shampoo for psoriasis: *see* CETRIMIDE, UNDECENOIC ACID.

Cedocard. Antianginal: *see* ISOSORBIDE NITRATE.

Celance. Antiparkinsonian: *see* PERGOLIDE.

Celebrex. Non-steroidal anti-inflammatory for osteoarthritis and rheumatoid arthritis: *see* CELECOXIB.

Celectol. Antihypertensive: *see* CELIPROLOL.

Celevac. Purgative: *see* METHYLCELLULOSE.

Cellcept. Immunosuppressant for prevention of rejection of kidney or heart transplants: *see* MYCOPHENOLATE.

Celluvisc. Tear substitute: *see* CARMELLOSE.

Ceporex. Antibiotic: *see* CEFALEXIN.

Cerazette. Progestogen-only contraceptive pill (POP): *see* DESOGESTREL.

Cernevit. Parenteral vitamin supplement: *see* BIOTIN, CHOLECALCIFEROL, CYANOCOBALAMIN, FOLIC ACID, GLYCINE, NICOTINAMIDE, PANTOTHENIC ACID, PYRIDOXINE, RIBOFLAVIN, THIAMINE, VITAMIN A, VITAMIN C, VITAMIN E.

Cerumol. Drops for removal of ear wax: *see* ARACHIS OIL, CHLOROBUTANOL, PARADICHLOROBENZENE.

Cetavlex. Topical anti-infective for minor abrasions: *see* CETRIMIDE.

Cetrotide. Hormone release antagonist used in infertility treatment: *see* CETRORELIX.

Chlorasol (d). Solution for cleansing and desloughing of skin ulcers: *see* SODIUM HYPOCHLORITE.

Choragon. Hormone: *see* GONADOTROPHIN.

Cialis (r). For treatment of erectile dysfunction: *see* TADALAFIL.

Cicatrin. Topical anti-infective: *see* BACITRACIN, CYSTEINE, GLYCINE, NEOMYCIN, THREONINE.

Cidomycin. Antibiotic for injection or topical use: *see* GENTAMICIN.

Cilest. Oral contraceptive: *see* ETHINYLESTRADIOL, NORGESTIMATE.

Ciloxan. Antibiotic for treatment of eye infections: *see* CIPROFLOXACIN.

Cipralex. Antidepressant also used for generalized anxiety disorder: *see* ESCITALOPRAM.

Cipramil. Antidepressant: *see* CITALOPRAM.

Ciproxin. Antibiotic: *see* CIPROFLOXACIN.

Citanest. Local anaesthetic for minor surgery: *see* PRILOCAINE.

Citanest with Octapressin. As Citanest plus vasoconstrictor to prolong action: *see* FELYPRESSIN.

Citramag. Purgative for use prior to surgery: *see* MAGNESIUM CITRATE.

Claforan. Antibiotic: *see* CEFOTAXIME.

Clarityn. Antihistamine: *see* LORATADINE.

Clexane. Anticoagulant to reduce the risk of thrombosis after surgery: *see* ENOXAPARIN.

Climagest. Hormone replacement therapy for treatment of menopausal symptoms: *see* ESTRADIOL, NORETHISTERONE.

Climaval. Hormone replacement therapy for relief of menopausal symptoms after hysterectomy: *see* ESTRADIOL.

Climesse. Sex hormone for postmenopausal symptoms and prophylaxis of postmenopausal osteoporosis: *see* ESTRADIOL, NORETHISTERONE.

Clinitar. Cream and shampoo for psoriasis and eczema: *see* COAL TAR.

Clinoril. Non-steroid anti-inflammatory/analgesic: *see* SULINDAC.

Clomid. Sex hormone: *see* CLOMIFENE.

Clopixol. Major tranquillizer administered as long-acting injection: *see* ZUCLOPENTHIXOL.

Clostet. Tetanus vaccine.

Clotam. A non-steroidal anti-inflammatory for migraine: *see* TOLFENAMIC ACID.

Clozaril. Antipsychotic: *see* CLOZAPINE.

CoAprovel. Antihypertensive: *see* HYDROCHLOROTHIAZIDE, IRBESARTAN.

Cobalin-H. Vitamin B$_{12}$ injection for treatment of B$_{12}$-deficient anaemia: *see* HYDROXOCOBALAMIN.

Co-Betaloc. Antihypertensive: *see* HYDROCHLOROTHIAZIDE, METOPROLOL.

Codafen continus (d). Combination analgesic with both rapid- and sustained-release properties: *see* CODEINE, IBUPROFEN.

Codalax. Laxative: *see* CO-DANTHRAMER.

Co-Diovan (r). Antihypertensive: *see* HYDROCHLOROTHIAZIDE, VALSARTAN.

Codipar. Analgesic: *see* CODEINE, PARACETAMOL.

Codis. Soluble analgesic: *see* CO-CODAPRIN.

Cogentin. Anticholinergic/antiparkinsonian: *see* BENZATROPINE.

Colazide. For ulcerative colitis: *see* BALSALAZIDE.

Colestid. For reduction of high blood cholesterol levels: *see* COLESTIPOL.

Colifoam. Corticosteroid in aerosol foam for topical treatment of inflammation of large bowel: *see* HYDROCORTISONE.

Colofac. Antispasmodic for abdominal colic: *see* MEBEVERINE.

Colomycin. Anti-infective: *see* POLYMYXIN B.

Colpermin. Used for intestinal colic: *see* PEPPERMINT OIL.

Combigan (r). Eye drops for chronic open-angle glaucoma or ocular hypertension: *see* BRIMONIDINE, TIMOLOL.

Combivent. For asthma: *see* IPRATROPIUM, SALBUTAMOL.

Combivir. Combination antiviral for use in HIV-positive patients with evidence of immunodeficiency: *see* LAMIVUDINE, ZIDOVUDINE.

Comploment. Sustained-release vitamin preparation for treatment of depression due to pyridoxine deficiency and the oral contraceptive: *see* PYRIDOXINE.

Comtess. Enzyme inhibitor used to control symptoms of Parkinson's disease: *see* ENTACAPONE.

Concavit. Vitamin mixture: *see* ANEURINE, CALCIFEROL, NICOTINAMIDE, PANTOTHENIC ACID, PYRIDOXINE, RIBOFLAVIN, VITAMIN A, VITAMIN C.

Concerta XL. Prolonged-release preparation for attention deficit hyperactivity disorder in children: *see* METHYLPHENIDATE.

Condyline. Topical treatment for genital warts: *see* PODOPHYLLOTOXIN.

Conotrane. Topical anti-infective: *see* BENZALKONIUM, DIMETICONE.

Contigen. Treatment for urinary stress incontinence: *see* COLLAGEN.

Convulex. Anticonvulsant: *see* VALPROIC ACID.

Copaxone. For reduction of frequency and severity of relapses in multiple sclerosis: *see* GLATIRAMER.

Coracten. Antianginal/antihypertensive: *see* NIFEDIPINE.

Cordarone X. Antidysrhythmic: *see* AMIODARONE.

Cordilox. Antianginal/antihypertensive: *see* VERAPAMIL.

Corgard

Corgard. Antihypertensive: *see* NADOLOL.

Corlan. Corticosteroid pellet for aphthous ulcers: *see* HYDROCORTISONE.

Coro-nitro. Oral spray for angina pectoris: *see* GLYCERYL TRINITRATE.

Corsodyl. Topical treatment for gingivitis: *see* CHLORHEXIDINE.

Cosalgesic. Analgesic: *see* CO-PROXAMOL.

Cosmegen Lyovac. Cytotoxic: *see* ACTINOMYCIN D.

Cosopt. Eye drops for glaucoma: *see* DORZOLAMIDE, TIMOLOL.

Cosuric. For gout: *see* ALLOPURINOL.

Covermark (b). Concealing cream: *see* TITANIUM DIOXIDE.

Coversyl. Antihypertensive: *see* PERINDOPRIL.

Coversyl Plus. Antihypertensive: *see* INDAPAMIDE, PERINDOPRIL.

Cozaar. Antihypertensive: *see* LOSARTAN.

Cozaar-comp. Antihypertensive: *see* HYDROCHLOROTHIAZIDE, LOSARTAN.

Cremalgin. Rubefacient: *see* CAPSICUM, GLYCOL SALICYLATE, METHYL NICOTINATE.

Creon. Used with food in pancreatic insufficiency: *see* PANCREATIC ENZYMES.

Crestor (r). To reduce blood cholesterol: *see* ROSUVASTATIN.

Crinone. A vaginal gel to treat infertility and menstrual disorders: *see* PROGESTERONE.

Crixivan. Antiviral for use in HIV-positive patients with evidence of immunodeficiency: *see* INDINAVIR.

Cromogen. For asthma: *see* SODIUM CROMOGLICATE.

Crystapen. Antibiotic: *see* BENZYLPENICILLIN.

Cubicin (r). Antibiotic injection: *see* DAPTOMYCIN.

Cuplex. Topical treatment for removal of warts, corns and callouses: *see* COPPER ACETATE, SALICYLIC ACID.

Curatoderm. Tropical treatment for psoriasis: *see* TACALCITOL.

Curosurf. Treatment for lung damage (respiratory distress syndrome) in premature babies requiring mechanical ventilation: *see* PORACTANT.

Cutivate. Topical treatment for eczema: *see* FLUTICASONE.

Cyclimorph (c). Narcotic analgesic: *see* CYCLIZINE, MORPHINE.

Cyclogest. Suppository for treatment of premenstrual symptoms: *see* PROGESTERONE.

Cyclo-Progynova. Sex hormones for menopausal symptoms: *see* ESTRADIOL, NORGESTREL.

Cyklokapron. Antifibrinolytic: *see* TRANEXAMIC ACID.

Cymbalta (r). Antidepressant also used for diabetic peripheral neuropathic pain: *see* DULOXETINE.

Cymevene. Antiviral: *see* GANCICLOVIR.

Cyprostat. Sex hormone for treatment of prostatic carcinoma: *see* CYPROTERONE.

Cystagon. Treatment for rare genetic kidney disorder (cystinosis): *see* MERCAPTAMINE.

Cystrin. Antispasmodic for treatment of urinary complaints: *see* OXYBUTININ.

Cytacon. For vitamin B_{12} deficiency: *see* CYANOCOBALAMIN.

Cytamen. For vitamin B_{12}-deficient anaemias: *see* CYANOCOBALAMIN.

Cytotec. For prophylaxis of gastric ulceration caused by non-steroid anti-inflammatory drugs: *see* MISOPROSTOL.

D

Daktacort. Topical anti-infective/corticosteroid: *see* HYDROCORTISONE, MICONAZOLE.

Daktarin. Topical antifungal for skin and nails: *see* MICONAZOLE.

Dalacin C. Antibiotic: *see* CLINDAMYCIN.

Dalivit. Multivitamin preparation: *see* ANEURINE, ASCORBIC ACID, CALCIUM PANTOTHENATE, ERGOCALCIFEROL, NICOTINAMIDE, PYRIDOXINE, RIBOFLAVIN, VITAMIN A, VITAMIN D.

Dalmane. Hypnotic: *see* FLURAZEPAM.

Danol. Semi-synthetic steroid used in endometriosis: *see* DANAZOL.

Dantrium. Muscle relaxant: *see* DANTROLENE.

Daonil. Oral hypoglycaemic: *see* GLIBENCLAMIDE.

Daraprim. Antimalarial: *see* PYRIMETHAMINE.

DDAVP. Synthetic antidiuretic hormone: *see* DESMOPRESSIN.

Debrisan. Powder used to aid healing of wounds: *see* DEXTRANOMER.

Deca-Durabolin. Anabolic steroid: *see* NANDROLONE.

Decapeptyl SR. Growth hormone analogue for treatment of advanced prostatic cancer and endometriosis: *see* TRIPTORELIN.

Deltacortril. Corticosteroid tablets or injection: *see* PREDNISOLONE.

Deltacortril Enteric. Corticosteroid. Enteric coating said to reduce gastric irritation: *see* PREDNISOLONE.

Deltastab. Corticosteroid tablets or injection: *see* PREDNISOLONE.

Demser. Antihypertensive: *see* METIROSINE.

De-Noltab. Antacid for treatment of peptic ulcer: *see* TRI-POTASSIUM DI-CITRATO BISMUTHATE.

Dentomycin. Topical antibiotic for dental use: *see* MINOCYCLINE.

Denzapine. Antipsychotic: *see* CLOZAPINE.

Depakote. To treat mania: *see* SODIUM VALPROATE.

Depixol. Major tranquillizer: *see* FLUPENTIXOL.

Depo-Medrone. Corticosteroid for intra-articular/intramuscular injection: *see* METHYLPREDNISOLONE.

Deponit 5. Prophylactic antianginal, formulated as a self-adhesive patch for transdermal absorption: *see* GLYCERYL TRINITRATE.

Depo-Provera. Progestogen, depot injection for endometriosis: *see* MEDROXYPROGESTERONE.

Dequacaine. Local anaesthetic lozenges: *see* BENZOCAINE, DEQUALINIUM.

Dequadin. Antiseptic throat lozenges: *see* DEQUALINIUM.

Dermovate. Topical steroid treatments: *see* CLOBETASOL.

Dermovate-NN (d). Topical corticosteroid/anti-infective: *see* CLOBETASOL, NEOMYCIN, NYSTATIN.

Deseril. Antiserotoninergic: *see* METHYSERGIDE.

Desferal. Chelating agent: *see* DESFERRIOXAMINE.

Desmospray. Metered nasal spray for treatment of diabetes insipidus and nocturnal enuresis: *see* DESMOPRESSIN.

Desmotabs. For nocturnal enuresis: *see* DESMOPRESSIN.

Destolit. Bile acid for dissolution of cholesterol gall stones: *see* URSODEOXYCHOLIC ACID.

Deteclo. Antibiotic: *see* CHLORTETRACYCLINE, DEMECLOCYCLINE, TETRACYCLINE.

Detrunorm. Smooth muscle relaxant with actions on bladder muscle. Reduces urinary incontinence in unstable bladder conditions: *see* PROPIVERINE.

Detrusitol. To control urinary incontinence: *see* TOLTERODINE.

Dettol. Topical antiseptic: *see* CHLOROXYLENOL.

Dexa-Rhinaspray. Nasal spray for allergic or chronic rhinitis: *see* DEXAMETHASONE, NEOMYCIN, TRAMAZOLINE.

Dexedrine (c). CNS stimulant: *see* DEXAMFETAMINE.

DF 118 Forte. Analgesic: *see* DIHYDROCODEINE.

DHC Continus. Sustained-release analgesic: *see* DIHYDROCODEINE.

Diamicron. Oral hypoglycaemic: *see* GLICLAZIDE.

Diamox. Diuretic: *see* ACETAZOLAMIDE.

Diamox SR. Sustained-release diuretic: *see* ACETAZOLAMIDE.

Dianette. Synthetic sex hormones for use in severe acne in women: *see* CYPROTERONE, ETHINYLESTRADIOL.

Diazemuls. Anxiolytic for injection, formulated as an oil-in-water emulsion. May be used in patients where injection of an aqueous solution causes thrombophlebitis or pain during injection: *see* DIAZEPAM.

Dibenyline. Alpha-adrenoceptor blocker: *see* PHENOXYBENZAMINE.

Dicloflex. Non-steroidal anti-inflammatory/analgesic: *see* DICLOFENAC.

Diclomax Retard. Sustained-release, non-steroid anti-inflammatory: *see* DICLOFENAC.

Diconal (c). Analgesic: *see* CYCLIZINE, DIPIPANONE.

Dicynene. Haemostatic: *see* ETAMSYLATE.

Didronel. Used in Paget's disease and osteoporosis: *see* ETIDRONATE DISODIUM.

Differin. Topical treatment for acne: *see* ADAPALENE.

Difflam. Topical, non-steroid anti-inflammatory/analgesic cream: *see* BENZYDAMINE.

Diflucan. Antifungal for oral and vaginal infection: *see* FLUCONAZOLE.

Digibind. Antidote for treatment of life-threatening digoxin toxicity: *see* DIGOXIN-SPECIFIC ANTIBODY.

Dijex. Antacid: *see* ALUMINIUM HYDROXIDE, MAGNESIUM CARBONATE.

Dilzem SR. Sustained-release antihypertensive: *see* DILTIAZEM.

Dimetriose. Synthetic steroid used in endometriosis: *see* GESTRINONE.

Dioctyl. Laxative: *see* DOCUSATE SODIUM.

Dioctyl ear drops. Oil for removal of ear wax: *see* DIOCTYL SODIUM SULPHOSUCCINATE.

Dioderm. Corticosteroid cream for inflammatory and allergic skin conditions: *see* HYDROCORTISONE.

Dioralyte. Electrolytes and dextrose supplied in a powder for reconstitution into a solution. Used orally to correct fluid and electrolyte balance (e.g. due to diarrhoea and vomiting).

Diovan. Antihypertensive: *see* VALSARTAN.

Diovol. Antacid: *see* ALUMINIUM HYDROXIDE, DIMETICONE, MAGNESIUM HYDROXIDE.

Dipentum. For ulcerative colitis: *see* OLSALAZINE.

Diprobase. Cream or ointment for topical application to dry skin: *see* CETOMACROGOL, CETOSTEARYL ALCOHOL, LIQUID PARAFFIN, SOFT PARAFFIN.

Diprosalic. Ointment and lotion for dermatitis: *see* BETAMETHASONE, SALICYLIC ACID.

Diprosone. Topical corticosteroid: *see* BETAMETHASONE.

Disipal. Anticholinergic/antiparkinsonian: *see* ORPHENADRINE.

Disprin CV (d). Sustained-release analgesic to reduce the risk of thrombosis: *see* ACETYLSALICYLIC ACID.

Distaclor. Antibiotic: *see* CEFACLOR.

Distaclor MR. Sustained-release antibiotic: *see* CEFACLOR.

Distalgesic. Analgesic: *see* DEXTROPROPOXYPHENE, PARACETAMOL.

Distamine. Chelating agent used in rheumatoid arthritis: *see* PENICILLAMINE.

Dithrocream. Cream for treatment of quiescent psoriasis: *see* DITHRANOL.

Ditropan. Antispasmodic for treatment of urinary complaints: *see* OXYBUTYNIN.

Diurexan. Diuretic/antihypertensive: *see* XIPAMIDE.

Dixarit. Migraine prophylactic: *see* CLONIDINE.

Dobovet. Topical treatment for psoriasis: *see* BETAMETHASONE, CALCIPOTRIOL.

Docusol. Laxative: *see* DOCUSATE SODIUM.

Dolmatil. Antipsychotic: *see* SULPIRIDE.

Dolobid. Analgesic: *see* DIFLUNISAL.

Doloxene (d). Analgesic: *see* DEXTROPROPOXYPHENE.

Domperamol (d). Antiemetic/analgesic for migraine: *see* DOMPERIDONE, PARACETAMOL.

Dopacard. Infusion for treatment of severe heart failure associated with cardiac surgery: *see* DOPEXAMINE.

Dopram. Respiratory stimulant: *see* DOXAPRAM.

Doralese. For relief of the symptoms of prostatic obstruction to urinary outflow: *see* INDORAMIN.

Dostinex. Dopamine agonist used to suppress lactation and other effects of hyperprolactinaemia: *see* CABERGOLINE.

Double Check. Spermicidal contraceptive: *see* NONOXYNOL.

Dovonex. Topical treatment for psoriasis: *see* CALCIPOTRIOL.

Dozic. Tranquillizer: *see* HALOPERIDOL.

Drapolene. Topical anti-infective: *see* BENZALKONIUM, CETRIMIDE.

Driclor. Topical antiperspirant for hyperhidrosis: *see* ALUMINIUM CHLORIDE.

Drogenil. Acts against male sex hormone (androgens) in treatment of carcinoma of the prostate gland: *see* FLUTAMIDE.

Dromadol. Analgesic: *see* TRAMADOL.

DTIC. Cytotoxic: *see* DACARBAZINE.

Duac. Topical gel to treat acne: *see* BENZOYL PEROXIDE, CLINDAMYIN.

Dubam. Rubefacient, pain-relieving spray: *see* ETHYL SALICYLATE, GLYCOL SALICYLATE, METHYL NICOTINATE, METHYL SALICYLATE.

Dulcolax. Laxative: *see* BISACODYL.

Duodopa (r). Intestinal gel for use with an enteral tube to control severe Parkinson's disease: *see* CO-CARELDOPA.

Duofilm. Topical treatment for warts: *see* LACTIC ACID, SALICYLIC ACID.

Duovent. Bronchodilator for inhalation: *see* FENOTEROL, IPRATROPIUM.

Duphalac. Purgative: *see* LACTULOSE.

Duphaston. For dysmenorrhoea and endometriosis: *see* DYDROGESTERONE.

Duragel (d). Spermicidal jelly used for contraception: *see* NONOXYNOL.

Durogesic Dtrans (c). Transdermal analgesic patch for treatment of chronic intractable pain: *see* FENTANYL.

Dyazide. Diuretic combination: *see* HYDROCHLOROTHIAZIDE, TRIAMTERENE.

Dynastat (r). An intravenous analgesic for short-term treatment of postoperative pain: *see* PARECOXIB.

Dynese. Antacid: *see* MAGALDRATE.

Dyspamet. Gastric histamine receptor blocker; reduces acid secretion: *see* CIMETIDINE.

Dysport. To treat spasms of muscles of the eye and face, focal spasticity in paediatric cerebral palsy patients and upper limb spasticity associated with stroke: *see* BOTULINUM TOXIN A.

Dytac. Diuretic: *see* TRIAMTERENE.

Dytide. Diuretic combination: *see* BENZTHIAZIDE, TRIAMTERENE.

E

E 45 cream. Skin-protective, paraffin-based cream.

Ebixa. To improve cognitive function in mild to moderate Alzheimer's dementia: *see* MEMANTINE.

Ebufac. Non-steroid anti-inflammatory/analgesic: *see* IBUPROFEN.

Econacort. Topical treatment of fungal/bacterial skin infections: *see* ECONAZOLE, HYDROCORTISONE.

Ecostatin. Antifungal for topical use: *see* ECONAZOLE.

Edronax. Antidepressant: *see* REBOXETINE.

Efcortelan. Topical corticosteroid: *see* HYDROCORTISONE.

Efcortesol inj. Intravenous corticosteroid: *see* HYDROCORTISONE.

Efexor. Antidepressant: *see* VENLAFAXINE.

Effercitrate. Effervescent formulation for treatment of cystitis: *see* POTASSIUM CITRATE.

Effico. 'Tonic': *see* ANEURINE, CAFFEINE, NICOTINAMIDE.

Efudix. Cytotoxic: *see* FLUOROURACIL.

Elantan. Antianginal: *see* ISOSORBIDE MONONITRATE.

Elantan LA. Sustained-release antianginal: *see* ISOSORBIDE MONONITRATE.

Elavil. Antidepressant: *see* AMITRIPTYLINE.

Eldepryl. Used with LEVODOPA in treatment of Parkinson's disease: *see* SELEGILINE.

Eldisine. Cytotoxic: *see* VINDESINE.

Electrolade. Oral replacement for electrolyte and fluid loss due to diarrhoea: *see* GLUCOSE, POTASSIUM CHLORIDE, SODIUM BICARBONATE, SODIUM CHLORIDE.

Elemental 028 (b). Dietary substitute for use in malabsorption states and undernourished patients.

Elidel (r). Topical cream for treatment of eczema (atopic dermatitis). Used short term (in flare-ups) or intermittently in the longer term but not approved for continuous use: *see* PIMECROLIMUS.

Elleste Duet. Hormone replacement therapy for postmenopausal symptoms and prophylaxis of postmenopausal osteoporosis: *see* ESTRADIOL, NORETHISTERONE.

Ellest Solo. Hormone replacement therapy for postmenopausal symptoms and prophylaxis of postmenopausal osteoporosis: *see* ESTRADIOL.

Elocon. Topical corticosteroid: *see* MOMETASONE.

Eloxatin. Cytotoxic: *see* OXALIPLATIN.

Eltroxin. Thyroid hormone: *see* LEVOTHYROXINE.

Eludril. Antiseptic solution/aerosol for oral infections: *see* CHLORHEXIDINE, CHLOROBUTANOL.

Elyzol. Antibiotic dental gel: *see* METRONIDAZOLE.

Emadine. Antihistamine eye drops to relieve hay fever symptoms: *see* EMEDASTINE.

Emcor. Antihypertensive, antianginal: *see* BISOPROLOL.

Emend (r). Antiemetic for use with cancer chemotherapy. Used only in combination with an antihistamine antiemetic (e.g. ONDANSETRON) and a corticosteroid (e.g. DEXAMETHASONE): *see* APREPITANT.

Emeside. Anticonvulsant: *see* ETHOSUXIMIDE.

Emflex. Non-steroid anti-inflammatory/analgesic: *see* ACEMETACIN.

Emla. Local anaesthetic cream for topical application in children to alleviate the pain of venepuncture: *see* LIDOCAINE, PRILOCAINE.

Emtriva (r). Oral antiviral for use in combination with other antiviral agents, in HIV-positive patients with evidence of immunodeficiency: *see* EMTRICITABINE.

Emulsiderm. Soothing, protective skin cream: *see* BENZALKONIUM, LIQUID PARAFFIN.

Enbrel (r). Antirheumatic, also used for severe psoriasis: *see* ETANERCEPT.

En-De-Kay. For prevention of dental caries: *see* SODIUM FLUORIDE.

Endoxana. Cytotoxic: *see* CYCLOPHOSPHAMIDE.

Engerix B. Genetically engineered vaccine for immunization against infective hepatitis (type B): *see* HEPATITIS B VACCINE.

Enrich (b). Liquid feed for enteral absorption.

Ensure (b). Liquid source of calories for oral nutrition in debilitating conditions.

Entocort CR. Controlled-release oral corticosteroid for treatment of Crohn's disease: *see* BUDESONIDE.

Epanutin. Anticonvulsant: *see* PHENYTOIN.

Ephynal. Vitamin preparation.

Epilim. Anticonvulsant: *see* SODIUM VALPROATE.

Epivir. Antiviral for use in HIV-positive patients with evidence of immunodeficiency: *see* LAMIVUDINE.

Eprex. Hormone treatment for anaemia in chronic renal failure or anaemia caused by chemotherapy: *see* EPOETIN ALFA.

Equasym (c). For attention deficit hyperactivity disorder: *see* METHYLPHENIDATE.

Erbitux (r). For the treatment of metastatic colorectal cancer in combination with IRINOTECAN: *see* CETUXIMAB.

Eryacne. Topical treatment for acne: *see* ERYTHROMYCIN.

Erymax. Antibiotic: *see* ERYTHROMYCIN.

Erythrocin. Antibiotic: *see* ERYTHROMYCIN.

Erythroped. Antibiotic: *see* ERYTHROMYCIN.

Eskamel. Cream for acne: *see* RESORCINOL, SULPHUR.

Eskornade. Anticholinergic/sympathomimetic/antihistamine mixture for symptomatic treatment of common

Esmeron

cold: *see* DIPHENYLPYRALINE, PHENYLPROPANOLAMINE.

Esmeron. Nondepolarizing skeletal muscle relaxant derived from VECURONIUM: *see* ROCURONIUM.

Estracombi. Transdermal patches for HRT: *see* ESTRADIOL, NORETHISTERONE.

Estracyt. Cytotoxic for carcinoma of the prostate: *see* ESTRAMUSTINE PHOSPHATE.

Estraderm. Oestrogen replacement therapy: *see* ESTRADIOL.

Estradot. Transdermal patches for menopausal symptoms and osteoporosis prophylaxis: *see* ESTRADIOL.

Estring. Hormone for vaginal application in postmenopausal vaginitis: *see* ESTRADIOL.

Ethyol. Cytoprotective used to reduce adverse effects of anticancer drugs: *see* AMIFOSTINE.

Eucardic (r). Antihypertensive and antianginal; also used for chronic cardiac failure: *see* CARVEDILOL.

Eudemine. Antihypertensive/ hyperglycaemic: *see* DIAZOXIDE.

Euglucon (d). Oral hypoglycaemic: *see* GLIBENCLAMIDE.

Eumovate. Corticosteroid eye drops: cream or ointment for skin: *see* CLOBETASONE.

Eumovate-N. As Eumovate plus: *see* NEOMYCIN.

Eurax. Topical antipruritic: *see* CROTAMITON.

Eurax-hydrocortisone. As Eurax plus: *see* HYDROCORTISONE.

Evista. Used to treat and prevent postmenopausal bone loss: *see* RALOXIFENE.

Evorel. Transdermal patch for HRT and prevention of osteoporosis: *see* ESTRADIOL.

Evorel Conti/Evorel Sequi. For hormone replacement therapy and prevention of osteoporosis: *see* ESTRADIOL, NORETHISTERONE.

Evra (r). Contraceptive transdermal patch: *see* ETHINYLESTRADIOL, NORELGESTROMIN.

Exelderm. Topical antifungal for skin infections: *see* SULCONAZOLE.

Exelon. To improve cognitive function in mild to moderate Alzheimer's dementia and dementia in idiopathic Parkinson's disease: *see* RIVASTIGMINE.

Exocin. Topical ophthalmic antibacterial: *see* OFLOXACIN.

Exorex. Topical treatment for psoriasis and other exezematous conditions: *see* COAL TAR.

Expulin. Cough linctus: *see* CHLORPHENAMINE, MENTHOL, PHOLCODINE, PSEUDOEPHEDRINE.

Exterol. Drops for removal of ear wax: *see* UREA HYDROGEN PEROXIDE.

Exubera. Fast-acting human INSULIN used by inhalation.

Ezetrol (r). Absorption inhibitor used to reduce blood cholesterol: *see* EZETIMIBE.

F

Famvir. Antiviral: *see* FAMCICLOVIR.

Fansidar. Antimalarial: *see* PYRIMETHAMINE, SULFADOXINE.

Fareston. For treatment of breast cancer: *see* TOREMIFENE.

Farlutal. Sex hormone for treatment of hormone-dependent malignancies: *see* MEDROXYPROGESTERONE.

Fasigyn. Antimicrobial: *see* TINIDAZOLE.

Faslodex (r). Cytotoxic drug for breast cancer: *see* FULVESTRANT.

Faverin. Antidepressant: *see* FLUVOXAMINE.

Fectrim. Antibacterial: *see* CO-TRIMOXAZOLE.

Fefol Spansule. Slow-release haematinic: *see* FERROUS SULPHATE, FOLIC ACID.

Fefol Z. Sustained-release haematinic: *see* FERROUS SULPHATE, FOLIC ACID, ZINC SULPHATE.

Feldene. Non-steroid anti-inflammatory/analgesic: *see* PIROXICAM.

Femara (r). For treatment of breast cancer: *see* LETROZOLE.

Fematrix. Transdermal patch for HRT and prevention of osteoporosis: *see* ESTRADIOL.

Femodene. Oral contraceptive: *see* ETHINYLESTRADIOL, GESTODENE.

Femoston. Sex hormones for postmenopausal symptoms and prophylaxis of postmenopausal osteoporosis: *see* DYDROGESTERONE, ESTRADIOL.

Femseven. Sex hormone for postmenopausal symptoms and prophylaxis of postmenopausal osteoporosis: *see* ESTRADIOL.

Femulen. Oral contraceptive: *see* ETYNODIOL.

Fenbid. Sustained-release non-steroid anti-inflammatory/analgesic: *see* IBUPROFEN.

Fenogal. For hyperlipidaemia: *see* FENOFIBRATE.

Fenopron. Non-steroid anti-inflammatory/analgesic: *see* FENOPROFEN.

Fentazin. Tranquillizer/antiemetic: *see* PERPHENAZINE.

Feospan Spansule. Slow-release haematinic: *see* FERROUS SULPHATE.

Ferfolic SV. Haematinic: *see* FERROUS GLUCONATE, FOLIC ACID.

Ferriprox. For iron overload in patients with thalassaemia: *see* DEFERIPRONE.

Ferrograd C. Slow-release haematinic/vitamin: *see* FERROUS SULPHATE, VITAMIN C.

Ferrograd Folic. Slow-release haematinic: *see* FERROUS SULPHATE, FOLIC ACID.

Fersaday. Slow-release haematinic: *see* FERROUS FUMARATE.

Fersamal. Haematinic: *see* FERROUS FUMARATE.

Filair. Steroid aerosol for asthma: *see* BECLOMETASONE.

Flagyl. Antibacterial: *see* METRONIDAZOLE.

Flagyl Compak. Anti-infective: *see* METRONIDAZOLE, NYSTATIN.

Flagyl-S. Antibacterial suspension: *see* BENZOYLMETRONIDAZOLE.

Flamazine. Anti-infective cream for burns: *see* SILVER SULFADIAZINE.

Flaxedil. Muscle relaxant: *see* GALLAMINE.

Fleet. Enema and oral purgative for use prior to surgery: *see* SODIUM ACID PHOSPHATE.

Fletcher's Phosphate Enema. Purgative: *see* SODIUM ACID PHOSPHATE, SODIUM PHOSPHATE.

Flexin continus (d). Sustained-release non-steroidal anti-inflammatory/ analgesic: *see* INDOMETACIN.

Flixonase. Intranasal steroid for allergic rhinitis and symptoms of nasal obstruction: *see* FLUTICASONE.

Flixotide. Corticosteroid inhalation for prevention of asthma: *see* FLUTICASONE.

Flolan (r). Anticoagulant: *see* EPOPROSTENOL.

Flomax MR (d). For treatment of benign hypertrophy of the prostate gland: *see* TAMSULOSIN.

Florinef. Adrenocorticosteroid: *see* FLUDROCORTISONE.

Floxapen. Antibiotic: *see* FLUCLOXACILLIN.

Fluanxol. Antidepressant/tranquillizer: *see* FLUPENTIXOL.

Fludara. Cytotoxic: *see* FLUDARABINE.

Fluor-a-Day. For prevention of dental caries: *see* SODIUM FLUORIDE.

Fluorigard. For prevention of dental caries: *see* SODIUM FLUORIDE.

Fluvirin (d). Influenza vaccine for immunization.

FML. Corticosteroid eye drops: *see* FLUOROMETHOLONE.

FML-Neo. Topical corticosteroid/ antibiotic: *see* FLUOROMETHOLONE, NEOMYCIN.

Foradil. Selective beta-adrenoceptor agonist for treatment of asthma: *see* FORMOTEROL.

Forceval. Multivitamin and mineral supplement.

Forceval protein (b). Protein, vitamin and mineral supplements for low sodium/ low-fat diets.

Forsteo (r). Recombinant fragment of PARATHYROID HORMONE used to increase bone strength in patients with osteoporosis: *see* TERIPARATIDE.

Fortipine LA. Antihypertensive, antianginal: *see* NIFEDIPINE.

Fortovase (d). Antiviral: *see* SAQUINAVIR.

Fortral (c). Analgesic: *see* PENTAZOCINE.

Fortum. Antibiotic: *see* CEFTAZIDIME.

Fosamax. Biphosphonate to reduce risk of bone fractures in osteoporosis: *see* ALENDRONIC ACID.

Fosavance (r). For postmenopausal osteoporosis: *see* ALENDRONIC ACID, COLECALCIFEROL.

Foscavir. Antiviral used to treat cytomegalovirus (CMV) retinitis in patients with AIDS: *see* FOSCARNET.

Fosfor. 'Tonic': *see* PHOSPHORYLCOLAMINE.

Fragmin. Anticoagulant used to prevent blood clotting during haemodialysis or haemofiltration and for treatment of patients with unstable coronary artery disease, deep vein thrombosis or pulmonary embolism: *see* HEPARIN.

Franol. Bronchodilator/sedative: *see* EPHEDRINE, THEOPHYLLINE.

Franol plus. As Franol.

Fre Amine. Amino acids and electrolytes for intravenous nutrition.

Fresubin (b). Liquid feed. Protein, fat and carbohydrate plus vitamins and electrolytes. For oral feeding when absorption of nutrients and vitamins is impaired.

Frisium. Anxiolytic/anticonvulsant: *see* CLOBAZAM.

Froben. Non-steroid anti-inflammatory analgesic: *see* FLURBIPROFEN.

Fru-Co. Diuretic combination: *see* CO-AMILOFRUSE.

Frumil. Diuretic combination: *see* AMILORIDE, FUROSEMIDE.

Frusene. Diuretic combination: *see* FUROSEMIDE, TRIAMTERENE.

Frusol. Diuretic: *see* FUROSEMIDE.

Fucibet. Topical cream for skin infections: *see* BETAMETHASONE, FUSIDIC ACID.

Fucidin. Antibiotic: *see* FUSIDIC ACID.

Fucidin H oint. and gel. Topical anti-infective/corticosteroid: *see* FUSIDIC ACID, HYDROCORTISONE.

Fucithalmic. Antibacterial eye drops: *see* GENTAMICIN.

Full Marks. Shampoo for head lice: *see* PHENOTHRIN.

Fungilin. Antifungal: *see* AMPHOTERICIN.

Fungizone intravenous. Antifungal injection: *see* AMPHOTERICIN.

Furadantin. Urinary anti-infective: *see* NITROFURANTOIN.

Fuzeon (r). Antiviral injection for use in combination with other antiviral agents in HIV-positive patients with evidence of immunodeficiency: *see* ENFUVIRTIDE.

Fybogel. Laxative for diverticular disease, constipation: *see* ISPAGHULA HUSK.

Fybogel mebeverine. Purgative/antispasmodic for treatment of bowel dysfunction and abdominal pain (e.g. irritable bowel syndrome): *see* ISPAGHULA, MEBEVERINE.

G

Gabitril. Anticonvulsant: *see* TIAGABINE.

Galactomin Preps (b). Low-lactose dietary supplement.

Galcodine. Cough suppressant: *see* CODEINE.

Galenphol. Cough suppressant: *see* PHOLCODINE.

Galfer and Galfer FA. For iron and folic acid-deficiency anaemias: *see* FERROUS FUMARATE, FOLIC ACID.

Galpseud. Linctus for hay fever and similar allergic conditions: *see* CHLORPHENAMINE, PSEUDOEPHEDRINE.

Gamanil. Antidepressant: *see* LOFEPRAMINE.

Gastrobid Continus (d). Sustained-release antiemetic: *see* METOCLOPRAMIDE.

Gastrocote. Antacid: *see* ALGINATE, ALUMINIUM HYDROXIDE, MAGNESIUM TRISILICATE, SODIUM BICARBONATE.

Gaviscon. Antacid: *see* ALGINATE, ALUMINIUM HYDROXIDE, MAGNESIUM TRISILICATE, SODIUM BICARBONATE.

Gaviscon advance. Antacid: *see* ALGINATES, POTASSIUM BICARBONATE.

Gaviscon Liquid. As Gaviscon with CALCIUM CARBONATE.

Gelofusine. Plasma expander: *see* GELATIN, SODIUM CHLORIDE.

Gelusil. Antacid: *see* ALUMINIUM HYDROXIDE, MAGNESIUM TRISILICATE.

Gemzar. Cytotoxic for treatment of lung cancer and breast cancer: *see* GEMCITABINE.

Genotropin. Synthetic growth hormone for treatment of short stature: *see* SOMATROPIN.

Genticin. Antibiotic for topical and parenteral use: *see* GENTAMICIN.

Genticin HC. As Genticin with HYDROCORTISONE.

Gentisone HC. Anti-inflammatory/anti-infective drops for outer ear: *see* GENTAMICIN, HYDROCORTISONE.

Gentran. Plasma expander: *see* DEXTRANS, SODIUM CHLORIDE.

Gentran 40/Gentran 70. Plasma expanders: *see* DEXTRANS.

Geref. Hormone: *see* SERMORELIN.

Givitol. Compound iron and vitamin preparation.

Glandosane. Solution of cellulose derivative and salts similar to saliva for dry mouth: *see* CARMELLOSE.

Glibenese. Oral hypoglycaemic: *see* GLIPIZIDE.

Glivec (r). Enzyme inhibitor which reduces proliferation in leukaemic cells. Used to treat chronic myeloid leukaemia: *see* IMATINIB.

Glucagen. Hyperglycaemic: *see* GLUCAGON.

Glucobay. Oral hypoglycaemic: *see* ACARBOSE.

Glucophage. Oral hypoglycaemic: *see* METFORMIN.

Glurenorm. Oral antidiabetic: *see* GLIQUIDONE.

Glutarol. Topical treatment for warts: *see* GLUTARALDEHYDE.

Glypressin. Hormone: *see* TERLIPRESSIN.

Glytrin. Antianginal: *see* GLYCERYL TRINITRATE.

Golden Eye. Antibacterial for eye infections: *see* DIBROMPROPAMIDINE.

Gopten. Antihypertensive: *see* TRANDOLAPRIL.

Graneodin. Antibiotic: *see* GRAMICIDIN, NEOMYCIN.

Granocyte. To raise neutrophil blood cell count in patients undergoing cytotoxic chemotherapy: *see* LENOGRASTIM.

Gregoderm (d). Topical anti-infective/corticosteroid: *see* HYDROCORTISONE, NEOMYCIN, NYSTATIN, POLYMYXIN B.

Grisol. Topical antifungal spray for athlete's foot: *see* GRISEOFULVIN.

GTN 300. Antianginal/vasodilator: *see* GLYCERYL TRINITRATE.

Gyno-Daktarin. Local application for vaginal and penile fungal infections: *see* MICONAZOLE.

Gynol II (d). Spermicidal jelly used for contraception: *see* NONOXYNOL.

Gyno-Pevaryl. Antifungal for topical treatment of vaginal infections: *see* ECONAZOLE.

H

Haelan. Topical corticosteroid: *see* FLUDROXYCORTIDE.

Haemaccel. Plasma expander: *see* GELATIN, SODIUM CHLORIDE.

Halciderm. Topical corticosteroid for skin disorders: *see* HALCINONIDE.

Haldol. Tranquillizer: *see* HALOPERIDOL.

Half Securon SR. Sustained-release antihypertensive and antianginal: *see* VERAPAMIL.

Halycitrol. Vitamins for injection: *see* VITAMIN A, VITAMIN D.

Havrix. Vaccine for immunization against infective hepatitis (type A): *see* HEPATITIS A VACCINE.

Haymine. For hay fever and similar allergic conditions: *see* CHLORPHENAMINE, EPHEDRINE.

Healonid. High-viscosity polymer solution for injection into eye during ophthalmic surgery: *see* SODIUM HYALURONATE.

Hedrin. For treatment of head lice: *see* DIMETICONE.

Hemabate. Synthetic prostaglandin used to treat maternal bleeding after birth: *see* CARBOPROST.

Heminevrin. Sedative/hypnotic: *see* CLOMETHIAZOLE.

Hepsal. Anticoagulant: *see* HEPARIN.

Hepsera (r). Antiviral to treat chronic hepatitis B: *see* ADEFOVIR.

Herceptin (r). Cytotoxic for treatment of breast cancer: *see* TRASTUZUMAB.

Herpetad. Antiviral: see ACICLOVIR.

Herpid. Antiviral: *see* DIMETHYL SULFOXIDE, IDOXURIDINE.

Hexalen. Cytotoxic: *see* ALTRETAMINE.

Hexopal. Peripheral vasodilator: *see* INOSITOL NICOTINATE.

Hibicet hospital concentrate. Antiseptic: *see* CETRIMIDE, CHLORHEXIDINE.

Hibiscrub. Antiseptic cleansing solution for pre-operative preparation of hands: *see* CHLORHEXIDINE.

Hibisol. Topical disinfectant used undiluted for hand and skin disinfection: *see* CHLORHEXIDINE.

Hibitane cream. Antiseptic for prevention of skin infection: *see* CHLORHEXIDINE.

HibTITER. Vaccine: *see* HAEMOPHILUS INFLUENZA TYPE B VACCINE.

Hioxyl (d). Antiseptic for cleaning infected wounds: *see* HYDROGEN PEROXIDE.

Hiprex. Urinary anti-infective: *see* METHENAMINE.

Hirudoid. Anticoagulant cream for bruising associated with superficial thrombophlebitis or trauma: *see* HEPARIN.

Histalix. Decongestant: *see* AMMONIUM CHLORIDE, DIPHENHYDRAMINE, MENTHOL, SODIUM CITRATE.

Hivid (d). Antiviral for use in advanced AIDS: *see* ZALCITABINE.

Hormonin. Sex hormones for menopausal symptoms: *see* ESTRADIOL, ESTRIOL, ESTRONE.

HRF. For diagnostic use in delayed sexual development and failure of pituitary gland function: *see* GONADORELIN.

Human Insulatard. Semi-synthetic human insulin made by biochemical conversion of porcine insulin: *see* INSULIN.

Human Mixtard 30/70. Semi-synthetic human insulin made by biochemical conversion of porcine insulin: *see* INSULIN.

Human Monotard. Long-acting synthetic human insulin (zinc suspension): *see* INSULIN.

Human Ultratard. Long-acting human insulin, prepared by modification of porcine insulin: *see* INSULIN.

Human Velosulin. Semi-synthetic human insulin made by biochemical conversion of porcine insulin: *see* INSULIN.

Humatrope. Synthetic human growth hormone used to treat growth failure due to growth hormone deficiency: *see* SOMATROPIN.

Humira (r). Cytokine injection used to treat symptoms of severe rheumatoid arthritis: *see* ADALIMUMAB.

Humulin. Human insulins manufactured by genetic engineering using bacteria. Humulin S – soluble insulin, Humulin I –

isophane insulin, Humulin M2, M3, M5 – mixed soluble and isophane insulins, Humulin Zn – insulin zinc suspension: *see* INSULIN.

Hyalgan. Intra-articular injection used to relieve pain of osteoarthritis of the knee: *see* HYALURONIC ACID.

Hycamtin. Cytotoxic for treatment of ovarian cancer: *see* TOPOTECAN.

Hydergine (d). For impaired mental function in the elderly: *see* CO-DERGOCRINE.

Hydrea. Cytotoxic: *see* HYDROXYCARBAMIDE.

Hydrocortistab. Corticosteroid for parenteral or topical use: *see* HYDROCORTISONE.

Hydromol. Water-dispersible bath additive for use on dry skin conditions: *see* LIQUID PARAFFIN.

Hygroton. Diuretic: *see* CHLORTALIDONE.

Hypnomidate. Intravenous anaesthetic: *see* ETOMIDATE.

Hypnovel. Intravenous sedative used before and during minor surgery: *see* MIDAZOLAM.

Hypotears (d). Eye drops for dry eyes: *see* POLYETHYLENE GLYCOL, POLYVINYL ALCOHOL.

Hypovase. Antihypertensive: *see* PRAZOSIN.

Hypurin Bovine. Purified beef insulin: *see* INSULIN.

Hypurin Isophane. Long-acting purified insulin: *see* INSULIN.

Hypurin Lente. Long-acting purified beef insulin (zinc suspension): *see* INSULIN.

Hypurin Neutral

Hypurin Neutral. Purified crystalline insulin: *see* INSULIN.

Hypurin Porcine. Purified pork insulin: *see* INSULIN.

Hypurin Protamine Zinc. Long-acting purified insulin: *see* INSULIN.

Hytrin. Antihypertensive: *see* TERAZOSIN.

I J K

Ibugel. Topical non-steroid anti-inflammatory/analgesic: *see* IBUPROFEN.

Ibuspray. Non-steroid analgesic in a metered-dose pump spray: *see* IBUPROFEN.

Icthaband. Topical treatment for eczema: *see* ZINC ICHTHAMMOL.

Ikorel. Antianginal: *see* NICORANDIL.

Ilosone (d). Antibiotic: *see* ERYTHROMYCIN.

Ilube. Eye drops for dry eyes: *see* ACETYLCYSTEINE, HYPROMELLOSE.

Imazin XL/Imazin XL Forte (d). Antianginal combined with analgesic to reduce the risk of thrombosis: *see* ASPIRIN, ISOSORBIDE MONONITRATE.

Imdur. Sustained-release antianginal: *see* ISOSORBIDE MONONITRATE.

Imigran. For acute migraine: *see* SUMATRIPTAN.

Immukin. For treatment of chronic granulomatous disease: *see* INTERFERON GAMMA.

Imodium. Antidiarrhoeal: *see* LOPERAMIDE.

Imunovir. For oral treatment of herpes simplex viral infections: *see* INOSINE PRANOBEX.

Imuran. Cytotoxic: *see* AZATHIOPRINE.

Inderal. Beta-adrenoceptor blocker: *see* PROPRANOLOL.

Inderal LA. Sustained-release antihypertensive: *see* PROPRANOLOL.

Indivina. HRT for treatment of menopausal symptoms and prophylaxis of postmenopausal symptoms: *see* ESTRADIOL, MEDROXYPROGESTERONE.

Indocid PDA. To treat heart defects in premature babies: *see* INDOMETACIN.

Indolar SR. Non-steroid anti-inflammatory/analgesic: *see* INDOMETACIN.

Indomod (d). Non-steroid anti-inflammatory/analgesic: *see* INDOMETACIN.

Inegy (r). For treatment of primary hypercholesterolaemia or mixed hyperlipidaemia: *see* EZETIMIBE, SIMVASTATIN.

Infacol. For relief of infantile colic: *see* SIMETICONE.

Infadrops. Antipyretic for infants: *see* PARACETAMOL.

Influvac. Inactivated influenza virus vaccine.

161

Innohep

Innohep. Anticoagulant to treat, or reduce the risk of, thrombosis after surgery: *see* TINZAPARIN.

Innovace. Antihypertensive: *see* ENALAPRIL.

Innozide. Antihypertensive: *see* ENALAPRIL, HYDROCHLOROTHIAZIDE.

Inspra (r). Used to reduce morbidity and mortality after myocardial infarction: *see* EPLERENONE.

Instillagel. Local anaesthetic/antiseptic gel for use in urethral catheterization and cystoscopy: *see* CHLORHEXIDINE, LIDOCAINE.

Insulatard. Long-acting purified pork (isophane) insulin: *see* INSULIN.

Intal. For asthma: *see* SODIUM CROMOGLICATE.

Integrilin. To prevent coronary thrombosis and myocardial infarction: *see* EPTIFIBATIDE.

Intralipid. High-energy source (fats) for intravenous feeding.

IntronA. For treatment of 'hairy cell' leukaemia, non-Hodgkin's lymphoma, malignant melanoma and chronic active hepatitis: *see* INTERFERON ALPHA-2B.

Invanz (r). Intravenous antibiotic: *see* ERTAPENEM.

Invirase. Antiviral: *see* SAQUINAVIR.

Iodosorb. Iodine-releasing preparation used as antiseptic in skin ulcers.

Iopidine. Alpha$_2$ agonist for control of raised intraocular pressure following laser surgery to the eye: *see* APRACLONIDINE.

Ipocol. For ulcerative colitis: *see* MESALAZINE.

Isib 60XL. Antianginal: *see* ISOSORBIDE MONONITRATE.

Ismelin. Antihypertensive: *see* GUANETHIDINE.

Ismo 20. Antianginal: *see* ISOSORBIDE MONONITRATE.

Isogel. Purgative: *see* ISPAGHULA.

Isoket retard. Vasodilator: *see* ISOSORBIDE DINITRATE.

Isomil (b). Milk-free replacement feed for milk-intolerant patients.

Isopto alkaline. Lubricant ('artificial tears') for dry eyes: *see* HYPROMELLOSE.

Isopto carbachol (d). Miotic eye drops for glaucoma: *see* CARBACHOL, HYPROMELLOSE.

Isopto frin (d). Lubricant/decongestant for inflamed (but not infected) eye: *see* METHYLCELLULOSE, PHENYLEPHRINE.

Isopto plain. Lubricant ('artificial tears') for dry eyes: *see* HYPROMELLOSE.

Isotard XL. Sustained-release antianginal: *see* ISOSORBIDE MONONITRATE.

Isotrex. Topical vitamin A derivative: *see* ISOTRETINOIN.

Isotrexin. Topical treatment for acne: *see* ERYTHROMYCIN, ISOTRETINOIN.

Isovorin (r). Reduces toxic effects of cytotoxic folic acid antagonists such as methotrexate drugs and 5-fluoruracil in treatment of colorectal cancer: *see* CALCIUM LEVOFOLINATE.

Ispagel. Laxative: *see* ISPAGHULA.

Istin. Antihypertensive/antianginal: *see* AMLODIPINE.

Juvela (b). GLUTEN-free bread/cake mix.

Kaletra. Antiviral: *see* LOPINAVIR, RITONAVIR.

Kalspare. Diuretic combination: *see* CHLORTALIDONE, TRIAMTERENE.

Kalten. Antihypertensive: *see* AMILORIDE, ATENOLOL, HYDROCHLOROTHIAZIDE.

Kamillosan oint. Topical preparation for sore skin: *see* CHAMOMILE OIL.

Kaodene. Antidiarrhoeal: *see* CODEINE, KAOLIN.

Kapake. Effervescent, soluble analgesic: *see* CODEINE, PARACETAMOL.

Karvol. Inhalation for nasal congestion: *see* MENTHOL.

Kay-Cee-L. Potassium supplement: *see* POTASSIUM CHLORIDE.

Kefadim. Antibiotic: *see* CEFTAZIDIME.

Keflex. Antibiotic: *see* CEFALEXIN.

Keftid. Antibiotic: *see* CEFACLOR.

Kelocyanor (d). Antidote for cyanide poisoning: *see* DICOBALT EDETATE.

Kemadrin. Antiparkinsonian: *see* PROCYCLIDINE.

Kenalog. Corticosteroid injection for allergic conditions: *see* TRIAMCINOLONE.

Kentera (r). For urinary frequency, urge frequency and urge incontinence: *see* OXYBUTYNIN.

Keppra (r). Anticonvulsant: *see* LEVETIRACETAM.

Keral. Non-steroid anti-inflammatory/analgesic: *see* DEXKETOPROFEN.

Keri. Lotion for dry skin: *see* MINERAL OIL.

Keromask (b). Concealing cream: *see* TITANIUM DIOXIDE.

Kest. Purgative: *see* MAGNESIUM SULPHATE, PHENOLPHTHALEIN.

Ketalar. Anaesthetic: *see* KETAMINE.

Ketek (r). Antibiotic: *see* TELITHROMYCIN.

Ketovite. Vitamin mixture: *see* ACETOMENAPHTHONE, ANEURINE, BIOTIN, FOLIC ACID, INOSITOL, NICOTINAMIDE, PANTOTHENIC ACID, PYRIDOXINE, RIBOFLAVIN, VITAMIN C, VITAMIN E.

Ketovite Liquid. As Ketovite with CYANOCOBALAMIN.

Kineret (r). Interleukin receptor antagonist used to treat signs and symptoms of rheumatoid arthritis: *see* ANAKINRA.

Kinidin Durules. Sustained-release antidysrhythmic: *see* QUINIDINE.

Kivexa (r). For HIV infection in combination with other antiretroviral treatment: *see* ABACAVIR, LAMIVUDINE.

Klaricid. Antibiotic: *see* CLARITHROMYCIN.

Klean-Prep. For rapid bowel clearance prior to examination or surgery: *see* POLYETHYLENE GLYCOL.

Kliofem. Female sex hormones for menopausal symptoms (HRT): *see* ESTRADIOL, NORETHISTERONE.

KLN. Antidiarrhoeal: *see* KAOLIN.

Kloref. Effervescent potassium supplement: *see* POTASSIUM BENZOATE, POTASSIUM BICARBONATE, POTASSIUM CHLORIDE.

Kogenate. Recombinant human clotting factor used in treatment of haemophilia: *see* FACTOR VIII.

Kolanticon. Antacid/antispasmodic: *see* ALUMINIUM HYDROXIDE, DICYCLOVERINE, MAGNESIUM OXIDE, SIMETICONE.

Konakion. For prothrombin deficiency: *see* PHYTOMENADIONE.

Konakion MM Paediatric (r). To prevent haemorrhagic disease in the newborn: *see* VITAMIN K.

Konsyl. Laxative: *see* ISPAGHULA.

Kytril. Antiemetic for treatment of nausea and vomiting induced by cytotoxic chemotherapy: *see* GRANISETRON.

L

Labiton. 'Tonic': *see* ANEURINE, CAFFEINE.

Labosept. Oral antiseptic: *see* DEQUALINIUM.

Lacri-Lube. Lubricant eye ointment for dry eyes: *see* HYDROUS WOOL FAT, LIQUID PARAFFIN.

Lacticare. Skin lotion: *see* LACTIC ACID, SODIUM PYRROLIDONE-CARBOXYLATE.

Ladropen. Antibiotic: *see* FLUCLOXACILLIN.

Lamictal. Anticonvulsant: *see* LAMOTRIGINE.

Lamisil. Antifungal: *see* TERBINAFINE.

Lanoxin. For cardiac failure: *see* DIGOXIN.

Lantus (r). Human insulin analogue to treat diabetes: *see* INSULIN.

Lanvis. Cytotoxic: *see* TIOGUANINE.

Largactil. Major tranquillizer/ antiemetic/ antivertigo: *see* CHLORPROMAZINE.

Lariam. Antimalarial: *see* MEFLOQUINE.

Lasikal. Diuretic with potassium supplement: *see* FUROSEMIDE, POTASSIUM CHLORIDE.

Lasilactone. Combination of two diuretics with different modes of action for use in refractory oedema: *see* FUROSEMIDE, SPIRONOLACTONE.

Lasix. Diuretic: *see* FUROSEMIDE.

Lasonil. Topical treatment for soft-tissue injury: *see* HEPARINOID, HYALURONIDASE.

Lasoride. Diuretic combination: *see* CO-AMILOFRUSE.

Laxoberal. Purgative: *see* SODIUM PICOSULFATE.

Ledclair. For heavy metal poisoning: *see* SODIUM CALCIUM EDETATE.

Lederfen. Non-steroid anti-inflammatory/ analgesic: *see* FENBUFEN.

Lederfolin. Antagonizes antifolate cytotoxic drugs: *see* FOLINIC ACID.

Ledermycin. Antibiotic: *see* DEMECLOCYCLINE.

Lescol. Used to reduce blood cholesterol levels: *see* FLUVOSTATIN.

Leukeran. Cytotoxic: *see* CHLORAMBUCIL.

Leustat. Cytotoxic used to treat leukaemia: *see* CLADRIBINE.

Levemire (r). Long-acting human INSULIN analogue.

Levitra (r). For treatment of erectile dysfunction: *see* VARDENAFIL.

Lexpec. Haematinic: *see* FOLIC ACID.

Lexpec with Iron. Haematinic: *see* FERRIC AMMONIUM CITRATE, FOLIC ACID.

Librium. Anxiolytic: *see* CHLORDIAZEPOXIDE.

Limclair. Increases calcium excretion: *see* SODIUM EDETATE.

Lioresal. Muscle relaxant: *see* BACLOFEN.

Lipantil. For hyperlipidaemia: *see* FENOFIBRATE.

Lipitor. To reduce blood cholesterol: *see* ATORVASTATIN.

Lipobase. Bland cream for dry skin, eczema and other itchy conditions: *see* CETOMACROGOL, CETOSTEARYL ALCOHOL, LIQUID PARAFFIN, SOFT PARAFFIN.

Lipofundin MCT/LCT and S. Fat emulsion for parenteral nutrition.

Lipostat. To reduce blood cholesterol: *see* PRAVASTATIN.

Liquifilm tears. Lubricant eye drops for dry eyes: *see* POLYVINYL ALCOHOL.

Liquigen (b). Milk substitute for malabsorption states containing medium-chain triglycerides.

Liskonum. Antidepressant: *see* LITHIUM SALTS.

Livial. Steroid with hormonal activity for menopausal disorders: *see* TIBOLONE.

Livostin (d). Antihistamine nasal spray/eye drops for relief of hay fever symptoms: *see* LEVOCABASTINE.

Locabiotal (d). Topical antibiotic for infections of upper respiratory tract: *see* FUSAFUNGINE.

Locasol (b). Low-calcium food substitute for calcium intolerance.

Loceryl. Antifungal nail lacquer: *see* AMOROLFINE.

Locoid. Topical corticosteroid for eczema and other skin conditions: *see* HYDROCORTISONE.

Locoid C. Topical corticosteroid/anti-infective: *see* CHLORQUINALDOL, HYDROCORTISONE.

Locoid Crelo. Steroid emulsion for eczema: *see* HYDROCORTISONE.

Locorten-Vioform. Topical corticosteroid/anti-infective for skin or ears: *see* CLIOQUINOL, FLUMETASONE.

Lodine. Non-steroid anti-inflammatory/analgesic: *see* ETODOLAC.

Loestrin 20. Oral contraceptive: *see* ETHINYLESTRADIOL, NORETHISTERONE.

Logynon. Oral contraceptive: *see* ETHINYLESTRADIOL, LEVONORGESTREL.

Lomexin (d). Antifungal for vaginal infection: *see* FENTICONAZOLE.

Lomont. Antidepressant: *see* LOFEPRAMINE.

Lomotil. Antidiarrhoeal: *see* ATROPINE SULPHATE, DIPHENOXYLATE.

Loniten. Antihypertensive: *see* MINOXIDIL.

Loperagen. Antidiarrhoeal: *see* LOPERAMIDE.

Lopid. Reduces lipid concentrations in the blood in hyperlipidaemias: *see* GEMFIBROZIL.

Lopresor. Beta-adrenoceptor blocker: *see* METOPROLOL.

Lopresor S.R. Sustained-release formulation of Lopresor: *see* METOPROLOL.

Loron. To treat hypercalcaemia induced by malignant disease: *see* SODIUM CLODRONATE.

Losec. For peptic ulcers and oesophageal reflux: *see* OMEPRAZOLE.

Lotriderm. Cream for topical treatment of cutaneous fungal infections: *see* BETAMETHASONE, CLOTRIMAZOLE.

Lubri-Tears. Lubricating ointment for dry eyes: *see* LIQUID PARAFFIN, SOFT PARAFFIN.

Ludiomil. Antidepressant: *see* MAPROTILINE.

Lumigan (r). Eye drops for treatment of glaucoma: *see* BIMATOPROST.

Lustral. Antidepressant: *see* SERTRALINE.

Lyclear. Topical treatment for head lice: *see* PERMETHRIN.

Lyrica (r). Used to treat neuropathic pain and intractable epilepsy: *see* PREGABALIN.

Lysodren. Oral antineoplastic for treatment of advanced adrenocortical cancer: *see* MITOTANE.

Lysovir. Antiviral fused for prophylaxis and treatment of influenza: *see* AMANTADINE.

M

Maalox. Antacid: *see* ALUMINIUM HYDROXIDE, MAGNESIUM HYDROXIDE.

Maalox Plus. As Maalox with SIMETICONE.

Mabcampath (r). Monoclonal antibody used in the treatment of chronic lymphocytic leukaemia: *see* ALEMTUZUMAB.

MabThera. For follicular lymphoma: *see* RITUXIMAB.

Macrobid. Urinary anti-infective: *see* NITROFURANTOIN.

Macrodantin. Antibacterial: *see* NITROFURANTOIN.

Madopar. Antiparkinsonian: *see* BENSERAZIDE, LEVODOPA.

Magnapen. Antibiotic: *see* AMPICILLIN, FLUCLOXACILLIN.

Malarone/Malarone Paediatric (r). Combination used for treatment of malaria which is resistant to single drug therapy: *see* ATOVAQUONE, PROGUANIL.

Manerix. Antidepressant: *see* MOCLOBEMIDE.

Manevac. Laxative: *see* ISPAGHULA, SENNOSIDE B.

Manusept. Topical antiseptic: *see* TRICLOSAN.

Marcain. Local anaesthetic injection: *see* BUPIVACAINE.

Marevan. Oral anticoagulant: *see* WARFARIN.

Marvelon. Oral contraceptive: *see* DESOGESTREL, ETHINYLESTRADIOL.

Maxalt. Selective 5-HYDROXYTRYPTAMINE (serotonin) agonist used to treat acute migraine: *see* RIZATRIPTAN.

Maxamaid (b). Phenylalanine-free mixture of AMINO ACIDS for phenylketonuric patients.

Maxepa. Mixture of fish oils used to reduce plasma lipids in patients with severe hypertriglyceridaemia.

Maxidex. Corticosteroid eye drops for non-infective, inflammatory conditions: *see* DEXAMETHASONE, HYPROMELLOSE.

Maxitrol. Corticosteroid/antibiotic eye drops/ointment: *see* DEXAMETHASONE, HYPROMELLOSE, NEOMYCIN, POLYMYXIN B.

Maxolon. Antiemetic: *see* METOCLOPRAMIDE.

Maxtrex. Cytotoxic: *see* METHOTREXATE.

MCT (1) and MCT Oil (b). Dietary substitutes containing triglycerides. For use in impaired fat absorption.

Medicoal (d). Oral adsorbent for treatment of acute poisoning and drug overdose: *see* ACTIVATED CHARCOAL.

Medinol Paediatric. Liquid antipyretic for children: *see* PARACETAMOL.

Medised. Analgesic/sedative: *see* PARACETAMOL, PROMETHAZINE.

Mifegyne

Medrone. Corticosteroid: *see* METHYLPREDNISOLONE.

Megace. Sex hormone: *see* MEGESTROL.

Menogon. Fertility treatment: *see* MENOTROPHIN.

Meptid. Analgesic: *see* MEPTAZINOL.

Merbentyl. Anticholinergic for gastro-intestinal colic: *see* DICYCLOVERINE.

Mercilon. Oral contraceptive: *see* DESOGESTREL, ETHINYLESTRADIOL.

Merocaine. Antiseptic/local anaesthetic lozenge for painful mouth conditions: *see* BENZOCAINE, CETYLPYRIDINIUM.

Merocet. Antiseptic mouthwash or lozenges: *see* CETYLPYRIDINIUM.

Meronem. Antibiotic: *see* MEROPENEM.

Mestinon. Anticholinesterase: *see* PYRIDOSTIGMINE.

Metabolic Mineral Mixture (b). Dietary mineral supplement.

Metalyse. To reduce the risk of thrombosis after suspected acute myocardial infarction: *see* TENECTEPLASE.

Metanium. Soothing, protective ointment and powder for nappy rash and other macerated skin conditions: *see* TITANIUM DIOXIDE.

Metatone. 'Tonic': *see* ANEURINE, MANGANESE, POTASSIUM GLYCEROPHOSPHATE, SODIUM GLYCEROPHOSPHATE.

Metenix 5. Diuretic: *see* METOLAZONE.

Metopirone. Used in test of pituitary function: *see* METYRAPONE.

Metosyn. Topical corticosteroid for skin disorders: *see* FLUOCINONIDE.

Metrogel. Topical antibiotic treatment for rosacea: *see* METRONIDAZOLE.

Metrolyl. Antimicrobial: *see* METRONIDAZOLE.

Metrotop. Topical gel for reducing smell of fungating tumours: *see* METRONIDAZOLE.

Mexitil. Antidysrhythmic: *see* MEXILETINE.

Mexitil Perlongets. Sustained-release form of Mexitil: *see* MEXILETINE.

Miacalcic. To treat hypercalcaemia associated with Paget's disease or bone cancer: *see* CALCITONIN.

Micardis. Antihypertensive: *see* TELMISARTAN.

Micardis Plus (r). Antihypertensive: *see* HYDROCHLOROTHIAZIDE, TELMISARTAN.

Micolette. Laxative enema: *see* GLYCEROL, SODIUM CITRATE, SODIUM LAURYL SULPHOACETATE.

Micralax. Purgative enema: *see* SODIUM ALKYL SULPHOACETATE, SODIUM CITRATE, SORBIC ACID.

Microgynon 30. Oral contraceptive: *see* ETHINYLESTRADIOL, NORGESTREL.

Micronor. Oral contraceptive: *see* NORETHISTERONE.

Microval (d). Oral contraceptive: *see* LEVONORGESTREL.

Mictral. For urinary tract infections: *see* CITRIC ACID, NALIDIXIC ACID, SODIUM CITRATE.

Midrid. For headache, migraine: *see* ISOMETHEPTENE, PARACETAMOL.

Mifegyne. For termination of intrauterine pregnancy: *see* MIFEPRISTONE.

169

Migard

Migard. For acute migraine: *see*
FROVATRIPTAN.

Migraleve. For migraine: *see* BUCLIZINE,
CODEINE, PARACETAMOL.

Migramax. For migraine: *see* ASPIRIN,
METOCLOPRAMIDE.

Migril. Vasoconstrictor for migraine: *see*
CAFFEINE, CYCLIZINE, ERGOTAMINE.

Mildison Lipocream. Topical
corticosteroid: *see* HYDROCORTISONE.

Mimpara (r). For treatment of high
calcium and phosphorus levels in
hyperparathyroidism: *see* CINACALCET.

Minihep. Subcutaneous injection for
thromboembolic disease: *see* HEPARIN.

Mini-i-jet. Sympathomimetic: *see*
ADRENALINE.

Minims. Single-dose ophthalmic
preparations.

Minitran. Prophylactic antianginal,
formulated as a self-adhesive patch for
transdermal absorption: *see* GLYCERYL
TRINITRATE.

Minocin. Antibiotic: *see* MINOCYCLINE.

Minodiab. Oral hypoglycaemic: *see*
GLIPIZIDE.

Mintec. Enteric-coated antispasmodic for
relief of pain in irritable bowel
syndrome: *see* PEPPERMINT OIL.

Minulet. Oral contraceptive: *see*
ETHINYLESTRADIOL, GESTODENE.

Miochol. Solution for intraocular
irrigation during eye surgery: *see*
ACETYLCHOLINE.

Mirapexin. Dopamine agonist used as
add-on treatment in Parkinson's disease

when L-dopa is not effective: *see*
PRAMIPEXOLE.

Mirena. Intrauterine progestogen-
releasing contraceptive system: *see*
LEVONORGESTREL.

Mithracin. Cytotoxic: *see* MITHRAMYCIN.

Mitomycin C Kyowa. Cytotoxic: *see*
MITOMYCIN.

Mitoxana. Cytotoxic: *see* IFOSFAMIDE.

Mivacron. Muscle relaxant: *see*
MIVACURIUM.

Mixtard 30/70. Long-acting purified pork
insulin mixture (30 per cent neutral,
70 per cent isophane): *see* INSULIN.

Mizollen. For hay fever and similar
allergic conditions: *see* MIZOLASTINE.

MMR II. Live vaccine for active
immunization against measles, mumps
and rubella.

Mobic. Non-steroidal anti-inflammatory
for acute osteoarthritis, chronic
rheumatoid arthritis and ankylosing
spondylitis: *see* MELOXICAM.

Mobiflex. Non-steroid anti-inflammatory/
analgesic: *see* TENOXICAM.

Modalim. Lipid-lowering drug: *see*
CIPROFIBRATE.

Modecate. Long-acting tranquillizer
injection: *see* FLUPHENAZINE.

Modisal XL/LA. Modified release
antianginal: *see* ISOSORBIDE
MONONITRATE.

Moditen. Tranquillizer: *see*
FLUPHENAZINE.

Moditen enanthate. Long-acting
tranquillizer injection: *see* FLUPHENAZINE.

Modrasone. Corticosteroid cream and ointment for application to skin: *see* ALCLOMETASONE.

Modrenal. Used to suppress secretion of adrenal cortical hormones: *see* TRILOSTANE.

Moducren. Antihypertensive: *see* AMILORIDE, HYDROCHLOROTHIAZIDE, TIMOLOL.

Moduret 25. Diuretic combination: *see* AMILORIDE, HYDROCHLOROTHIAZIDE.

Moduretic. Diuretic combination. Available as solution for patients who cannot swallow tablets: *see* AMILORIDE, HYDROCHLOROTHIAZIDE.

Mogadon. Hypnotic: *see* NITRAZEPAM.

Molcer. Drops to soften ear wax: *see* DIOCTYL SODIUM SULPHOSUCCINATE.

Molipaxin. Antidepressant: *see* TRAZODONE.

Monocor (d). Antihypertensive: *see* BISOPROLOL.

Monomax SR. Antianginal: *see* ISOSORBIDE MONONITRATE.

Mononine. Clotting factor concentrate for treatment of haemophilia B or Christmas disease: *see* FACTOR IX.

Monoparin. Anticoagulant: *see* HEPARIN.

Monotrim (d). Antimicrobial: *see* TRIMETHOPRIM.

Monovent (d). Sympathomimetic bronchodilator: *see* TERBUTALINE.

Monozide 10. Antihypertensive: *see* BISOPROLOL, HYDROCHLOROTHIAZIDE.

Monphytol. Topical antifungal: *see* CHLOROBUTANOL, METHYL SALICYLATE, SALICYLIC ACID, UNDECENOIC ACID.

Morcap SR (c) (d). Sustained-release oral narcotic analgesic: *see* MORPHINE.

Morhulin. Topical preparation for abrasions, skin ulcers: *see* ZINC OXIDE.

Morphgesic SR (c). Analgesic: *see* MORPHINE.

Motens. Antihypertensive: *see* LACIDIPINE.

Motifene. Rapid-release and sustained-release non-steroidal, anti-inflammatory analgesic: *see* DICLOFENAC.

Motilium. Antiemetic: *see* DOMPERIDONE.

Motival. Sedative/antidepressant: *see* FLUPHENAZINE, NORTRIPTYLINE.

Motrin (d). Non-steroid anti-inflammatory/ analgesic: *see* IBUPROFEN.

Movelat. Rubefacient: *see* CORTICOSTEROID, HEPARINOID, SALICYLIC ACID.

Movicol. Laxative for chronic constipation: *see* POLYETHYLENE GLYCOL, POTASSIUM CHLORIDE, SODIUM BICARBONATE, SODIUM CHLORIDE.

MST continus (c). Sustained-release oral narcotic analgesic: *see* MORPHINE.

MSUD Aid (b). Dietary aid for maple syrup urine disease.

Mucodyne. Mucolytic: *see* CARBOCISTEINE.

Mucogel. Antacid: *see* ALUMINIUM HYDROXIDE, MAGNESIUM HYDROXIDE.

Multibionta. Intravenous vitamins: *see* ANEURINE, NICOTINAMIDE, PANTOTHENIC ACID, PYRIDOXINE, RIBOFLAVIN, VITAMIN A, VITAMIN C, VITAMIN E.

Multiparin. Anticoagulant: *see* HEPARIN.

MXL (c). Sustained-release oral narcotic analgesic: *see* MORPHINE.

Mycobutin

Mycobutin. Antibiotic: *see* RIFABUTIN.

Mycota. Topical antifungal: *see*
UNDECENOIC ACID.

Mydriacyl. Mydriatic/cycloplegic eye
drops: *see* TROPICAMIDE.

Mydrilate. Mydriatic/cycloplegic eye
drops: *see* CYCLOPENTOLATE.

Myfortic. Immunosuppressant for
prevention of rejection of kidney, liver
or heart transplants: *see*
MYCOPHENOLATE.

Myleran. Cytotoxic: *see* BUSULFAN.

Myocrisin. Gold injection for
rheumatoid arthritis: *see*
AUROTHIOMALATE SODIUM.

Myotonine chloride. Produces gut and
bladder emptying: *see* BETHANECHOL.

Mysoline. Anticonvulsant: *see*
PRIMIDONE.

N

Nalcrom. For ulcerative colitis: *see* SODIUM CROMOGLICATE.

Nalorex. Narcotic antagonist: *see* NALTREXONE.

Napratec. Non-steroid anti-inflammatory/ analgesic combined with prophylaxis of gastric ulceration: *see* MISOPROSTOL, NAPROXEN.

Naprosyn. Non-steroid anti-inflammatory/ analgesic: *see* NAPROXEN.

Naprosyn SR. Sustained-release non-steroid anti-inflammatory/analgesic: *see* NAPROXEN.

Naramig. For migraine: *see* NARATRIPTAN.

Narcan (d). Narcotic antagonist: *see* NALOXONE.

Nardil. Antidepressant (monoamine oxidase inhibitor): *see* PHENELZINE.

Naropin. Local anaesthetic injection: *see* ROPIVACAINE.

Narphen (c) (d). Analgesic: *see* PHENAZOCINE.

Nasacort. Nasal spray for relief of hay fever symptoms: *see* TRIAMCINOLONE.

Naseptin. Antiseptic/antibacterial cream for topical use in nasal carriers of staphylococci: *see* CHLORHEXIDINE, NEOMYCIN.

Nasobec. Nasal spray for relief of hay fever symptoms: *see* BECLOMETASONE.

Nasofan. Topical intranasal steroid spray for allergic rhinitis: *see* FLUTICASONE.

Nasonex. Nasal spray for relief of hay fever symptoms: *see* MOMETASONE.

Natrilix. Antihypertensive: *see* INDAPAMIDE.

Navelbine. For treatment of breast cancer: *see* VINORELBINE.

Navidrex. Diuretic: *see* CYCLOPENTHIAZIDE.

Navispare. Diuretic: *see* AMILORIDE, CYCLOPENTHIAZIDE.

Navoban. Antiemetic: *see* TROPISETRON.

Nebcin (d). Antibiotic: *see* TOBRAMYCIN.

Nebido (r). Hormone replacement therapy: *see* TESTOSTERONE.

Nebilet. Antihypertensive: *see* NEBIVOLOL.

Negram (d). Antibacterial: *see* NALIDIXIC ACID.

Neoclarityn. Antihistamine: *see* DESLORATADINE.

Neo-cortef. Topical corticosteroid/ antibacterial ointment/lotion/drops: *see* HYDROCORTISONE, NEOMYCIN.

Neo-Cytamen. Vitamin: *see* HYDROXOCOBALAMIN.

Neo-Mercazole. Antithyroid: *see* CARBIMAZOLE.

Neo-Naclex

Neo-Naclex. Diuretic: *see*
BENDROFLUMETHIAZIDE.

Neo-Naclex-K. As Neo-Naclex plus
POTASSIUM CHLORIDE in slow-release
matrix.

Neoral. Immunosuppressant formulated
for improved bioavailability: *see*
CICLOSPORIN.

Neorecormon. Hormone treatment for
anaemia in chronic renal failure in
patients on chronic dialysis: *see* EPOETIN
BETA.

Neosporin. Antibacterial eye drops: *see*
GRAMICIDIN, NEOMYCIN, POLYMYXIN B.

Neotigason. Used to treat psoriasis: *see*
ACITRETIN.

Nerisone. Corticosteroid cream for skin
conditions: *see* DIFLUCORTOLONE.

Netillin. Antibiotic: *see* NETILMICIN.

Neulactil. Antipsychotic: *see* PERICYAZINE.

Neulasta (r). Granulocyte stimulating
factor used to treat neutropenia occurring
as a complication of cytotoxic
chemotherapy: *see* PEGFILGRASTIM.

Neupogen. To raise neutrophil blood cell
count in patients undergoing cytotoxic
chemotherapy: *see* FILGRASTIM.

Neupro (r). Transdermal patches for
treatment of Parkinson's disease: *see*
ROTIGOTINE.

Neurontin. Anticonvulsant used for
epilepsy and neuralgia: *see* GABAPENTIN.

Nexium. For gastro-oesophageal reflux
and duodenal and peptic ulcers: *see*
ESOMEPRAZOLE.

Niaspan. To reduce blood cholesterol and
triglyceride: *see* NICOTINIC ACID.

Nicam. Topical gel for acne: *see*
NICOTINAMIDE.

Nicef. Antibiotic: *see* CEFRADINE.

Nicorette. Anti-smoking preparations: *see*
NICOTINE.

Nicotinell. Transdermal patch for treatment
of dependence during withdrawal from
cigarette smoking: *see* NICOTINE.

Niferex. Haematinic: *see*
POLYSACCHARIDE–IRON COMPLEX.

Nimbex. Nondepolarizing muscle
relaxant: *see* CISATRACURIUM.

Nimotop. Intravenous vasodilator used to
reduce ischaemia after subarachnoid
haemorrhage: *see* NIMODIPINE.

Nipent. Cytotoxic: *see* PENTOSTATIN.

Nitrocine. Antianginal/vasodilator
injection. Used as infusion to prevent
myocardial ischaemia (e.g. in cardiac
surgery or unstable angina): *see*
GLYCERYL TRINITRATE.

Nitrolingual. Vasodilator oral spray for
symptomatic relief of angina: *see*
GLYCERYL TRINITRATE.

Nitromin. Antianginal in spray
formulation: *see* GLYCERYL TRINITRATE.

Nitronal. Vasodilator (antianginal) for
intravenous use in intractable cardiac
failure and unstable angina: *see*
GLYCERYL TRINITRATE.

Nivaquine. Antimalarial: *see* CHLOROQUINE.

Nivemycin. Antibiotic for oral and topical
use: *see* NEOMYCIN.

Nizoral. Antifungal: *see* KETOCONAZOLE.

Nocutil. Nasal spray for treatment of
nocturnal enuresis in children and

diabetes insipidus in adults and children: *see* DESMOPRESSIN.

Nolvadex. For treatment of anovular infertility and breast cancer: *see* TAMOXIFEN.

Nolvadex-D. As Nolvadex formulated for once-daily dosage: *see* TAMOXIFEN.

Nootropil. Anticonvulsant: *see* PIRACETAM.

Norcuron. Muscle relaxant: *see* VECURONIUM.

Norditropin. Synthetic human growth hormone used to treat growth failure due to growth hormone deficiency: *see* SOMATROPIN.

Norgalax. Laxative: *see* DOCUSATE SODIUM.

Norgeston. Oral contraceptive: *see* LEVONORGESTREL.

Noriday. Oral contraceptive: *see* NORETHISTERONE.

Norimin. Oral contraceptive: *see* ETHINYLESTRADIOL, NORETHISTERONE.

Norimode. Antidiarrhoeal: *see* LOPERAMIDE.

Norinyl-1/Norinyl-1/28. Oral contraceptives: *see* MESTRANOL, NORETHISTERONE.

Noristerat. Depot contraceptive: *see* NORETHISTERONE.

Noritate. Topical treatment for rosacea: *see* METRONIDAZOLE.

Normacol. Purgative: *see* FRANGULA, STERCULIA.

Normasol Undine. Single-dose ophthalmic preparation of SODIUM CHLORIDE.

Normax. Purgative: *see* CO-DANTHRUSATE.

Norprolac. Dopamine antagonist used in suppression of the effects of hyperprolactinaemia, e.g. galactorrhoea: *see* QUINAGOLIDE.

Norvir. Antiviral: *see* RITONAVIR.

Novantrone. Cytotoxic: *see* MITOXANTRONE.

Novofem. Hormone replacement therapy for treatment of menopausal symptoms and prevention of postmenopausal osteoporosis: *see* ESTRADIOL, NORETHISTERONE.

Novonorm. Oral antidiabetic: *see* REPAGLINIDE.

Novoseven. Recombinant human clotting factor used in treatment of haemophilia: *see* FACTOR VIIA.

Noxafil (r). Oral antifungal used to treat invasive fungal infections: *see* POSACONAZOLE.

Noxyflex S. Anti-infective for instillation in bladder or other body cavities: *see* NOXYTIOLIN.

Nozinan. Antipsychotic: *see* LEVOMEPROMAZINE.

Nuelin. Bronchodilator: *see* THEOPHYLLINE.

Nulacin. Antacid: *see* CALCIUM AND MAGNESIUM ANTACIDS.

Nupercainal. Topical skin anaesthetic: *see* CINCHOCAINE.

Nurofen. Non-prescription analgesic: *see* IBUPROFEN.

Nu-Seals Aspirin. Enteric-coated analgesic: *see* ACETYLSALICYLIC ACID.

Nutramigen (b). Dietary aid for lactose intolerance, galactosaemia.

Nutraplus. Topical cream for dry skin: *see* UREA.

Nutrizym

Nutrizym. For use in pancreatic deficiency: *see* PANCREATIC ENZYMES.

NutropinAq. For growth failure: *see* SOMATROPIN.

Nuvelle. Hormone replacement therapy: *see* ESTRADIOL, LEVONORGESTREL.

Nuvelle continuous. Non-bleed continuous hormone replacement therapy: *see* ESTRADIOL, NORETHISTERONE.

Nystaform. Cream or ointment for topical treatment of fungal skin infections due to *Candida* spp: *see* CHLORHEXIDINE, NYSTATIN.

Nystaform-HC. Topical anti-infective/anti-inflammatory: *see* CHLORHEXIDINE, HYDROCORTISONE, NYSTATIN.

Nystan. Antifungal: *see* NYSTATIN.

Nytol. Hypnotic: *see* DIPHENHYDRAMINE.

O

Occlusal. Wart remover: *see* SALICYLIC ACID.

Ocufen. Eye drops to prevent trauma-induced pupil constriction during eye surgery: *see* FLURBIPROFEN.

Oculotect. Lubricant 'artificial tears' for dry eyes: *see* POVIDONE.

Odrik (d). Antihypertensive: *see* TRANDOLAPRIL.

Oestrogel. Sex hormone for postmenopausal symptoms and prevention of osteoporosis: *see* ESTRADIOL.

Olbetam. Reduces raised blood lipids: *see* ACIPIMOX.

Olmetec (r). Antihypertensive: *see* OLMESARTAN MEDOXOMIL.

Olmetec Plus (r). Antihypertensive: *see* HYDROCHLOROTHIAZIDE, OLMESARTAN.

Oncovin. Cytotoxic: *see* VINCRISTINE.

One-Alpha. Vitamin D derivative: *see* ALFACALCIDOL.

Opatanol (r). Antiallergic antihistamine eye drops to relieve symptoms of hay fever: *see* OLOPATADINE.

Opilon. Peripheral vasodilator: *see* MOXISYLYTE.

Opticrom. Eye drops for allergic conjunctivitis: *see* SODIUM CROMOGLICATE.

Optilast. Antihistamine eye drops for allergic conjunctivitis: *see* AZELASTINE.

Optimax. Antidepressant: *see* TRYPTOPHAN.

Orabase. Topical inert protective application for skin and mucosae.

Orahesive. Topical inert protective powder for skin and mucosae.

Oraldene. Rinse for oral infections: *see* HEXETIDINE.

Oramorph (c). Liquid, oral analgesic: *see* MORPHINE.

Orap. Tranquillizer: *see* PIMOZIDE.

Orelox. Antibiotic: *see* CEFPODOXIME.

Orgalutran. Hormone release antagonist used in infertility treatment: *see* GANIRELIX.

Orgaran. Anticoagulant: *see* DANAPAROID SODIUM.

Orovite. Vitamin mixture: *see* ANEURINE, NICOTINAMIDE, PYRIDOXINE, RIBOFLAVIN, VITAMIN C.

Orovite 7. Vitamin mixture for deficiency: *see* ANEURINE, CALCIFEROL, NICOTINAMIDE, PYRIDOXINE, RIBOFLAVIN, VITAMIN A, VITAMIN C.

Ortho-Creme. Spermicidal cream: *see* NONOXYNOL, RICINOLEIC ACID, SODIUM LAURYL SULPHATE.

Ortho-Forms. Spermicidal pessary.

Ortho-Gynest. Vaginal pessary for vaginal inflammation and irritation: *see* ESTRIOL.

177

Orudis. Non-steroid anti-inflammatory/ analgesic: *see* KETOPROFEN.

Oruvail. Sustained-release non-steroid anti-inflammatory/analgesic: *see* KETOPROFEN.

Osmolite (b). Liquid feed for enteral absorption.

Otomize. Spray for treatment of external ear inflammation/infection: *see* DEXAMETHASONE, NEOMYCIN.

Otosporin. Antibiotic/anti-inflammatory ear drops: *see* HYDROCORTISONE, NEOMYCIN, POLYMYXIN B.

Otrivine. Nasal decongestant: *see* XYLOMETAZOLINE.

Ovestin. Female sex hormone for deficiency states: *see* ESTRIOL.

Ovranette. Oral contraceptive: *see* ETHINYLESTRADIOL, NORGESTREL.

Ovysmen. Oral contraceptive: *see* ETHINYLESTRADIOL, NORETHISTERONE.

Oxanid. Anxiolytic: *see* OXAZEPAM.

Oxis. Selective beta-adrenoceptor blocker for treatment of asthma: *see* FORMOTEROL.

OxyContin (c). Opioid analgesic given orally or by injection (r) for severe pain: *see* OXYCODONE.

Oxymycin. Antibiotic: *see* OXYTETRACYCLINE.

OxyNorm (c). Sustained-release opioid analgesic for severe pain: *see* OXYCODONE.

P

Pabrinex. Vitamin injection: *see* VITAMIN B, VITAMIN C.

Paediasure (b). Oral dietary supplement for children up to six years old.

Paldesic. Analgesic elixir: *see* PARACETAMOL.

Palfium (c) (d). Narcotic analgesic: *see* DEXTROMORAMIDE.

Palladone (c). Opioid analgesic for severe pain: *see* HYDROMORPHONE.

Paludrine. Antimalarial: *see* PROGUANIL.

Pamergan P100 (c). Premedication combination containing narcotic analgesic: *see* PETHIDINE, PROMETHAZINE.

Panadeine. Non-prescription analgesic: *see* CODEINE, PARACETAMOL.

Panadol. Analgesic: *see* CODEINE, PARACETAMOL.

Pancrease. *See* PANCREATIC ENZYMES.

Pancrex/Pancrex V/Pancrex V Forte. For use in pancreatic deficiency: *see* PANCREATIN.

Panoxyl 5 and 10. Topical treatment for acne: *see* BENZOYL PEROXIDE.

Paracodol. Effervescent analgesic/antipyretic: *see* CODEINE, PARACETAMOL.

Paradote. Analgesic with antidote against overdose: *see* METHIONINE, PARACETAMOL.

Parake. Analgesic/antipyretic: *see* CO-CODAMOL.

Paramax. Analgesic/antiemetic for migraine. METOCLOPRAMIDE aids drug absorption by relief of the gastric stasis which can occur during a migraine attack as well as acting as an antiemetic: *see* METOCLOPRAMIDE, PARACETAMOL.

Paramol. Analgesic: *see* DIHYDROCODEINE, PARACETAMOL.

Paraplatin. Cytotoxic: *see* CARBOPLATIN.

Pariet. For peptic ulcer and oesophageal reflux: *see* RABEPRAZOLE.

Parlodel. Dopamine agonist: *see* BROMOCRIPTINE.

Parnate. Antidepressant monoamine oxidase inhibitor: *see* TRANYLCYPROMINE.

Paroven. Vitamin derivative for symptomatic treatment of aching associated with varicose veins: *see* TROXERUTIN.

Parvolex. Injection for treatment of paracetamol overdosage: *see* ACETYLCYSTEINE.

Pavacol-D. Cough suppressant: *see* ESSENTIAL OILS, PHOLCODINE.

PegIntron. Interferon for treatment of chronic hepatitis C: *see* PEGINTERFERON ALFA-2B.

Penbritin. Antibiotic: *see* AMPICILLIN.

Pennsaid. Topical non-steroidal anti-inflammatory analgesic: *see* DICLOFENAC.

Pentacarinat. Antiprotozoal: *see* PENTAMIDINE.

Pentasa. Enema to treat ulcerative colitis: *see* MESALAZINE.

Pentostam. Antimony derivative: *see* STIBOGLUCONATE SODIUM.

Pepcid PM. Gastric histamine blocker; reduces acid secretions: *see* FAMOTIDINE.

Peptac. For oesophagitis due to gastric reflux: *see* ALGINATE, CALCIUM CARBONATE, SODIUM BICARBONATE.

Peptamen (b). Peptide-based liquid food for use when gastrointestinal function is impaired. Contains carbohydrate (maltodextrin and starch), protein (whey protein hydrolysate), fat (MCT, sunflower oil, lecithin and residual milk fat), vitamins, minerals and trace elements.

Percutol. Vasodilator gel for application to skin in prophylaxis of angina: *see* GLYCERYL TRINITRATE.

Perdix. Antihypertensive: *see* MOEXIPRIL.

Perfalgan (r). Intravenous preparation for injection used for short-term treatment of pain after surgery and fever: *see* PARACETAMOL.

Perfan. For relief of cardiac failure: *see* ENOXIMONE.

Periactin. Serotonin antagonist for allergic conditions and migraine: *see* CYPROHEPTADINE.

Perinal. For itching and pain from haemorrhoids: *see* HYDROCORTISONE, LIDOCAINE.

Persantin. For ischaemic heart disease: *see* DIPYRIDAMOLE.

Pevaryl. Topical antifungal for skin infections: *see* ECONAZOLE, TRIAMCINOLONE.

Pharmalgen. Insect venom, prepared from bees or wasps for desensitization in allergic individuals.

Pharmorubicin. Cytotoxic: *see* EPIRUBICIN.

Phenergan. Antihistamine for topical and systemic use: *see* PROMETHAZINE.

Phosphate-Sandoz. Effervescent phosphate supplement for hyperparathyroidism and other bone disease.

Photofrin (r). Cytotoxic for treatment of non-small cell lung cancer and oesophageal cancer: *see* PORFIMER.

Phyllocontin. For asthma and cardiac failure: *see* AMINOPHYLLINE.

Physeptone (c). Narcotic analgesic: *see* METHADONE.

Physiotens. Antihypertensive: *see* MOXONIDINE.

Phytex. Topical antifungal paint: *see* BORIC ACID, METHYL SALICYLATE, SALICYLIC ACID, TANNIC ACID.

Picolax. Saline purgative: *see* MAGNESIUM CITRATE, SODIUM PICOSULFATE.

Pilogel. Miotic eye gel for glaucoma: *see* PILOCARPINE.

Piportil depot. Long-acting tranquillizer injection: *see* PIPOTIAZINE.

Piriton. Antihistamine: *see* CHLORPHENAMINE.

Pitressin. Hormone: *see* VASOPRESSIN.

PK Aid 1 (b). Dietary aid for phenylketonuria.

Plaquenil. Anti-inflammatory: *see* HYDROXYCHLOROQUINE.

Plavix. Antiplatelet drug used to prevent ischaemic vascular disease: *see* CLOPIDOGREL.

Plendil. Antianginal/antihypertensive: *see* FELODIPINE.

Plesmet (d). For iron-deficiency anaemia: *see* FERROUS SULPHATE.

Pletal (r). To improve blood flow in patients with arterial disease, and enable them to walk further: *see* CILOSTAZOL.

Pneumovax II. Vaccine for immunization against pneumococcal infections, e.g. lobar pneumonia, meningitis or endocarditis.

Polycal (b). Source of carbohydrate for kidney, liver and various metabolic diseases.

Polycose (b). Lactose- and GLUTEN-free polysaccharide mixture.

Polyfax. Antibiotic: *see* BACITRACIN, POLYMYXIN B.

Polytar (b). Topical treatment for psoriasis: *see* COAL TAR.

Ponstan. Anti-inflammatory/analgesic: *see* MEFENAMIC ACID.

Posalfilin. Topical treatment for warts: *see* PODOPHYLLUM, SALICYLIC ACID.

Posiject (d). Infusion for treatment of severe heart failure: *see* DOBUTAMINE.

postMI. Enteric-coated aspirin to reduce the risk of thrombosis: *see* ACETYLSALICYLIC ACID.

Potaba. Nutrient used for skin disorders: *see* POTASSIUM *para*-AMINOBENZOATE.

Powergel. Topical anti-inflammatory analgesic: *see* KETOPROFEN.

Pragmatar (d). Topical treatment for seborrhoea: *see* COAL TAR, SALICYLIC ACID, SULPHUR.

Praxilene. Peripheral vasodilator: *see* NAFTIDROFURYL.

Precortisyl. Corticosteroid: *see* PREDNISOLONE.

Predenema. Corticosteroid enema: *see* PREDNISOLONE.

Predfoam. Corticosteroid aerosol foam for rectal administration. Used to treat ulcerative colitis and similar inflammatory bowel conditions: *see* PREDNISOLONE.

Pred Forte. Topical corticosteroid eye drops for use in inflammatory non-infective eye conditions: *see* PREDNISOLONE.

Predsol. Corticosteroid: *see* PREDNISOLONE.

Predsol-N. Corticosteroid/antibiotic ear drops: *see* NEOMYCIN, PREDNISOLONE.

Pregaday. For anaemia of pregnancy: *see* FERROUS FUMARATE, FOLIC ACID.

Pregestimil (b). Dietary aid for glucose, lactose, protein intolerance.

Premarin. Natural oestrogens from a pregnant mare's urine for deficiency states.

Premique. Sex hormones for postmenopausal symptoms: *see* MEDROXYPROGESTERONE, OESTROGEN.

Prempak-C. Sex hormones for replacement therapy at and after menopause: *see* NORGESTREL, OESTROGEN.

Prescal. Antihypertensive: *see* ISRADIPINE.

Preservex. Non-steroidal anti-inflammatory analgesic: *see* ACECLOFENAC.

Presinex. Antidiuretic hormone formulated as a nasal spray for treatment

Prestim

of nocturnal enuresis associated with multiple sclerosis: *see* DESMOPRESSIN.

Prestim. Antihypertensive: *see* BENDROFLUMETHIAZIDE, TIMOLOL.

Prexige (r). Non-steroidal anti-inflammatory for relief of pain in osteoarthritis and short-term relief of pain due to orthopaedic surgery, dental surgery or dysmenorrhoea: *see* LUMIRACOXIB.

Priadel. Antidepressant: *see* LITHIUM SALTS.

Primacor. Phosphodiesterase inhibitor for treatment of severe congestive cardiac failure: *see* MILRINONE.

Primaxin. Antibiotic for intravenous use: *see* CILASTIN, IMIPENEM.

Primolut N. To reduce or postpone menstruation: *see* NORETHISTERONE.

Primoteston depot. Male sex hormone for deficiency states: *see* TESTOSTERONE.

Primperan. Antiemetic. Promotes gastric emptying: *see* METOCLOPRAMIDE.

Prioderm. Topical treatment for lice: *see* MALATHION.

Pripsen. For threadworms, roundworms: *see* PIPERAZINE.

Pro-Banthine. Anticholinergic used for antispasmodic and antacid effects: *see* PROPANTHELINE.

Procorlan (r). Antianginal: *see* IVABRADINE.

Proctofoam HC. Topical treatment for ano-rectal conditions: *see* HYDROCORTISONE, PRAMOCAINE.

Proctosedyl. Local treatment for haemorrhoids: *see* CINCHOCAINE, HYDROCORTISONE.

Pro-epanutin. Anticonvulsant for intravenous use: *see* FOSPHENYTOIN.

Proflex. Non-steroidal anti-inflammatory analgesic for topical use: *see* IBUPROFEN.

Progynova. Female sex hormone for deficiency states: *see* ESTRADIOL.

Proleukin. Cytotoxic: *see* ALDESLEUKIN.

Pronestyl. Antidysrhythmic: *see* PROCAINAMIDE.

Propaderm. Topical corticosteroid: *see* BECLOMETASONE.

Propaderm A and C. Topical corticosteroid/anti-infective: *see* BECLOMETASONE, CHLORTETRACYCLINE, CLIOQUINOL.

Propain. Analgesic/antihistamine for headache and muscular pain: *see* CAFFEINE, CODEINE, DIPHENHYDRAMINE, PARACETAMOL.

Propecia. Oral treatment for male pattern baldness: *see* FINASTERIDE.

Propine. Eye drops for chronic open-angle glaucoma: *see* DIPIVEFRINE.

Proscar. For treatment of benign hypertrophy of the prostate gland: *see* FINASTERIDE.

Prosobee (b). Dietary aid for lactose intolerance.

Prostap. Hormone used to treat prostate cancer and endometriosis and before surgery of the uterus: *see* LEUPRORELIN.

Prostin E2. Prostaglandin: *see* DINOPROSTONE.

Prostin VR. Prostaglandin: *see* ALPROSTADIL.

Protelos (r). For treatment of postmenopausal osteoporosis: *see* STRONTIUM RANELATE.

Prothiaden. Antidepressant: *see* DOSULEPIN.

Protifar. Dietary aid. High-protein source from skimmed milk for use in low-protein states.

Protium. For peptic ulcers and oesophageal reflux: *see* PANTOPRAZOLE.

Protopic (r). Topical treatment for severe atopic dermatitis: *see* TACROLIMUS.

Provera. For menstrual disorders: *see* MEDROXYPROGESTERONE.

Provera 100 mg. High-dose MEDROXYPROGESTERONE for treatment of endometrial, prostate and renal cancer.

Provigil (r). To reduce sedation caused by narcolepsy or other pathological conditions: *see* MODAFINIL.

Pro-Viron. Male sex hormone for deficiency states: *see* MESTEROLONE.

Prozac. Antidepressant: *see* FLUOXETINE.

Psoriderm preps. Topical treatments for psoriasis: *see* COAL TAR, LECITHINS.

Psoriderm-S. As Psoriderm plus SALICYLIC ACID.

Psorin. For topical treatment of psoriasis and eczema: *see* COAL TAR, DITHRANOL, SALICYLIC ACID.

Pulmicort. Steroid aerosol for asthma: *see* BUDESONIDE.

Pulmozyme. Synthetic enzyme used to reduce sputum viscosity in cases of cystic fibrosis: *see* DORNASE ALFA.

Pump-Hep. Anticoagulant for continuous infuson: *see* HEPARIN.

Puri-Nethol. Cytotoxic: *see* MERCAPTOPURINE.

Pylorid. For treatment of peptic ulcers where there is evidence of bacterial infection due to *Helicobacter pylori*: *see* RANITIDINE BISMUTH CITRATE.

Pyralvex. Topical anti-inflammatory for mouth ulcers: *see* ANTHRAQUINONE GLYCOSIDES, SALICYLIC ACID.

Q R

Quellada M. Topical treatment for scabies and lice: *see* MALATHION.

Questran. For hypercholesterolaemia: *see* COLESTYRAMINE.

Quinaband. Impregnated bandage: *see* CALAMINE, CLIOQUINOL, ZINC OXIDE.

Quinoderm. Topical treatment for acne: *see* BENZOYL PEROXIDE, HYDROXYQUINOLINE.

Qvar. CFC-free aerosol for asthma: *see* BECLOMETASONE.

Radian B. Rubefacient: *see* CAMPHOR, MENTHOL, METHYL SALICYLATE.

Rapamune (r). Immunosuppressant for use after kidney transplant: *see* SIROLIMUS.

Rapifen (c). Narcotic analgesic: *see* ALFENTANIL.

Rapitil. Eye drops for allergic conjunctivitis: *see* NEDOCROMIL.

Raptiva (r). Immunosupressant for treatment of severe psoriasis: *see* EFALIZUMAB.

RBC. Topical antihistamine: *see* ANTAZOLINE, CALAMINE, CAMPHOR, CETRIMIDE.

Rebetol. Antiviral for chronic hepatitis: *see* RIBAVIRIN.

Rebif. For reduction of frequency and severity of relapses in multiple sclerosis: *see* INTERFERON BETA-1A.

Recombinate (d). Clotting factor for treatment of haemophilia: *see* FACTOR VIII.

Rectogesic (r). Analgesic ointment for pain associated with anal fissures: *see* GLYCERYL TRINITRATE.

Reductil. Anti-obesity agent: *see* SIBUTRAMINE.

ReFacto. Recombinant human clotting factor used in treatment of haemophilia: *see* FACTOR VIII.

Refludan. Anticoagulant: *see* LEPIRUDIN.

Refolinon. Antagonizes antifolate cytotoxic drugs: *see* FOLINIC ACID.

Regaine. Topical treatment for male pattern baldness: *see* MINOXIDIL.

Regranex. Topical treatment for diabetic ulcers: *see* BECAPLERMIN.

Regulan. Purgative: *see* ISPAGHULA.

Regurin. To control urinary incontinence: *see* TROSPIUM.

Relaxit. Enema for constipation: *see* GLYCEROL, SODIUM CITRATE, SODIUM LAURYL SULPHATE, SORBIC ACID, SORBITOL.

Relenza. Antiviral for inhalation; used to treat influenza: *see* ZANAMIVIR.

Relestat (r). Antihistamine eye drops to alleviate the ocular symptoms of hay fever: *see* EPINASTINE.

Relifex. Non-steroid anti-inflammatory analgesic: *see* NABUMETONE.

Remedeine. Analgesic: *see* DIHYDROCODEINE, PARACETAMOL.

Remicade (r). For treatment of Crohn's disease, rheumatoid arthritis, ankylosing spondylitis, ulcerative colitis and plaque psoriasis: *see* INFLIXIMAB.

Reminyl. To improve cognitive function in mild to moderate Alzheimer's dementia: *see* GALANTAMINE.

Remnos. Hypnotic: *see* NITRAZEPAM.

Reopro. Monoclonal antibody used to reduce risk of blood clotting after heart surgery and as an antianginal: *see* ABCIXIMAB.

Replax. Oral treatment for acute migraine headaches: *see* ELETRIPTAN.

Requip. Dopamine agonist for treatment of Parkinson's disease: *see* ROPINIROLE.

Resonium-A. Ion exchange resin: *see* SODIUM POLYSTYRENE SULPHONATE.

Respontin Nebules. Bronchodilator nebulizer: *see* IPATROPIUM.

Restandol. Male sex hormone: *see* TESTOSTERONE.

Retin-A. Topical treatment for acne: *see* TRETINOIN.

Retinova. Topical treatment used to improve appearance of skin affected by long-term exposure to sun: *see* TRETINOIN.

Retrovir. Antiviral: *see* ZIDOVUDINE.

Revanil. Dopamine agonist for use in Parkinson's disease: *see* LISURIDE.

Revatio (r). For treatment of pulmonary arterial hypertension: *see* SILDENAFIL.

Reyataz (r). Oral antiviral for use in combination with other antiviral agents in treatment of HIV-positive patients with evidence of immunodeficiency: *see* ATAZANAVIR.

Rheomacrodex. Plasma expander: *see* DEXTRANS.

Rheumacin LA. Sustained-release, non-steroid anti-inflammatory/analgesic: *see* INDOMETACIN.

Rhinocort. Corticosteroid nasal spray for treatment of nasal symptoms, hay fever and other nasal allergies: *see* BUDESONIDE.

Rhinolast. Antihistamine nasal spray: *see* AZELASTINE.

Riamet (r). Antimalarial combination: *see* ARTEMETHER/LUMEFANTRINE.

Ridaura. Orally active gold compound for treatment of rheumatoid arthritis: *see* AURANOFIN.

Rifadin. Antituberculosis: *see* RIFAMPICIN.

Rifater. Antituberculosis: *see* ISONIAZID, PYRAZINAMIDE, RIFAMPICIN.

Rifinah. Antituberculosis: *see* ISONIAZID, RIFAMPICIN.

Rilutek. To slow the progression of motor neurone disease: *see* RILUZOLE.

Rimactane. Antituberculosis: *see* RIFAMPICIN.

Rimactazid. Antituberculosis: *see* ISONIAZID, RIFAMPICIN.

Rimso-50. Used in bladder inflammation: *see* DIMETHYL SULFOXIDE.

Rinatec. Nasal spray for relief of watery nasal discharge: *see* IPRATROPIUM.

Risperdal. Antipsychotic: *see* RISPERIDONE.

Risperdal Consta

Risperdal Consta (r). Antipsychotic formulated for depot injection: *see* RISPERIDONE.

Rite-Diet gluten-free (b). Dietary substitute for GLUTEN sensitivity.

Rite-Diet protein-free (b). Dietary substitute for protein intolerance (e.g. renal failure).

Rivotril. Anticonvulsant: *see* CLONAZEPAM.

Roaccutane. VITAMIN A derivative: *see* ISOTRETINOIN.

Robaxin. Muscle relaxant: *see* METHOCARBAMOL.

Robinul. Anticholinergic for peptic ulcers: *see* GLYCOPYRRONIUM.

Robinul neostigmine. As Robinul with NEOSTIGMINE.

Rocaltrol. Vitamin used for correction of calcium and phosphate metabolism in renal osteodystrophy and in postmenopausal osteoporosis: *see* CALCITRIOL.

Rocephin. Antibiotic: *see* CEFTRIAXONE.

Roferon-A. Antiviral agent used to treat an AIDS-associated tumour, chronic myelogenous leukaemia, malignant melanomA and chronic hepatitis C: *see* INTERFERON ALPHA-2A.

Rogitine. For diagnostic test/treatment of phaeochromocytoma: *see* PHENTOLAMINE.

Rohypnol (c) (d). Hypnotic: *see* FLUNITRAZEPAM.

Roter. Antacid: *see* BISMUTH SUBNITRATE, FRANGULA, MAGNESIUM CARBONATE, SODIUM BICARBONATE.

Rowachol. For biliary disorders: *see* CAMPHOR, EUCALYPTUS, MENTHOL.

Rowatinex. For biliary disorders. Mixture of ESSENTIAL OILS (e.g. ANETHOLE, CAMPHOR, EUCALYPTUS).

Rozex. Topical antibiotic treatment for rosacea: *see* METRONIDAZOLE.

Rynacrom. Topical insufflation for allergic rhinitis: *see* SODIUM CROMOGLICATE.

Rynacrom compound. As Rynacrom with XYLOMETAZOLINE.

Rythmodan. Antidysrhythmic: *see* DISOPYRAMIDE.

Rythmodan retard. Sustained-release formulation of Rythmodan.

S

Sabril. Anticonvulsant: *see* VIGABATRIN.

Saizen. Synthetic human growth hormone used to treat growth failure in children due to growth hormone deficiency or chronic renal failure: *see* SOMATROPIN.

Salactol. Topical treatment for warts: *see* LACTIC ACID, SALICYLIC ACID.

Salagen. To treat dry mouth and dry eyes associated with radiotherapy or chronic inflammatory autoimmune disease: *see* PILOCARPINE.

Salamol. Inhaler for asthma: *see* SALBUTAMOL.

Salatac. Topical treatment for warts: *see* LACTIC ACID, SALICYLIC ACID.

Salazopyrin. For ulcerative colitis: *see* SULFASALAZINE.

Salofalk. For ulcerative colitis: *see* MESALAZINE.

Salonair. Rubefacient: *see* BENZYL NICOTINATE, CAMPHOR, GLYCOL SALICYLATE, MENTHOL, METHYL SALICYLATE, SQUALANE.

Salzone. Analgesic: *see* PARACETAMOL.

Sandimmun. Immunosuppressant: *see* CICLOSPORIN.

Sandocal. Effervescent supplement for calcium deficiency states.

Sandoglobulin. Concentrate of IMMUNOGLOBULIN for patients with deficiency of this protein.

Sando-K. Effervescent potassium supplement. Mixture of POTASSIUM CHLORIDE and POTASSIUM BICARBONATE. Provides potassium and chloride ions for absorption. Gastric irritation much less than with simple POTASSIUM CHLORIDE solution. Some irritation may still occur. Danger of hyperkalaemia if used in renal failure, treated by haemodialysis and ion exchange resins.

Sandostatin. For relief of symptoms of gastroenteropancreatic insulin secreting tumours and endocrine tumours, e.g. carcinoid syndrome, and for acromegaly: *see* OCTREOTIDE.

Sandrena. Hormone replacement therapy for postmenopausal symptoms: *see* ESTRADIOL.

Sanomigran. Migraine prophylactic: *see* PIZOTIFEN.

Scheriproct. Topical treatment for haemorrhoids: *see* CINCHOCAINE, PREDNISOLONE.

Scopoderm TTS. Antiemetic for travel sickness. Absorbed through the skin from a self-adhesive patch: *see* HYOSCINE HYDROBROMIDE.

Secadrex (d). Antihypertensive: *see* ACEBUTOLOL, HYDROCHLOROTHIAZIDE.

Seconal sodium (c). Sedative/hypnotic: *see* SECOBARBITAL.

Sectral. Beta-adrenoceptor blocker: *see* ACEBUTOLOL.

187

Securon

Securon. Antianginal/antihypertensive: *see* VERAPAMIL.

Selexid. Antibiotic: *see* PIVMECILLINAM.

Selsun (b). Shampoo for seborrhoeic dermatitis: *see* SELENIUM SULPHIDE.

Semi-Daonil. Oral hypoglycaemic: *see* GLIBENCLAMIDE.

Senokot. Purgative: *see* SENNA.

Septrin. Antibacterial: *see* CO-TRIMOXAZOLE.

Seractil (r). Analgesic: *see* DEXIBUPROFEN.

Serc. For Ménière's syndrome: *see* BETAHISTINE.

Serenace. Tranquillizer: *see* HALOPERIDOL.

Seretide. Inhaled beta-stimulant and corticocosteroid combination for regular treatment of asthma: *see* FLUTICASONE, SALMETEROL.

Serevent. Bronchodilator: *see* SALMETEROL.

Seroquel. Antipsychotic for treatment of schizophrenia: *see* QUETIAPINE.

Seroxat. Antidepressant: *see* PAROXETINE.

Sevredol (c). Analgesic: *see* MORPHINE.

Simeco. Antacid: *see* ALUMINIUM HYDROXIDE, MAGNESIUM CARBONATE, MAGNESIUM HYDROXIDE, SIMETICONE.

Sinemet preparations. Antiparkinsonian containing varying doses of LEVODOPA plus CARBIDOPA.

Sinequan (d). Anxiolytic/antidepressant: *see* DOXEPIN.

Singulair. Antiasthmatic: *see* MONTELUKAST.

Sinthrome. Anticoagulant: *see* ACENOCOUMAROL.

Siopel. Soothing, antiseptic cream for skin rashes: *see* CETRIMIDE, DIMETICONE.

Skelid. Used in Paget's disease: *see* TILUDRONIC ACID.

Skinoren. Topical treatment for acne: *see* AZELAIC ACID.

Skin testing solutions. Allergen extracts used in skin testing for allergies.

Slo-Indo. Anti-inflammatory analgesic: *see* INDOMETACIN.

Slophyllin. Sustained-release bronchodilator: *see* THEOPHYLLINE.

Slow-K. Slow-release POTASSIUM CHLORIDE.

Slow Sodium. Slow-release SODIUM CHLORIDE.

Slow-Trasicor. Antihypertensive. Sustained-release formulation of OXPRENOLOL.

Slozem. Sustained-release antihypertensive, antianginal: *see* DILTIAZEM.

Sno-Pro. Milk replacement for patients with phenylketonuria.

Sno Tears. Lubricant eye drops for dry eyes: *see* POLYVINYL ALCOHOL.

Sodium Amytal (c). Hypnotic/sedative: *see* AMOBARBITAL.

Sofradex. Corticosteroid/anti-infective drops for use in eyes or ears: *see* DEXAMETHASONE, FRAMYCETIN, GRAMICIDIN.

Soframycin. Topical anti-infective: *see* FRAMYCETIN, GRAMICIDIN.

Soframycin inj. and tabs. Antibiotic: *see* FRAMYCETIN.

Solaraze. Topical non-steroidal anti-inflammatory analgesic: *see* DICLOFENAC.

Solarcaine. Local anaesthetic cream: *see* BENZOCAINE, TRICLOSAN.

Solian. Antipsychotic for treatment of schizophrenia: *see* AMISULPRIDE.

Solivito N. Vitamins for injection: *see* ANEURINE, BIOTIN, CYANOCOBALAMIN, FOLIC ACID, NICOTINAMIDE, PANTOTHENIC ACID, PYRIDOXINE, RIBOFLAVIN, VITAMIN C.

Solpadeine. Soluble, effervescent analgesic: *see* CAFFEINE, CODEINE, PARACETAMOL.

Solpadol. Analgesic: *see* CODEINE, PARACETAMOL.

Solu-Cortef. Corticosteroid injection: *see* HYDROCORTISONE.

Solu-Medrone. Corticosteroid injection: *see* METHYLPREDNISOLONE.

Solvazinc. Soluble zinc supplements for zinc-deficiency states: *see* ZINC SULPHATE.

Somatuline. Treatment for acromegaly: *see* LANREOTIDE.

Somavert (r). Growth hormone antagonist for treatment of acromegaly: *see* PEGVISOMANT.

Sominex. Antihistamine hypnotic: *see* PROMETHAZINE.

Somnite. Hypnotic: *see* NITRAZEPAM.

Somnwell. Hypnotic: *see* CLORAL BETAINE.

Sonata. Hypnotic: *see* ZALEPLON.

Soneryl (c). Hypnotic/sedative: *see* BUTOBARBITAL.

Sotacor. Beta-adrenoceptor blocker: *see* SOTALOL.

Spasmonal. Antispasmodic for gastro-intestinal or uterine spasm: *see* ALVERINE.

Spectraban (b). Topical application for protection of skin from ultraviolet light.

Spiriva (r). Inhaled bronchodilator for chronic obstructive lung disease: *see* TIOTROPIUM.

Spiroctan. Diuretic: *see* SPIRONOLACTONE.

Spirolone. Diuretic: *see* SPIRONOLACTONE.

Sporanox. Oral antifungal for vulvovaginal candidiasis, pityriasis versicolour and dermatophytoses: *see* ITRACONAZOLE.

Sprilon. Barrier preparation to protect skin as a spray application: *see* DIMETICONE, ZINC OXIDE.

Stalevo (r). Fixed combinations of the amino acid, LEVODOPA, with two enzyme inhibitors. Used to treat the later stages of Parkinson's disease where there are problems with the 'on–off' variation in response to the existing treatment: *see* CARBIDOPA, ENTACAPONE, LEVODOPA.

Staril. Antihypertensive: *see* FOSINOPRIL.

Starlix. Oral hypoglycaemic: *see* NATEGLINIDE.

STD inj. Scleroses varicose veins: *see* SODIUM TETRADECYL SULPHATE.

Stelazine. Tranquillizer: *see* TRIFLUOPERAZINE.

Stemetil. Tranquillizer/antiemetic/antivertigo: *see* PROCHLORPERAZINE.

Ster-Zac (b). Topical anti-infective: *see* HEXACHLOROPHENE.

Stesolid. Anticonvulsant: *see* DIAZEPAM.

Stiemycin. Antibiotic solution for topical application in acne: *see* ERYTHROMYCIN.

Stilnoct

Stilnoct. Hypnotic: *see* ZOLPIDEM.

Strattera (r). For attention deficit hyperactivity disorder: *see* ATOMOXETINE.

Strefen. Non-steroidal anti-inflammatory analgesic lozenge for sore throat: *see* FLURBIPROFEN.

Streptase. Fibrinolytic: *see* STREPTOKINASE.

Striant SR. Hormone replacement formulated as a buccal tablet allowing slow release and absorption through gums and cheeks. *see* TESTOSTERONE.

Stugeron. Antiemetic/antivertigo: *see* CINNARIZINE.

Sublimaze (c). Narcotic analgesic: *see* FENTANYL.

Sudafed. Decongestant: *see* PSEUDOEPHEDRINE.

Sudafed Co. As Sudafed with PARACETAMOL.

Sudafed Expectorant. As Sudafed with GUAIFENESIN.

Sudafed Linctus. As Sudafed with DEXTROMETHORPHAN.

Sudafed Plus. As Sudafed with TRIPROLIDINE.

Sudocrem. Bland topical cream for bed sores, nappy rash and burns: *see* BENZYLBENZOATE, LANOLIN, ZINC OXIDE.

Suleo-M. Topical treatment for lice: *see* MALATHION.

Sulpitil. Antipsychotic: *see* SULPIRIDE.

Sulpor. For chronic schizophrenia: *see* SULPIRIDE.

Sultrin vaginal preps (d). Local antibacterial combination: *see*
SULFABENZAMIDE, SULFACETAMIDE, SULFATHIAZOLE.

Supralip. For hyperlipidaemia: *see* FENOFIBRATE.

Suprax. Antibacterial: *see* CEFIXIME.

Suprecur. Clotting factor concentrate for treatment of haemophilia B or Christmas disease: *see* FACTOR IX.

Suprefact. Hormone: *see* BUSERELIN.

Surgam. Non-steroid anti-inflammatory/ analgesic: *see* TIAPROFENIC ACID.

Surmontil. Antidepressive: *see* TRIMIPRAMINE.

Survanta. Treatment for lung damage (respiratory distress syndrome) in premature babies requiring mechanical ventilation: *see* BERACTANT.

Suscard buccal. Vasodilator tablets for buccal absorption: *see* GLYCERYL TRINITRATE.

Sustac. Antianginal: *see* GLYCERYL TRINITRATE.

Sustanon. Male sex hormone for deficiency states or inoperable breast carcinoma: *see* TESTOSTERONE.

Sustiva (r). Antiretroviral for use in combination with other drugs in HIV-infected patients: *see* EFAVIRENZ.

Symbicort. Inhalant for asthma: *see* BUDESONIDE, FORMOTEROL.

Symmetrel. Antiparkinsonian and antiviral agent: *see* AMANTADINE.

Synacthen. Synthetic corticotrophic injection: *see* TETRCOSACTIDE.

Synagis (r). Antiviral to prevent lower respiratory tract infections in infants: *see* PALIVIZUMAB.

Synalar. Corticosteroid: *see* FLUOCINOLONE.

Synalar C and N. Topical corticosteroid/ anti-infective: *see* CLIOQUINOL, FLUOCINOLONE, NEOMYCIN.

Synarel. Synthetic hormone for intranasal treatment of endometriosis: *see* NAFARELIN.

Syndol. Analgesic: *see* CAFFEINE, CODEINE, DOXYLAMINE, PARACETAMOL.

Synercid. Antibiotic: *see* DALFOPRISTIN, QUINUPRISTIN.

Synflex. Non-steroid anti-inflammatory/ analgesic: *see* NAPROXEN.

Synphase. Oral contraceptive: *see* ETHINYLESTRADIOL, NORETHISTERONE.

Syntaris. Topical corticosteroid spray for nasal allergies: *see* FLUNISOLIDE.

Synthamin. AMINO ACIDS and electrolyte sources for intravenous feeding.

Syntocinon. Synthetic pituitary hormone: *see* OXYTOCIN.

Syntometrine. Contracts uterine muscle: *see* ERGOMETRINE, OXYTOCIN.

Syprol. Beta-adrenoceptor blocker to treat arrhythmia, hypertension, angina, migraine, and anxiety: *see* PROPRANOLOL.

Syscor MR. Antianginal, antihypertensive: *see* NISOLDIPINE.

Sytron. For iron-deficiency anaemia: *see* SODIUM FEREDETATE.

T

Tagamet. Gastric histamine receptor blocker; reduces acid secretion: *see* CIMETIDINE.

Tambocor. Antiarrhythmic: *see* FLECAINIDE.

Tamiflu (r). Oral antiviral for prevention and treatment of influenza: *see* OSELTAMIVIR.

Tanatril. Long-acting antihypertensive/ ACE inhibtor: *see* IMIDAPRIL.

Tarceva (r). Oral antineoplastic used to treat advanced non-small cell lung cancer: *see* ERLOTINIB.

Targocid. Antibiotic: *see* TEICOPLANIN.

Targretin (r). Cytotoxic: *see* BEXAROTENE.

Tarivid. Antibacterial: *see* OFLOXACIN.

Tarka. Antihypertensive: *see* TRANDOLAPRIL, VERAPAMIL.

Tasmar (r). To treat Parkinson's disease: *see* TOLCAPONE.

Tavanic. Antibiotic: *see* LEVOFLOXACIN.

Tavegil. Antihistamine: *see* CLEMASTINE.

Taxol. Cytotoxic: *see* PACLITAXEL.

Taxotere. Cytotoxic to treat breast cancer and prostate cancer: *see* DOCETAXEL.

Tazocin. Antibiotic: *see* PIPERACILLIN, TAZOBACTAM.

Tears Naturale. Drops for dry eyes: *see* DEXTRANS, HYPROMELLOSE.

Tegretol. Anticonvulsant: *see* CARBAMAZEPINE.

Telfast. Antihistamine: *see* FEXOFENADINE.

Telzir (r). Antiviral for treatment of HIV-1 infection: *see* FOSAMPRENAVIR.

Temgesic (c). Analgesic: *see* BUPRENORPHINE.

Tenif. Antihypertensive: *see* ATENOLOL, NIFEDIPINE.

Tenoret-50. Antihypertensive: *see* ATENOLOL, CHLORTALIDONE.

Tenoretic. Antihypertensive combination identical to Tenoret-50 but double dose of both drugs.

Tenormin. Beta-adrenoceptor blocker: *see* ATENOLOL.

Tensipine MR. Antianginal/ antihypertensive: *see* NIFEDIPINE.

Tensium. Anxiolytic: *see* DIAZEPAM.

Teoptic. Eye drops for glaucoma: *see* CARTEOLOL.

Teril Retard (d). Sustained-release anticonvulsant also used for prophylactic treatment of manic depression, and in trigeminal neuralgia: *see* CARBAMAZEPINE.

Tertroxin. Thyroid hormone: *see* LIOTHYRONINE.

Testim (r). Topical, transdermal gel for replacement therapy of male sex hormone: *see* TESTOSTERONE.

Tetralysal. Antibiotic: *see* LYMECYCLINE.

Teveten. Antihypertensive: *see* EPROSARTAN.

T-Gel. Shampoo for psoriasis, dandruff, eczema: *see* COAL TAR.

Thovaline. Skin protective: *see* ZINC OXIDE.

Tilade (r). Aerosol inhalation for preventive treatment of asthma and bronchitis with reversible obstruction of the airways: *see* NEDOCROMIL.

Tildiem. Antianginal and antihypertensive: *see* DILTIAZEM.

Tilolec. Antiparkinsonian: *see* CO-CARELDOPA.

Tiloryth. Antibiotic: *see* ERYTHROMYCIN.

Timentin. Antibacterial: *see* CLAVULANIC ACID, TICARCILLIN.

Timodine. Antifungal/corticosteroid cream: *see* BENZALKONIUM, DIMETICONE, HYDROCORTISONE, NYSTATIN.

Timoptol. Eye drops for glaucoma: *see* TIMOLOL.

Tinaderm M. Topical antifungal: *see* NYSTATIN, TOLNAFTATE.

Tisept. Topical disinfectant: *see* CETRIMIDE, CHLORHEXIDINE.

Tixylix. Cough suppressant mixture: *see* PHOLCODINE, PROMETHAZINE.

Tobi. Antibiotic for chronic lung infection: *see* TOBRAMYCIN.

Tobradex. Eye drops to reduce inflammation and control infection after cataract surgery: *see* DEXAMETHASONE, TOBRAMYCIN.

Tofranil (d). Antidepressant: *see* IMIPRAMINE.

Tomudex. Cytotoxic for treatment of large bowel cancer: *see* RALTITREXED.

Topal. Antacid: *see* ALGINIC ACID, ALUMINIUM HYDROXIDE, MAGNESIUM CARBONATE.

Topamax. Anticonvulsant also used for prophylaxis of migraine headache: *see* TOPIRAMATE.

Topicycline. Antibiotic for topical application in acne: *see* TETRACYCLINE.

Toradol. Non-steroidal anti-inflammatory analgesic for postoperative pain: *see* KETOROLAC.

Torem. Diuretic: *see* TORASEMIDE.

Tracleer (r). Endothelin receptor antagonist: *see* BOSENTAN.

Tracrium. Muscle relaxant: *see* ATRACURIUM.

Tractocile. Uterine relaxant: *see* ATOSIBAN.

Tramacet (r). Combination analgesic for moderate to severe pain: *see* PARACETAMOL, TRAMADOL.

Tramake Insts. Analgesic: *see* TRAMADOL.

Trandate. Antihypertensive: *see* LABETALOL.

Transiderm-Nitro. Transdermal preparation for prophylactic treatment of angina pectoris whereby the drug is applied to the skin on a self-adhesive patch: *see* GLYCERYL TRINITRATE.

Transtec (c). Patch for relief of chronic pain and moderate to severe cancer pain: *see* BUPRENORPHINE.

Transvasin. Rubefacient: *see* ETHYL NICOTINATE.

Tranxene (d). Tranquillizer: *see* CLORAZEPATE.

Trasicor

Trasicor. Beta-adrenoceptor blocker: *see* OXPRENOLOL.

Trasidrex. Antihypertensive: *see* CYCLOPENTHIAZIDE, OXPRENOLOL.

Trasylol. Used in acute pancreatitis: *see* APROTININ.

Travasept. Disinfectant: *see* CETRIMIDE, CHLORHEXIDINE.

Travasept 30. Topical disinfectant to be used undiluted for wound and skin disinfection: *see* CETRIMIDE, CHLORHEXIDINE.

Travatan (r). Eye drops for glaucoma: *see* TRAVOPROST.

Traxam. Fibrinolytic: *see* FELBINAC.

Trental. Peripheral vasodilator: *see* PENTOXIFYLLINE.

Treosulfan. Cytotoxic: *see* THREITOL DIMETHANE SULPHONATE.

TRH. Hormone: *see* PROTIRELIN.

Tri-Adcortyl. Topical corticosteroid/ antibiotic: *see* GRAMICIDIN, NEOMYCIN, NYSTATIN, TRIAMCINOLONE.

Triadene. Oral contraceptive: *see* ETHINYLESTRADIOL, GESTODENE.

Triamco. Diuretic: *see* HYDROCHLOROTHIAZIDE, TRIAMTERENE.

Triapin/Triapin Mite (r). Antihypertensive combination: *see* FELODIPINE, RAMIPRIL.

Tridestra. Sex hormones for postmenopausal symptoms: *see* ESTRADIOL, MEDROXYPROGESTERONE.

Trimopan. Antimicrobial: *see* TRIMETHOPRIM.

Trimovate. Topical corticosteroid/anti-infective: *see* CLOBETASONE, NYSTATIN, OXYTETRACYCLINE.

Trinordiol. Oral contraceptive: *see* ETHINYLESTRADIOL, LEVONORGESTREL.

TriNovum. Oral contraceptive with three different strengths for use at different stages of the menstrual cycle: *see* ETHINYLESTRADIOL, NORETHISTERONE.

Triperidol. Antipsychotic: *see* TRIFLUPERIDOL.

Triptafen M. Antidepressant/ tranquillizer: *see* AMITRIPTYLINE, PERPHENAZINE.

Trisenox (r). Intravenous treatment for acute leukaemia that has relapsed or not responded to standard chemotherapy: *see* ARSENIC TRIOXIDE.

Trisequens. Female sex hormones for menopausal symptoms: *see* ESTRADIOL, NORETHISTERONE.

Tritace. Antihypertensive: *see* RAMIPRIL.

Trizivir. Antiviral: *see* ABACAVIR, LAMIVUDINE, ZIDOVUDINE.

Tropium. Anxiolytic: *see* CHLORDIAZEPOXIDE.

Trosyl. Topical antifungal for nail infections: *see* TIOCONAZOLE.

Trusopt. Topical treatment for glaucoma: *see* DORZOLAMIDE.

Truvada (r). Antiviral: *see* EMTRICITABINE, TENOFOVIR.

Tuberculin Tine Test. Intradermal injection test for tuberculosis: *see* TUBERCULIN.

Tuinal (c). Hypnotic: *see* AMOBARBITAL, SECOBARBITAL.

Twinrix. Combined vaccine for hepatitis A and hepatitis B.

Tylex. Analgesic: *see* CODEINE, PARACETAMOL.

Typhim Vi. Inactivated typhoid vaccine for injection: *see* TYPHOID VACCINE.

Tyrozets. Local anaesthetic throat lozenges: *see* BENZOCAINE, TYROTHRICIN.

U V

Ubretid. Anticholinesterase: *see* DISTIGMINE.

Ucerax. Antihistamine used as an anxiolytic and antipruritic: *see* HYDROXYZINE.

Uftoral (r). To treat colorectal cancer. TEGAFUR, a prodrug of FLUOROURACIL, combined with uracil to produce higher levels of FLUOROURACIL without toxic levels of TEGAFUR.

Ultiva. Analgesic for use in general anaesthesia: *see* REMIFENTANIL.

Ultrabase. Bland, protective cream recommended for use when topical steroids are withdrawn: *see* LIQUID PARAFFIN, SOFT PARAFFIN, STEARYL ALCOHOL.

Ultralanum. Topical corticosteroid/anti-infective: *see* FLUOCORTOLONE.

Ultraproct. Local treatment for haemorrhoids: *see* CINCHOCAINE, FLUOCORTOLONE.

Ultratard (d). Long-acting purified beef insulin (zinc suspension): *see* INSULIN.

Unguentum. Protective cream for use on skin. May be used as vehicle for drugs.

Uniflu. For symptomatic treatment of common cold: *see* CAFFEINE, CODEINE, DIPHENHYDRAMINE, PARACETAMOL, PHENYLEPHRINE, VITAMIN C.

Uniphyllin. Sustained-release bronchodilator: *see* THEOPHYLLINE.

Uniroid. Local treatment for haemorrhoids: *see* CINCHOCAINE, HYDROCORTISONE, NEOMYCIN, POLYMIX B.

Unisept. Topical disinfectant: *see* CHLORHEXIDINE.

Univer. Antianginal/antihypertensive: *see* VERAPAMIL.

Uprima (d). For treatment of erectile dysfunction: *see* APOMORPHINE.

Urdox. Bile acid for dissolution of cholesterol gall stones: *see* URSODEOXYCHOLIC ACID.

Uriben. Antibiotic: *see* NALIDIXIC ACID.

Urispas. Anticholinergic antispasmodic for urinary tract colic: *see* FLAVOXATE.

Uromitexan. Used to prevent bladder toxicity resulting from cyclophosphamide treatment: *see* CYCLOPHOSPHAMIDE, MESNA.

Uro-Tainer. Sterile solution for maintenance of urinary catheters: *see* CHLORHEXIDINE, MAGNESIUM CITRATE, MANDELIC ACID, SODIUM CHLORIDE.

Ursofalk. Bile acid for dissolution of cholesterol gall stones: *see* URSODEOXYCHOLIC ACID.

Utinor. Antibacterial: *see* NORFLOXACIN.

Utovlan. Hormone: *see* NORETHISTERONE.

Uvistat (b). Topical applications for protection of skin from ultraviolet light: *see* MEXENONE.

Vagifem. Hormone for vaginal application in menopausal conditions: *see* ESTRADIOL.

Valclair. Anxiolytic suppository: *see* DIAZEPAM.

Valcyte. Antiviral: *see* VALGANCICLOVIR.

Valium (d). Anxiolytic: *see* DIAZEPAM.

Vallergan. Antihistamine: *see* ALIMEMAZINE.

Valoid. Antihistamine: *see* CYCLIZINE.

Valtrex. Antiviral: *see* VALACICLOVIR.

Vamin. Amino acids and carbohydrate for intravenous nutrition.

Vancocin. Antibiotic: *see* VANCOMYCIN.

Vaniqa (r). Topical treatment for facial hirsutism in women: *see* EFLORNITHINE.

Varidase. Enzymes for topical use in the removal of fibrinous or blood clots: *see* STREPTODORNASE, STREPTOKINASE.

Vascace. Antihypertensive: *see* CILAZAPRIL.

Vasogen. Soothing, protective cream for sore skin: *see* CALAMINE, DIMETICONE, ZINC OXIDE.

Vasoxine. Vasoconstrictor: *see* METHOXAMINE.

Vectavir. Topical antiviral: *see* PENCICLOVIR.

Veganin. Analgesic: *see* ACETYLSALICYLIC ACID, CODEINE, PARACETAMOL.

Velbe. Cytotoxic: *see* VINBLASTINE.

Velcade (r). For the treatment of multiple myeloma: *see* BORTEZOMIB.

Velosef. Antibiotic: *see* CEFRADINE.

Velosulin. Purified crystalline pork insulin: *see* INSULIN.

Ventavis (r). Prostacyclin analogue used by inhalation to treat pulmonary hypertension: *see* ILOPROST.

Ventmax. Sustained release bronchodilator: *see* SALBUTAMOL.

Ventodisks. Inhalation system for bronchodilation: *see* SALBUTAMOL.

Ventolin. Sympathomimetic bronchodilator: *see* SALBUTAMOL.

Ventolin Evohaler. CFC-free aerosol for asthma: *see* SALBUTAMOL.

Vepesid. Cytotoxic: *see* ETOPOSIDE.

Veracur. Topical treatment for warts: *see* FORMALDEHYDE.

Vermox. For threadworms, whipworms, roundworms, hookworms: *see* MEBENDAZOLE.

Verrugon. Ointment for warts: *see* SALICYLIC ACID.

Vertab SR. Sustained-release antianginal, antihypertensive: *see* VERAPAMIL.

Vesanoid. Used with chemotherapy in treatment of leukaemia: *see* TRETINOIN.

Vesicare (r). For treatment of urinary incontinence: *see* SOLIFENACIN.

Vexol. Eye drops to treat postoperative inflammation: *see* RIMEXOLONE.

Vfend. Antifungal: *see* VORICONAZOLE.

Viagra. For treatment of erectile dysfunction: *see* SILDENAFIL.

Viazem XL. Sustained-release antianginal/antihypertensive: *see* DILTIAZEM.

Vibramycin

Vibramycin. Antibiotic: *see* DOXYCYCLINE.

Vibramycin-D. Water-dispersible antibiotic tablets, avoids the danger of oesophageal damage which may occur with capsules: *see* DOXYCYCLINE.

Videne. Disinfectant: *see* POVIDONE-IODINE.

Videx. Antiviral for use in advanced AIDS: *see* DIDANOSINE.

Vigranon B. Vitamin syrup: *see* ANEURINE, NICOTINAMIDE, PANTHENOL, PYRIDOXINE, RIBOFLAVIN.

Vioform-Hydrocortisone. Topical anti-infective: *see* CLIOQUINOL, HYDROCORTISONE.

Viracept. Antiviral for use in HIV-positive patients with evidence of immunodeficiency: *see* NELFINAVIR.

Viraferon. Treatment for hepatitis B and C: *see* INTERFERON ALPHA-2B.

Viramune. Antiviral for use in HIV-positive patients with evidence of immunodeficiency: *see* NEVIRAPINE.

Virazid. Antiviral: *see* RIBAVIRIN.

Virazole. Antiviral for severe respiratory tract infections in children: *see* RIBAVIRIN.

Viread (r). Antiviral for use in HIV-infected patients: *see* TENOFOVIR.

Virgan. Topical transparent gel to treat acute viral infection of the cornea (surface of the eye): *see* GANCICLOVIR.

Virormone. Hormone injection: *see* TESTOSTERONE.

Visclair. Reduces mucous viscosity: *see* MECYSTEINE.

Viscopaste. Impregnated bandage: *see* ZINC OXIDE.

Viscotears. Tear substitute: *see* POLYACRYLIC ACID.

Viskaldix. Antihypertensive: *see* CLOPAMIDE, PINDOLOL.

Visken. Beta-adrenoceptor blocker: *see* PINDOLOL.

Vista-Methasone N. Corticosteroid/antibiotic nasal drops: *see* BETAMETHASONE, NEOMYCIN.

Vistide. Antiviral: *see* CIDOFOVIR.

Vitlipid. Fat-soluble vitamins for parenteral nutrition with fat solutions: *see* CALCIFEROL, PHYTOMENADIONE, VITAMIN A.

Vividrin. For prevention and treatment of allergic conjunctivitis: *see* SODIUM CROMOGLICATE.

Vivotif. Live oral vaccine for typhoid: *see* TYPHOID VACCINE.

Volmax. Sustained-release bronchodilator: *see* SALBUTAMOL.

Volraman. Non-steroidal anti-inflammatory/analgesic: *see* DICLOFENAC.

Volsaid Retard. Sustained-release anti-inflammatory: *see* DICLOFENAC.

Voltarol. Non-steroid anti-inflammatory/analgesic: *see* DICLOFENAC.

Voltarol Emugel. Topical non-steroidal anti-inflammatory/analgesic: *see* DICLOFENAC.

Voltarol ophtha. Eye drops for use after cataract surgery: *see* DICLOFENAC.

W X Y Z

Warticon. Topical treatment for genital warts: *see* PODOPHYLLOTOXIN.

Waxsol. Drops to soften ear wax: *see* DIOCTYL SODIUM SULPHOSUCCINATE.

Welldorm. Hypnotic: *see* CLORAL BETAINE.

Wellvone. Antiprotozoal: *see* ATOVAQUONE.

Wilzin (r). To prevent absorption of copper in Wilson's disease: *see* ZINC ACETATE.

Wright's vaporizer. Inhalation for nasal, bronchial congestion: *see* CHLOROCRESOL.

Xagrid (r). For reduction of elevated blood platelet counts in myeloproliferative disease: *see* ANAGRELIDE.

Xalacom (r). Eye drops for glaucoma: *see* LATANOPROST, TIMOLOL.

Xalatan. Eye drops for treatment of glaucoma: *see* LATANOPROST.

Xanax. Anxiolytic: *see* ALPRAZOLAM.

Xatral. Alpha$_1$ antagonist used for symptomatic treatment of benign prostatic hypertrophy: *see* ALFUZOSIN.

Xeloda (r). Noncytotoxic precursor for treatment of colorectal cancer and breast cancer: *see* CAPECITABINE.

Xenazine. To treat movement disorders: *see* TETRABENAZINE.

Xenical. Anti-obesity: *see* ORLISTAT.

Xepin. Topical treatment for pruritis: *see* DOXEPIN.

Xolair (r). Monoclonal antibody used to counteract the inflammatory response in severe persistent asthma: *see* OMALIZUMAB.

Xylocaine. Local anaesthetic: *see* LIDOCAINE.

Xyloproct. Local anaesthetic/ corticosteroid for anal conditions: *see* HYDROCORTISONE, LIDOCAINE, ZINC OXIDE.

Xylotox preps. Local anaesthetic: *see* ADRENALINE, LIDOCAINE.

Xyzal (r). Antihistamine: *see* LEVOCETIRIZINE.

Yasmin. Oral contraceptive. *see* DROSPIRENONE, ETHINYLESTRADIOL.

Yentreve (r). For stress urinary incontinence in women: *see* DULOXETINE.

Yutopar. Uterine relaxant: *see* RITODRINE.

Zacin. Topical analgesic cream for use in osteoarthritis: *see* CAPSAICIN.

Zaditen. Antihistamine for prevention of asthma, also available as eye drops (r) for seasonal allergic conjunctivitis: *see* KETOTIFEN.

Zamadol. Analgesic for moderate to severe pain: *see* TRAMADOL.

Zanaflex. Muscle relaxant: *see* TIZANIDINE.

Zanidip. Antihypertensive: *see* LERCANIDIPINE.

Zantac. Gastric histamine receptor blocker. Reduces acid secretion: *see* RANITIDINE.

Zapain. Analgesic: *see* CODEINE, PARACETAMOL.

Zaponex. Antipsychotic: *see* CLOZAPINE.

Zarontin. Anti-epileptic: *see* ETHOSUXIMIDE.

Zavedos. Cytotoxic antibiotic used to treat leukaemia: *see* IDARUBICIN.

Zeasorb. Powder for excessive perspiration: *see* CHLOROXYLENOL.

Zeffix. Treatment for chronic hepatitis B: *see* LAMIVUDINE.

Zelapar. For Parkinson's disease; may be given as a rapid-release formulation to be dissolved on the tongue at a reduced dose with fewer adverse effects: *see* SELEGILINE.

Zemplar (r). For prevention and treatment of secondary hyperparathyroidism associated with chronic renal failure: *see* PARICALCITOL.

Zemtard XL. Antianginal/ antihypertensive: *see* DILTIAZEM.

Zenapax (r). Immunosuppressant to prevent rejection of kidney transplants: *see* DACLIZUMAB.

Zerit. Antiviral for treatment of HIV infection: *see* STAVUDINE.

Zestoretic. Antihypertensive: *see* HYDROCHLOROTHIAZIDE, LISINOPRIL.

Zestril. Antihypertensive: *see* LISINOPRIL.

Ziagen. Antiviral for use in HIV-positive patients with evidence of immunodeficiency: *see* ABACAVIR.

Zidoval. Antibacterial: *see* METRONIDAZOLE.

Zimbacol XL. For hyperlipidaemia: *see* BEZAFIBRATE.

Zimovane. Hypnotic for insomnia: *see* ZOPICLONE.

Zinacef. Antibiotic: *see* CEFUROXIME.

Zincaband. Zinc paste bandage.

Zincomed. For zinc deficiency: *see* ZINC SULPHATE.

Zindaclin. Antibiotic gel for acne: *see* CLINDAMYCIN.

Zineryt. Topical antibiotic for treatment of acne: *see* ERYTHROMYCIN, ZINC ACETATE.

Zinga. Gastric histamine receptor blocker; reduces acid secretion: *see* NIZATIDINE.

Zinnat. Antibiotic: *see* CEFUROXIME.

Zirtek. Antihistamine: *see* CETIRIZINE.

Zispin. Antidepressant: *see* MIRTAZAPINE.

Zisprin SolTab. Antidepressant formulated as a tablet that disintegrates on the tongue and can be swallowed without water: *see* MIRTAZAPINE.

Zita. Gastric histamine receptor blocker that reduces acid secretion: *see* CIMETIDINE.

Zithromax. Antibiotic: *see* AZITHROMYCIN.

Zocor. For hypercholesterolaemia: *see* SIMVASTATIN.

Zocor Heart Pro. For hypercholesterolaemia; available over the counter: *see* SIMVASTATIN.

Zofran. Antiemetic for treatment of vomiting caused by cytotoxic chemotherapy, radiotherapy and surgery: *see* ONDANSETRON.

Zoladex. Hormone for treatment of cancer of the prostate gland, breast cancer and endometriosis: *see* GOSERELIN.

Zoleptil. Antipsychotic for treatment of schizophrenia: *see* ZOTEPINE.

Zolvera. Antianginal/antihypertensive/antiarrythmic: *see* VERAPAMIL.

Zomacton. Synthetic human growth hormone used to treat growth failure in children due to growth hormone deficiency: *see* SOMATROPIN.

Zomig. For acute migraine, available for oral treatment and as a nasal spray (r): *see* ZOLMITRIPTAN.

Zomorph (c). Sustained-release analgesic: *see* MORPHINE.

Zonegran (r). Anticonvulsant: *see* ZONISAMIDE.

Zorac. Topical treatment for psoriasis: *see* TAZAROTENE.

Zoton. For peptic ulcers, acid-related indigestion and oesophageal reflux: *see* LANSOPRAZOLE.

Zovirax. Antiviral: *see* ACICLOVIR.

Z Span Spansule. Sustained-release zinc for zinc deficiency: *see* ZINC SULPHATE.

Zumenon. For relief of menopausal symptoms: *see* ESTRADIOL.

Zyban. Anti-smoking preparation: *see* BUPROPION.

Zydol. Analgesic: *see* TRAMADOL.

Zyloric. For gout: *see* ALLOPURINOL.

Zyprexa. Antipsychotic for oral treatment or intramuscular injection (r): *see* OLANZAPINE.

APPENDIX
Common Slang Names for Misused Drugs

This list of names has been compiled from several sources. Please note that the information given here cannot be as accurate as that provided elsewhere in the *Drugs Handbook,* because slang names change according to fashion. Some slang names refer to preparations that are mixtures of drugs. When names may be used to refer to one individual drug or another, rather than a mixture, the drugs are listed as alternatives (e.g. CANNABIS *or* COCAINE).

A. *see* AMFETAMINE

Acapulco. *see* CANNABIS

Ace. *see* AMFETAMINE *or* CANNABIS

Acid. *see* LSD *or* MDMA

Adam. *see* MDMA

Adam & Eve. *see* MDA *or* MDEA

Afghan. *see* CANNABIS

Afghan black. *see* CANNABIS

African bush. *see* CANNABIS

Amph. *see* AMFETAMINE

Amphets. *see* AMFETAMINE

Angels. *see* AMOBARBITAL *or* AMYL NITRITE

Angel dust. *see* PHENCYCLIDINE

Bananas. *see* LSD

Barbs. *see* Barbiturates *e.g.* AMOBARBITAL

Base. *see* COCAINE

Basuco. *see* CANNABIS

Beam me up Scotty. *see* COCAINE, PHENCYCLIDINE (mix)

Bernice. *see* COCAINE

Bhang. *see* CANNABIS

Big brownies. *see* MDMA

Big C. *see* COCAINE

Big H. *see* HEROIN

Billy. *see* AMFETAMINE

Billy Whizz. *see* AMFETAMINE

Birds. *see* AMOBARBITAL

Biscuits. *see* MDMA

Black. *see* CANNABIS

Black and whites. *see* AMFETAMINE *or* MDMA

Black beauties. *see* AMFETAMINE, DEXAMFETAMINE

Black bomber. *see* AMFETAMINE

Black busters. *see* Barbiturates *e.g.* AMOBARBITAL

Appendix

Black gum. *see* HEROIN

Black lightening. *see* LSD

Black pearls. *see* DIAZEPAM

Black rings. *see* LSD

Black rock. *see* AMFETAMINE *or* CANNABIS *or* COCAINE

Black Russian. *see* CANNABIS

Black stuff. *see* OPIUM

Black tar. *see* HEROIN

Blackbirds. *see* AMFETAMINE

Blast. *see* CANNABIS

Blockers. *see* Barbiturates *e.g.* AMOBARBITAL

Blotter. *see* LSD

Blow. *see* CANNABIS *or* COCAINE

Blue bullets. *see* Barbiturates *e.g.* AMOBARBITAL

Blue devils. *see* Barbiturates *e.g.* AMOBARBITAL

Blue dolls. *see* Barbiturates *e.g.* AMOBARBITAL

Blue heaven. *see* AMOBARBITAL *or* AMYL NITRATE

Blue star. *see* LSD

Blue unicorn. *see* LSD

Bluebirds. *see* Barbiturates *e.g.* AMOBARBITAL

Blues. *see* AMFETAMINE, DEXAMFETAMINE *or* DIETHYLPROPION

Blunts. *see* CANNABIS

Bomber. *see* CANNABIS

Bombido. *see* AMFETAMINE

Boo. *see* CANNABIS

Boy. *see* HEROIN

Brass. *see* CANNABIS

Brick. *see* CANNABIS

Broccoli. *see* CANNABIS

Brown. *see* HEROIN

Brown sugar. *see* HEROIN

Brown tar. *see* HEROIN

Brownies. *see* MDMA

Bubblegum. *see* CANNABIS *or* COCAINE

Burgers. *see* MDMA

Bush. *see* CANNABIS

C. *see* COCAINE

California sunrise. *see* AMFETAMINE *or* CAFFEINE

Californian sunshine. *see* LSD *or* MDMA

Candy. *see* COCAINE *or* HEROIN *or* Barbiturates *e.g.* AMOBARBITAL

Carrie. *see* COCAINE

Cartwheels. *see* AMFETAMINE

Cecil. *see* COCAINE

Charas. *see* CANNABIS

Charge. *see* CANNABIS

Chalk. *see* AMFETAMINE

Charlie. *see* COCAINE

Cheer. *see* LSD

Chewies. *see* AMOBARBITAL, SECOBARBITAL (TUINAL)

Chi. *see* HEROIN

China white. *see* FENTANYL *or* HEROIN

China whites. *see* MDA

Chinese H. *see* HEROIN

Chinese reds. *see* HEROIN

Chitari. *see* CANNABIS

Chocolate. *see* HEROIN

Cholly. *see* COCAINE

Christal. *see* METHAMFETAMINE

Cities. *see* MDMA

Clarity. *see* MDMA

Cloud 9. *see* COCAINE

Cocoa. *see* HEROIN

Coke. *see* COCAINE

Co-pilots. *see* AMFETAMINE

Colombian. *see* CANNABIS

Corine. *see* COCAINE

Crack. *see* COCAINE

Crank. *see* METHAMFETAMINE

Crap. *see* HEROIN

Crazy medicine. *see* METHAMFETAMINE

Cristy. *see* METHAMFETAMINE

Crystal. *see* COCAINE *or* METHAMFETAMINE *or* PHENCYCLIDINE

Crystals. *see* AMFETAMINE

Dagga (Dhaga). *see* CANNABIS

Dennis the Menace. *see* MDMA

Dexies. *see* DEXAMFETAMINE (DEXEDRINE)

DFs. *see* DIHYDROCODEINE

Diet pills. *see* AMFETAMINE

Dike. *see* DICONAL

Dirt. *see* HEROIN

Dirty. *see* CANNABIS

Disco biscuits. *see* MDMA

Doctor. *see* MDMA

Dog vitamins. *see* DIAZEPAM

Dog food. *see* HEROIN

Dollies. *see* METHADONE

Dolls. *see* METHADONE *or* Barbiturates *e.g.* AMOBARBITAL

Dominoes. *see* AMFETAMINE, DEXAMFETAMINE

Dope. *see* CANNABIS

Dots. *see* LSD

Double cross. *see* AMFETAMINE

Double dreads. *see* AMFETAMINE, LSD (mix)

Double 'O's. *see* MORPHINE

Double trouble. *see* AMOBARBITAL, SECOBARBITAL (TUINAL)

Double zero. *see* CANNABIS

Dove. *see* MDMA

Appendix

Downers. *see* Barbiturates
e.g. AMOBARBITAL

Dragon. *see* HEROIN

Draw. *see* CANNABIS

Dream. *see* COCAINE

Drop. *see* LSD

Dummy dust. *see* CAFFEINE, EPHEDRINE,
METHAMFETAMINE (mix)

Dust. *see* COCAINE *or* HEROIN *or*
PHENCYCLIDINE

Dynamite. *see* COCAINE, MORPHINE (mix)

E. *see* MDMA *or* CANNABIS

Ecstasy. *see* MDMA

Edward. *see* MDMA

Elephant. *see* HEROIN *or* MDMA

Essence. *see* MDMA

Eye openers. *see* AMFETAMINE

Fantasia. *see* MDMA

Fantasy. *see* LSD, MDMA (mix) *or* LSD,
MESCALINE (mix)

Fast. *see* AMFETAMINE

Flake. *see* COCAINE

Flash. *see* LSD

Flatliners. *see* MDMA

Freebase. *see* COCAINE

French blues. *see* AMFETAMINE

Ganja. *see* CANNABIS

Gear. *see* HEROIN

Girl. *see* COCAINE

Glass. *see* METHAMFETAMINE

Go fast. *see* METHAMFETAMINE

Gold dust. *see* COCAINE

Gold star. *see* COCAINE

Golden haze. *see* CANNABIS

Goofballs. *see* AMFETAMINE *or*
Barbiturates *e.g.* AMOBARBITAL

Gorillas. *see* Barbiturates
e.g. AMOBARBITAL

Grass. *see* CANNABIS

Gravel. *see* COCAINE

Green. *see* KETAMINE

Green eggs. *see* TEMAZEPAM

Grey biscuits. *see* MDMA

Gum. *see* OPIUM *or* HEROIN

H. *see* HEROIN *or* CANNABIS

Happy dust. *see* COCAINE

Hard stuff. *see* MORPHINE

Harry. *see* HEROIN

Hash. *see* CANNABIS

Hay. *see* CANNABIS

Hawk. *see* LSD

Haze. *see* LSD

Hearts. *see* AMFETAMINE

Heaven dust. *see* COCAINE

Hemp. *see* CANNABIS

Herb. *see* CANNABIS

Horse. *see* HEROIN *or* CANNABIS

Ice. *see* COCAINE *or* METHAMFETAMINE

Idiot pills. *see* Barbiturates
e.g. AMOBARBITAL

Jack. *see* HEROIN

Jam/Jelly. *see* COCAINE

Jane. *see* CANNABIS

Jellies. *see* TEMAZEPAM

Jelly beans. *see* AMFETAMINE *or*
TEMAZEPAM

Joint. *see* CANNABIS

Joy. *see* HEROIN

Junk. *see* DIAMORPHINE

K. *see* KETAMINE

Kermits. *see* MDMA

Kief. *see* CANNABIS

Kif. *see* CANNABIS

King Kong pills. *see* Barbiturates
e.g. AMOBARBITAL

King's habit. *see* COCAINE

Kit kat. *see* KETAMINE

Knife. *see* LSD

L. *see* LSD

LA. *see* METHAMFETAMINE

Lady. *see* COCAINE

Lebanese. *see* CANNABIS

Leaf. *see* CANNABIS

Liberty cap. *see* PSILOCYBIN

Lightning. *see* AMFETAMINE

Lightning flash. *see* LSD

Liquid acid. *see* LSD

Liquid E. *see* KETAMINE

Liquid gold. *see* AMYL NITRITE

Liquid red. *see* AMFETAMINE

Locker room. *see* AMYL NITRITE

Loco weed. *see* CANNABIS

Love doves. *see* MDMA

Love drug. *see* MDA *or* MDMA *or*
METHAQUALONE

Love pills. *see* METHAQUALONE

Love weed. *see* CANNABIS

Lucy. *see* LSD

M&Ms. *see* MDMA

M25s. *see* MDMA

Magic mushrooms. *see* PSILOCYBIN

Malawi grass. *see* CANNABIS

Man Uniteds. *see* MDMA

Mandies. *see* METHAQUALONE (MANDRAX)

Marijuana. *see* CANNABIS

Marshmallow. *see* Barbiturates
e.g. AMOBARBITAL

Mary. *see* CANNABIS

Mary Jane. *see* AMFETAMINE *or* CANNABIS

Mescal. *see* MESCALINE

Appendix

Meth. *see* METHADONE *or* METHAMFETAMINE

Mexican brown. *see* HEROIN

Mexican green. *see* CANNABIS

Mexican Lebanese gold. *see* CANNABIS

Mexican mud. *see* HEROIN

Mexican reds. *see* Barbiturates *e.g.* AMOBARBITAL

Mexican valium. *see* ROHYPNOL

Micro dot. *see* LSD

Mind, body and soul. *see* LSD

Miss Emma. *see* MORPHINE

Misties. *see* MORPHINE

Moggies. *see* NITRAZEPAM (MOGADON)

Monkey. *see* MORPHINE

Morf. *see* MORPHINE

Moroccan. *see* CANNABIS

Mosaic. *see* LSD

Mushies. *see* PSILOCYBIN

Neb. *see* Barbiturates *e.g.* AMOBARBITAL

Nemmies. *see* Barbiturates *e.g* AMOBARBITAL

Nepalese. *see* CANNABIS

New Yorkers. *see* MDMA

Nimbies. *see* Barbiturates *e.g.* AMOBARBITAL

Northern lights. *see* CANNABIS

Nose candy. *see* COCAINE

Nuggets. *see* COCAINE *or* AMFETAMINE

Nutties. *see* MDMA

O. *see* OPIUM

Orange roughies. *see* MORPHINE

Orange sunshine. *see* LSD

Oranges. *see* AMFETAMINE *or* DEXAMFETAMINE *or* MORPHINE

'P'. *see* AMFETAMINE

Paki black. *see* CANNABIS

Palf. *see* DEXTROMORAMIDE (PALFIUM)

Panama red. *see* CANNABIS

Paper mushrooms. *see* LSD

Parachute. *see* COCAINE, HEROIN (mix)

Paradise. *see* COCAINE

PCP. *see* PHENCYCLIDINE

Peace pill. *see* PHENCYCLIDINE

Peach. *see* PALFIUM

Peanut. *see* HEROIN

Peanuts. *see* Barbiturates *e.g.* AMOBARBITAL

Penguins. *see* LSD

Pep pills. *see* AMFETAMINE

Percy. *see* CANNABIS

Persian white. *see* HEROIN

Peter Pan. *see* MDMA *or* PHENCYCLIDINE

Phase 4, Phase 5, Phase 7. *see* MDMA

Phyamps. *see* METHADONE

208

Pills. *see* MDMA

Pink ladies. *see* Barbiturates
e.g. AMOBARBITAL

Pinks. *see* SECOBARBITAL

Poke. *see* SILDENAFIL

Poor man's cocaine. *see* AMFETAMINE

Poppers. *see* AMYL NITRITE

Pot. *see* CANNABIS

Powder. *see* HEROIN *or* AMFETAMINE

Power pack. *see* MDMA

Product. *see* AMFETAMINE

Puff. *see* CANNABIS

Purple haze. *see* CANNABIS *or* LSD

Purple hearts. *see* DEXAMFETAMINE

Quick. *see* KETAMINE

R2. *see* ROHYPNOL

Rainbows. *see* LSD *or* AMOBARBITAL,
SECOBARBITAL (TUINAL)

Ram. *see* AMYL NITRITE

Red and whites. *see* MDMA

Red devil. *see* AMFETAMINE *or* CAFFEINE *or*
MDEA *or* PSEUDOEPHEDRINE

Red devils. *see* Barbiturates
e.g. AMOBARBITAL *or* AMFETAMINE

Red rock. *see* METHADONE

Red seal. *see* CANNABIS

Reds/Red birds. *see* Barbiturates
e.g. AMOBARBITAL

Reds and blues. *see* AMOBARBITAL,
SECOBARBITAL (TUINAL)

Reefer. *see* CANNABIS

Resin. *see* CANNABIS

Rhubarb & custard. *see* MDMA

Roach. *see* ROHYPNOL

Rocks. *see* COCAINE

Rocky. *see* CANNABIS

Roofies. *see* ROHYPNOL

Rope. *see* CANNABIS *or* ROHYPNOL

Rugby balls. *see* TEMAZEPAM

Rush. *see* AMYL NITRITE

Scag. *see* HEROIN

Scat. *see* HEROIN

Scooby-snack. *see* MDMA

Seggy. *see* SECOBARBITAL

Shabu. *see* METHAMFETAMINE

Shamrocks. *see* MDMA *or* MDEA

Shrooms. *see* PSILOCYBIN

Silver haze. *see* CANNABIS

Silver pearl. *see* CANNABIS

Sinsemilla. *see* CANNABIS

Skag. *see* DIAMORPHINE

Skunk. *see* CANNABIS

Sleepers. *see* Barbiturates
e.g. AMOBARBITAL

Sleigh-ride. *see* COCAINE

Appendix

Smack. *see* DIAMORPHINE *or* COCAINE

Smilies. *see* LSD

Smoke. *see* CANNABIS

Snapper. *see* AMYL NITRITE

Snow. *see* COCAINE

Snowball. *see* MDA

Softballs. *see* Barbiturates
e.g. AMOBARBITAL

Special K. *see* KETAMINE

Speed. *see* AMFETAMINE

Splash. *see* AMFETAMINE

Spliff. *see* CANNABIS

Sputnik. *see* CANNABIS, OPIUM (mix)

Stag. *see* AMYL NITRITE

Stardust. *see* COCAINE

Stars. *see* LSD

Sticks. *see* CANNABIS

Stones. *see* COCAINE

Strawberries. *see* LSD

Strawberry fields. *see* LSD

Stud. *see* AMYL NITRITE

Stuff. *see* CANNABIS *or* HEROIN

Sugar. *see* LSD

Sulph. *see* AMFETAMINE *or* MORPHINE

Super K. *see* KETAMINE

Sweeties. *see* MDMA

Sweets. *see* AMFETAMINE

Syrup. *see* METHADONE

Tar. *see* MORPHINE *or* OPIUM

Tea. *see* CANNABIS

Tem. *see* TEMGESIC

Temazzies. *see* TEMAZEPAM

Temmies. *see* TEMAZEPAM *or* TEMGESIC

Temple balls. *see* CANNABIS

Thai sticks. *see* CANNABIS

Tibetan gold. *see* CANNABIS

Tiger. *see* HEROIN

TNT. *see* AMYL NITRITE

Toot. *see* COCAINE

Tripper. *see* LSD

Trips. *see* LSD

Truck drivers. *see* AMFETAMINE

Tulips. *see* MDMA

Uppers. *see* AMFETAMINE

Vitamin K. *see* KETAMINE

Wacky baccy. *see* CANNABIS

Wake ups. *see* AMFETAMINE

Wash rock. *see* COCAINE

Weed. *see* CANNABIS

White burger sauce. *see* MDA *or* MDEA
or MDMA

White cap. *see* MDA

White cloud. *see* COCAINE

White dynamite. *see* HEROIN

White girl. *see* COCAINE

White lady. *see* COCAINE

White stuff. *see* MORPHINE *or* COCAINE

Whites. *see* AMFETAMINE *or* MDMA

Whizz. *see* AMFETAMINE

Whizz bomb. *see* AMFETAMINE, LSD (mix) *or* MDMA

Window (panes). *see* LSD

Woodpeckers. *see* AMFETAMINE

XTC. *see* MDMA

Ya ba. *see* AMFETAMINE

Yellow eggs. *see* TEMAZEPAM

Yellow submarines. *see* TEMAZEPAM

Yellows. *see* Barbiturates
e.g. AMOBARBITAL

Zip. *see* METHAMFETAMINE

Zoom. *see* AMFETAMINE, COCAINE, HEROIN (mix)

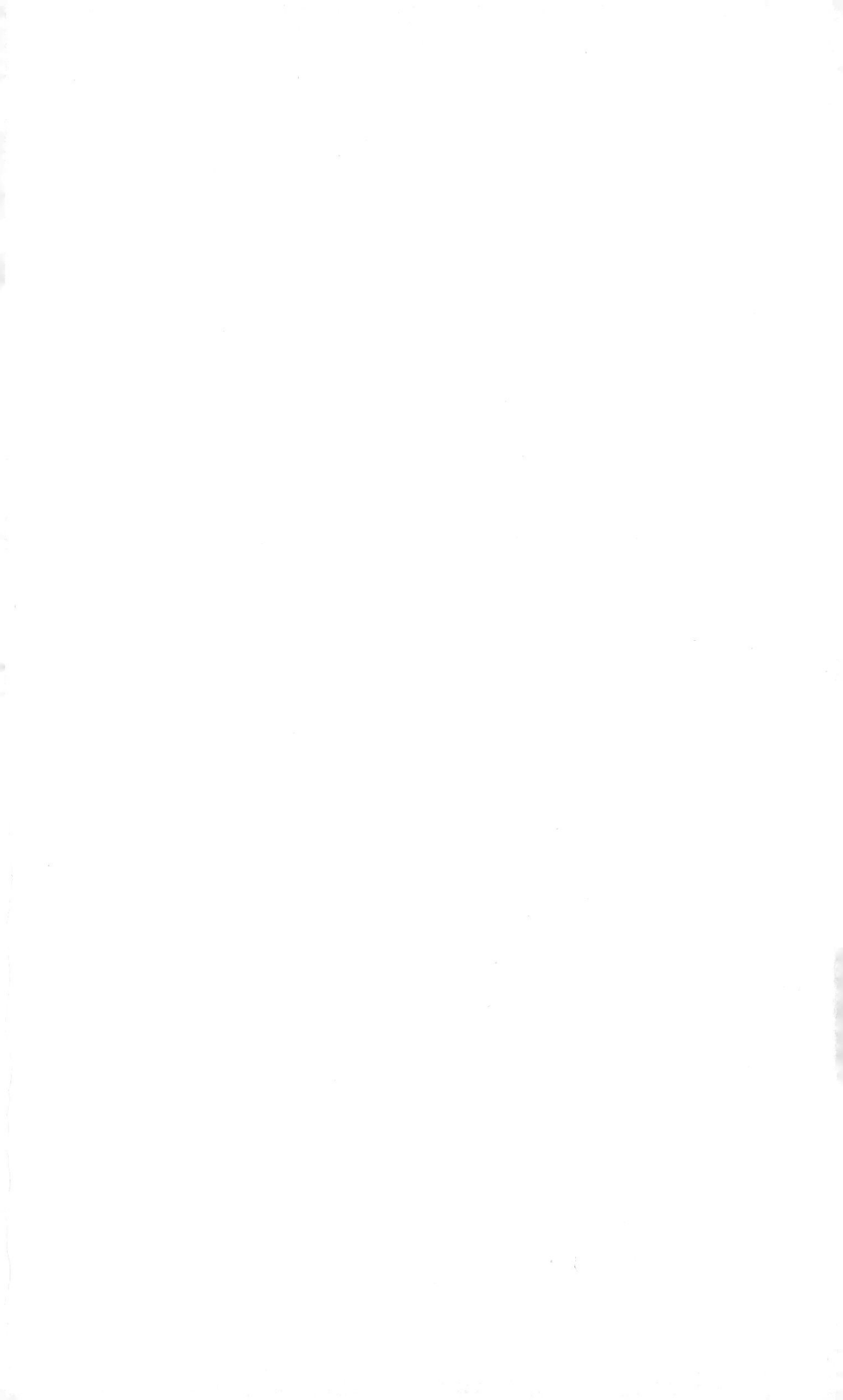